FOURTH EDITIO

Communication and Communication Disorders

A Clinical Introduction

ELENA PLANTE
The University of Arizona

PÉLAGIE M. BEESON
The University of Arizona

PEARSON

Boston   Columbus   Indianapolis   New York   San Francisco   Upper Saddle River
Amsterdam   Cape Town   Dubai   London   Madrid   Milan   Munich   Paris   Montréal   Toronto
Delhi   Mexico City   São Paulo   Sydney   Hong Kong   Seoul   Singapore   Taipei   Tokyo

Executive Editor and Publisher: Stephen D. Dragin
Editorial Assistant: Michelle Hochberg
Marketing Manager: Joanna Sabella
Production Editor: Paula Carroll
Editorial Production Service: Walsh & Associates, Inc.
Manufacturing Buyer: Megan Cochran
Electronic Composition: Jouve
Interior Design: Jouve
Cover Designer: Jennifer Hart

Credits and acknowledgments borrowed from other sources and reproduced, with permission, in this textbook appear on page 390.

Many of the designations by manufacturers and sellers to distinguish their products are claimed as trademarks. Where those designations appear in this book, and the publisher was aware of a trademark claim, the designations have been printed in initial caps or all caps.

Library of Congress Cataloging-in-Publication Data

Plante, Elena
  Communication and communication disorders : a clinical introduction / Elena Plante, Pélagie M. Beeson. — 4th ed.
    p. cm.
  Includes bibliographical references and index.
  ISBN-13: 978-0-13-265812-6
  ISBN-10: 0-13-265812-7
  1. Communicative disorders. 2. Communicative disorders in children.
I. Beeson, Pelagie M. II. Title.

RC423.P59 2013
616.85'5—dc23

2012020353

10 9 8 7 6 5 4 3 2 1

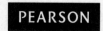

www.pearsonhighered.com

ISBN 10: 0-13-265812-7
ISBN 13: 978-0-13-265812-6

To our patients, who continue to teach us.

To our colleagues, who share our enjoyment of the science and service of our profession.

To our students, for whom this book is written.

CONTENTS

PREFACE TO THE FOURTH EDITION

New to This Edition

We would like to thank our academic colleagues who strive to inspire the next generation of professionals working in the field of communication disorders and sciences. We have received positive feedback from many of you over the past few years and have endeavored to provide an even better tool for students with the fourth edition of this book. In this edition, we have retained many of the features that so many of you have told us are great teaching tools. These include the liberal use of case illustrations, and clinical problem solving questions at the end of chapters. We have updated all the chapters to be sure that they reflect current concepts or to better represent concepts we have found to be difficult for students new to this area of study. Certain chapters have undergone substantial changes and we have included other features that are new to this edition. These include the following:

- All chapters now include textboxes that highlight salient points in the text and encourage students to become engaged with the text. These textboxes also provide instructors with topical mappings of the text that can guide development of lectures or selection of exam questions that are drawn from the book.
- The majority of chapters (nine of the thirteen) include new and updated figures. Many of these include photographs designed to give students a better sense of what practice in the field looks like. Photos in Chapters 3 and 7 are designed to help students link developmental milestones in speech and language with the physical development of children as they go through these stages. Chapters 4, 8, and 9 contain photos depicting speech and language therapy. Chapters 10 through 12 include new photos that demonstrate common audiologic procedures.
- We have expanded discussion of language acquisition in Chapter 7 to illustrate the both the learning capabilities of infants and the later stages of language acquisition that continue after children have mastered the basics around age 4. This is intended to provide a more complete view of language development for students.
- Chapter 8, Language Disorders in Children, contains new sections on Attention Deficit Disorders and Intellectual Impairments. These new sections expand these topics relative to previous editions in order to provide an up-to-date treatment of these topics. However, we strived to present this information in a way that remains accessible to students, providing an introduction to these topics rather than comprehensive coverage.

■ We have added to Chapter 10, The Biological Foundations of Hearing, to provide information concerning how the structures and functions of the hearing system can be measured clinically. The chapter introduces concepts like otoscopy, impedance audiometry, otoacoustic emissions testing, ABR, and MRI as clinical measures and the text is accompanied by illustrative photographs. This is intended to help students link audiometric procedures revisited in later chapters with the anatomical and physiological phenomena that they examine.

■ We have included an entirely new chapter on Disorders of Hearing in Children (Chapter 11), authored by James Dean, AuD. This chapter presents information on the etiologic basis of hearing loss and current hearing technologies in use with children today. It also uses the case presentation format to give readers the sense of practice as a pediatric audiologist in a number of contexts.

We would like to thank the following reviewers for their time and suggestions for this edition: Yu-Kyong Choe, University of Massachusetts-Amherst; Jennifer Garrett, University of Northern Iowa; and Iona Johnson, Towson University.

We hope that this fourth edition continues to reflect the real love that both practitioners and researchers in the field of communication sciences have for the work they do. We are proud to be able to represent the field to those who may not know much about the work of audiologists and speech-language pathologists. We hope that many of our readers will be inspired to join the professions to serve and learn from those with communication disorders, as we have through the years.

PREFACE TO THE THIRD EDITION

When we wrote the first edition of this textbook, our intention was to speak to the undergraduate student encountering speech, language, and hearing sciences for the first time. We strove to present concepts in a simplified yet interesting manner. As we taught from the textbook and received feedback from others who used the book, we found that we hit the mark in many respects. In our second and third editions, we directed our efforts to improve the book by further simplifying difficult concepts, removing excess detail, and strengthening the clarity of writing. We updated the content for this edition to make it consistent with the science and evidence-based practice of the professions, and also included a number of new figures to further illustrate the concepts. We have retained a clinical emphasis by introducing communication disorders with case examples, which have proved effective in bringing the reality of the disorders and the professions to life. We added to the lists of books from the popular literature that include personal accounts of individuals with communication disorders as the reading of this literature has been a valuable and enjoyable activity for our students.

As we worked to revise this text, we were again impressed by the breadth and depth of our field. We continue to be fascinated by the science within and outside our field and within and outside our respective specialties. We feel fortunate to have the privilege to work with such impressive and delightful colleagues in the process. We thank Drs. Julie Barkmeier-Kraemer, Anne Marie Tharpe, Linda Norrix, Fran Harris, and Ted Glattke for their excellent chapters and gracious responses to our editorial efforts to unify the tone of the book. We also appreciate the generous contributions of other faculty in our department, including Brad Story and Barbara Cone-Wesson, who help to keep our knowledge current. We appreciate the time and input of reviewers Patricia Mercaitis (University of Massachusetts, Amherst) and Benjamin Munson (University of Minnesota). Finally, we are indebted to Susan Carnahan, who provided significant editorial assistance for this revision, and we thank Celeste Connelly, HyeSuk Cho, and Jennifer Parrott for their support as well. We are pleased with the outcome of the combined efforts in this editorial process, and look forward to teaching from this new edition. We hope that others will find it useful as well.

Elena Plante, PhD, CCC-SLP

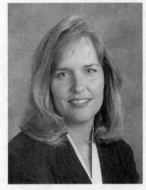

Elena Plante completed her bachelor's and master's degrees in speech-language pathology at Loyola University in Maryland. Before completing her doctorate at the University of Arizona, she worked as a speech-language pathologist in the public schools. Since completing her doctorate and postdoctoral studies, she has been on the faculty in the Department of Speech, Language, and Hearing Sciences at the University of Arizona. Her research has focused on the biological basis of specific language impairment and she was one of the early adopters of magnetic resonance imaging as a research tool in speech-language pathology. Her clinical research focuses on improving both assessment and treatment methods for those with developmental language disorder. She is a co-author of the *Pediatric Test of Brain Injury*, the first of its kind for children with traumatic brain injury. She has received support for her research from grants from the National Institutes of Health. Dr. Plante is a Fellow of the American Speech-Language-Hearing Association and the University of Arizona College of Science. She speaks regularly at national and international conferences on the topic of developmental language disorders.

Elena Plante, PhD, CCC-SLP

Pélagie M. Beeson, PhD, CCC-SLP

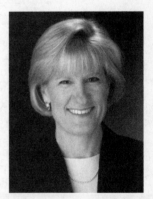

Pélagie (Pagie) Maritz Beeson received her bachelor's and master's degrees in speech-language pathology from the University of Kansas. She began her clinical career at a community speech and language center in Fairbanks, Alaska, where she provided service to a diverse clinical population. She later completed her doctoral work at the University of Arizona, where she also served as the coordinator of the American Indian Professional Training Program in Speech-Language Pathology and Audiology. Currently, Dr. Beeson is Professor and Head of the Department of Speech, Language, and Hearing Sciences at the University of Arizona. Her research and clinical work have been devoted to neurogenic communication disorders in adults, with a particular emphasis on the nature and treatment of aphasia, alexia, and agraphia, as well as the cognitive mechanisms and neural substrates of written language. Dr. Beeson's research has been supported for many years by the National Institute on Deafness and Other Communication Disorders (NIH/NIDCD). She is board certified in Adult Neurogenic Communication Disorders by the Academy of Neurologic Communication Disorders

Pélagie M. Beeson, PhD, CCC-SLP

and Sciences. Dr. Beeson is a Fellow of the American Speech-Language-Hearing Association and previously served as coordinator of the ASHA Special Interest Division 2: Neurophysiology and Neurogenic Speech and Language Disorders. She frequently speaks at national and international conferences on the topic of acquired language impairments in adults.

Julie Barkmeier-Kraemer, PhD

Julie Barkmeier-Kraemer has extensive experience with assessment and treatment of voice and swallowing problems. She worked in the Department of Otolaryngology–Head and Neck Surgery at the University of Iowa Hospitals and Clinics for seven years, where she initiated assessment and treatment services for patients with dysphagia. In addition, she coordinated and participated in the assessment and treatment of individuals with voice problems in the University of Iowa Voice Clinic. After completing her doctoral studies in speech pathology at the University of Iowa in 1994, Dr. Barkmeier-Kraemer worked as a research scientist in the Voice and Speech Section of the National Institute on Deafness and Other Communication Disorders (NIDCD). Her research at the NIDCD focused on modulation of laryngeal reflexes during swallowing as well as studying long-term effects of botulinum toxin treatment on adductor-type spasmodic dysphonia. Her clinical work while at the NIDCD focused on assessment and treatment of neurogenic voice disorder. Julie Barkmeier-Kraemer is currently a professor in the Department of Otolaryngology at the University of California - Davis Voice and Swallowing Center.

James Dean, AuD

Dr. James Dean is a Senior Lecturer in Audiology and Pediatric Audiologist in the Department of Speech Language and Hearing Sciences at the University of Arizona. He also serves as a faculty member for the Arizona Leadership and Education in Neurodevelopment and Related Disabilities program. He received his Master of Science degree in audiology from the University of Wisconsin and his Doctor of Audiology degree from the Arizona School of Health Sciences. He also has a master's degree in Education for the Deaf from the Clark School-Smith College Teacher for the Deaf program. Dr. Dean has over twenty-five years of experience providing audiologic assessment and habilitation services to hearing impaired children and their families. He also has extensive experience working with children who have developmental disabilities.

Theodore J. Glattke, PhD

Theodore Glattke is an emeritus professor in the Department of Speech, Language, and Hearing Sciences and the Department of Surgery at the University of Arizona. He is the former editor of the *Journal of Speech and Hearing Research* and the *Journal of Communication Disorders*. During his distinguished career, Dr. Glattke provided clinical serviced in the areas of diagnostic audiology and electronystagmography and conducted research in noninvasive physiological measures of the auditory system. Dr. Glattke is a recipient of the Honors of the American Speech-Language-Hearing Association, as well as the American Academy of Audiology's Distinguished Achievement Award.

Frances P. Harris, PhD

Fran Harris is a practicing audiologist and clinical faculty member in the Department of Speech, Language, and Hearing Sciences at the University of Arizona, where she holds the James S. and Dyan Pignatelli chair in Audiologic Rehabilitation for Adults. She has over twenty years' experience as a clinical audiologist, with particular expertise in rehabilitation of hearing loss in adults. She runs the Living with Hearing Loss Program and is involved in a wide range of community outreach activities that improve the lives of adults with hearing loss. In addition to her clinical expertise, she has also conducted research on the characteristics of otoacoustic emissions in adults with and without impaired hearing. She has published numerous scientific articles, primarily on otoacoustic emissions, and has presented her work nationally and internationally.

Linda Norrix, PhD

Linda Norrix is an ASHA certified audiologist. After completing her doctoral studies in 1995, she was a research scientist at the Center for Neurogenic Communication Disorders at the University of Arizona. Her primary research involved examining the perception of auditory and visual speech. Dr. Norrix is currently a clinical assistant professor in the Department of Speech, Language, and Hearing Sciences at the University of Arizona, where she mentors students who are learning to evaluate and manage individuals with hearing impairments. Her current research interests are in the areas of auditory processing disorders, the use of FM systems with open-fit amplification, and the auditory brainstem response.

CHAPTER 1

Introduction to the Professions of Audiology and Speech-Language Pathology

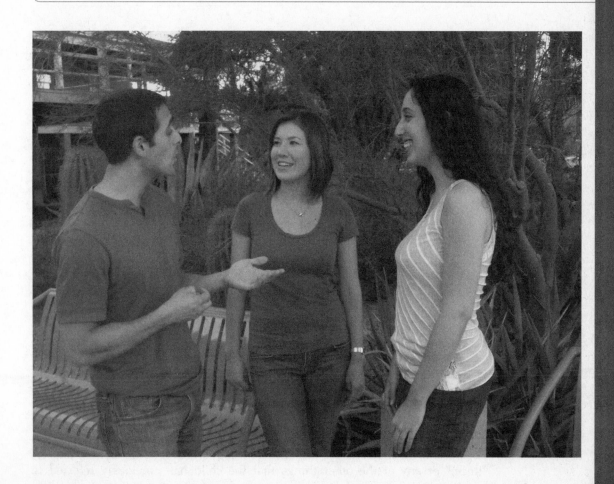

PREVIEW   Communication is so pervasive in daily life that we typically take it for granted until something goes awry. In this chapter, we introduce the field of communication disorders, starting with an examination of normal communication in its various modalities. Then we profile six individuals with disorders of speech, language, or hearing. These cases represent the estimated 10 percent of the population for whom communication is impaired. We can begin to understand the bases of these disorders by determining where normal communication breaks down and what aspects of speech, language, and hearing are affected. Later chapters examine these processes in detail. For individuals with communication impairments, the services of a speech-language pathologist or audiologist may significantly improve the quality of daily life. We will meet some professionals in communication disorders and sciences who share their perspectives regarding the rewards and challenges of this broad, dynamic field.

Normal Communication

Human communication embodies a rich tapestry of information conveyed through vocalizations, gesture, and emotional expression. **Communication** includes all means by which information is transmitted between a sender and a receiver. By this definition, we know that animals communicate through posture, movement, facial gestures, scent, and sound production. Humans are unique among animals in that we have a highly developed system of symbolic communication that we call **language**. Language may be spoken, written, or signed. Although all forms of language are used to communicate ideas, not all forms of communication involve language (see Figure 1.1). A look at some real-life examples of human communication illustrates that language and communication can take many forms.

> A father carried his 18-month-old son in his arms as he walked through a public park. His son leaned over and excitedly extended his arms into the air. "Da?" the toddler asked. The father looked to see what had caught his son's attention. A young girl from the neighborhood was walking her dog. "Oh, it's a dog," the father replied. "Da! Da!" the son exclaimed, bouncing with excitement.

With the use of a "word," tone of voice, and gestures, this child begins to use language to ask a question, make a statement, and indicate interest. The father accepts the attempt at language as meaningful, even though it only approximates a word in its adult form. He uses the situational context and the child's gestures and emotional tone to support his interpretation of his son's meaning. It becomes obvious that the child is using "da" to mean "dog" and not "dad," "man," "teddy," "juice," or any of the other things that the child has previously referred to with those sounds. The father's response to his son turns an attempt at a word

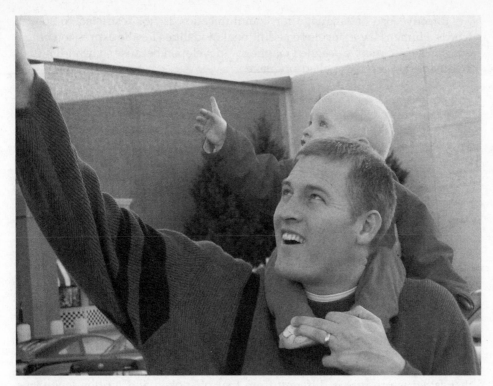

FIGURE 1.1 Communication develops before children use their first words.

into a conversation, to the enjoyment of both. As we will see, not all attempts at communication are equally successful, leading to frustrating or amusing outcomes.

> Sixty-four students sat in a lecture room, one with no windows, listening to their instructor. The professor, who had taught the course nine times before, droned on: "One might question, uh, the relational meanings that best describe, uh, the language of young children. Remember, that Bloom said (as well as Sinclair or, uh, and Bowerman) that it is possible to put in a logical order the kind of language experiences that occur in a typical order of uh, let us say, emergence."

It is sad to admit that some of the poorest communication may occur in the classroom. This lecturer's convoluted word order and interruptions due to word-retrieval pauses interfere with effective communication. The meaning of the subject matter may be difficult for the students to comprehend even without the teacher's poor sentence formulation. The students may not be listening for many reasons, including the instructor's poor narrative, fatigue from a previous activity, worry about upcoming exams, or even the lack of ventilation in the room.

Effective use of language for communication is not restricted to spoken words. Humans have developed additional modalities for the expression of language. One alternative—signed language—developed because some individuals are unable to perceive spoken language.

A 23-year-old student was hired as a classroom interpreter for a 19-year-old deaf engineering student. The interpreter had limited knowledge of the highly technical content of the engineering classes. To this was added the strain of translating the heavily accented and often broken English, spoken by the foreign-born instructor, into the completely different grammatical organization of American Sign Language. The engineering student, who had a pronounced playful streak, took advantage of these conditions for a little good-natured ribbing of the interpreter. At one point during the lecture, a fly was buzzing around the interpreter's nose and she swatted at it in mid-sentence. The student leaned forward, looked at her face, and repeated the gesture of swatting the fly, indicating he needed the gesture defined as if it were a word he did not know. When the interpreter ignored this obviously facetious request, the student only repeated it with increasing elaborations of the gesture and facial expression. This act finally caught the attention of the instructor, who stopped the class to see if there was a problem. Thoroughly embarrassed, the student and interpreter finished out the lecture without further interruption.

American Sign Language (ASL) uses a system of manual gestures instead of spoken words to convey information. In ASL, hand and arm positions, facial expressions, and movements in space are used to express vocabulary and a grammatical structure that is different from that of spoken and written languages. Like other languages, however, ASL has a normal developmental sequence when learned as a first language. No matter the mode, all languages can be used for a variety of purposes, such as communicating, thinking, and learning, as well as teasing and humor.

Like signed language, written language also uses the visual modality for communication. The written word may be used to inform, entertain, and regulate behavior.

While traveling in the Southwest, we had occasion to visit the Ghost Ranch Living Museum in northern New Mexico. This center includes a small zoo of animals indigenous to the area. Signs in front of each animal habitat warned, "Do not feed your fingers to the animals. Their diet is carefully monitored."

This clever sign conveyed at least two important pieces of information. Visitors should not feed the animals, and the animals will bite. In this case, the sign's creator used a humorous approach and indirect language to convey the message. The tone of the written message was particularly appropriate to the setting, because it contributed to, rather than detracted from, the visitor's enjoyment of the sights. The use of indirect language is interesting here, in that much more is communicated than the words actually denote.

Normal communication encompasses verbal and nonverbal elements that, in combination, are used for a variety of purposes. Communication is successful when information is accurately transmitted from a sender to a receiver. Some aspects of communication, such as nonverbal elements, are not always intentional. Sometimes our bodies "give us away." For example, our posture, facial expression, and vocal quality may combine to indicate fatigue, even when we may be very interested in the topic of conversation. Other elements, such as proximity and gestures, communicate the speaker's status, attitudes, and emotions.

Many of the nonverbal elements of communication are culturally regulated. For example, Anglo listeners tend to provide speakers with periodic feedback by nods and vocalized signals of affirmation. A Navajo audience provides fewer overt signs of attention; polite listeners attend unobtrusively. Some cultures maintain constant eye contact when listening; for others, "staring" at a speaker is rude. Even subtle variations, such as the length of pauses between utterances, are culturally determined. Although this may seem to be a minor aspect of communication, violations may have profound effects on the listener. A speaker who pauses too long may appear to be withholding and unsociable. One whose pauses are too short may appear to be impertinent and domineering. Most individuals are able to monitor and use an ongoing stream of nonverbal information for effective communication. However, these nonverbal skills are dependent on normal development and can be disrupted in some individuals, just as spoken and written communication can be impaired.

> Communication disorders can result from conditions that
> - are present at birth
> - emerge as a child develops
> - result from an acquired loss or impairment

Six Individuals with Communication Impairment

The need or desire to communicate permeates much of our daily lives, including family interactions, written and spoken communication at work, and recreational activities. However, those who have difficulty making themselves understood or understanding others may be acutely aware of their limitations. To appreciate the impact of these limitations, we review a few stories of individuals with various forms of communication impairment.

As we will see from these cases, communication disorders affect both children and adults, and they do not discriminate by ethnic background or economic status.

> *Beth Feldman*[1] is a 23-year-old student teacher who developed bilateral vocal nodules, or bumps, on both vocal folds. By noon every day, she lost her voice completely, making it impossible to control the twenty-six children in her fourth-grade class. Her supervising teacher warned her that she could not continue as a student teacher if she did not improve her voice. Seeking help in a voice clinic at a university hospital, Beth learned that she speaks at the bottom of her pitch range, clears her throat excessively, speaks with excessive effort and tension in her throat, and

---

[1]We have changed the names of all individuals whose communication disorders are described in this book. In some instances the case history reflects a blend of several individuals.

exhibits other behaviors detrimental to her vocal health. She consulted two ear-nose-throat physicians (otolaryngologists), and each of them told her that she had two small nodules, one on each vocal fold, that were not big enough to explain the severe voice symptoms she was experiencing. Both doctors recommended voice therapy. Ms. Feldman's initial attempts to schedule voice therapy were thwarted by her busy schedule, and her voice problem persisted. After several months, she finally made a return visit to the voice clinic to initiate treatment.

Jim Fields is a 43-year-old promoter who arranges concerts for rock and pop musicians. His wife convinced him to have his hearing checked when she noticed that he was no longer hearing his wristwatch alarm and that he had difficulty understanding her over the telephone. His evaluation by an audiologist revealed a moderate to severe hearing loss of the type associated with noise exposure. The audiologist learned that his history of noise exposure dated back to his teens, when he sang in a band that in his words "substituted volume for talent." Since that time, there had been many occasions when he remembered leaving a performance with "ringing ears" or "fuzzy hearing." The audiologist explained the relationship between exposure to loud sound and the hearing loss Mr. Fields was experiencing. Mr. Fields now uses hearing protection when exposed to loud music (and other loud sounds) to slow further hearing loss. He enrolled in a speechreading (lipreading) course to help compensate for his hearing loss. In addition, he returns for regular hearing checkups to monitor his hearing acuity. He elected to forgo a hearing aid at this time but understands that one may become a necessity in the future.

Rodolfo Torres, age 13 months, was evaluated by team members of a university oro-facial disorders clinic. He was born in Mexico with a bilateral cleft lip and palate. Although his cleft lip was surgically repaired within a few weeks of his birth, the roof of his mouth remained unrepaired. All of his attempts at speech sounds appeared to come out of his nose because of the coupling of his oral and nasal cavities. He was examined by a plastic surgeon, who recommended immediate surgery to complete the repair of his cleft. Both the audiologist and otolaryngologist found that the boy had a middle-ear infection, which was producing a moderate hearing loss. The speech-language pathologist determined that Rodolfo exhibited normal language comprehension for Spanish and urged surgical intervention to help reduce his severe hypernasality. The boy and his mother made plans to live temporarily with his uncle in Tucson so the first stage of surgery could be started. The social worker on the team met with the speech-language pathologist, the plastic surgeon, and the boy's mother to coordinate the surgery and follow-up speech services.

Bruce Murrich, age 69, is a retired executive who suffered a stroke in his sleep, awakening with right-side paralysis (hemiplegia) and aphasia (loss of language). His sudden symptoms transformed him from a golf-playing, fun-loving retiree to a man unable to speak except for occasional profanity. He was also powerless to move his right arm and leg. He and his wife reacted initially to the severe disability with disbelief and denial, hoping that, with proper medical attention, his symptoms would go away after a few days. After several weeks of persistent impairment, Mr. and Mrs. Murrich sought rehabilitation, including speech-language pathology services. Mr. Murrich began receiving individual speech-language therapy (plus physical and occupational therapies), and participated in group treatment with other individuals with aphasia. His wife attended a weekly spouse group and received individual counseling from a social worker in the rehabilitation center. As Mr. Murrich's language improved to the point where he could communicate many thoughts and needs in two- to three-word utterances, his spirits improved dramatically. Now, about eighteen months after the stroke, Mr. Murrich and his wife continue to be encouraged by his improvements, but also accept the relative permanence of his disability.

Devon Douglas was 17 when we first met him. His younger brother, Andrew, had been diagnosed with a rare genetic condition that often affects development. The family lived in a remote town and traveled two hours each way to reach our clinic, where they participated in a research study to determine the communication aspects of Andrew's genetic disorder. When we first talked with the boy's mother, she had more concerns about Devon than about Andrew, despite the fact that Devon did not have the genetic disorder. She reported that he had struggled throughout his school history to maintain average grades. Over the years, starting when Devon was in second grade, she had repeatedly asked the school system to evaluate him for a learning disability. Each time, the school staff indicated that they did not see Devon as having any educational handicaps, so he was never evaluated. Devon reported that teachers had told him that he was lazy and could do better if he tried. His mother was now worried that school was such a struggle that he might drop out before graduation. As part of our research program, we evaluated Devon's cognitive and linguistic skills. Testing revealed that his general cognitive abilities were in the high-average range. However, he had great difficulty putting together grammatically correct sentences, following spoken directions, and understanding what he read. In fact, his overall language skills were quite weak. At age 17, we diagnosed a language-based learning disability for the first time in this young man's life.

Mary Kim is an animated 5-year-old girl, the youngest of three children. When she was born in a Los Angeles hospital, she appeared healthy in all respects, but she did not pass the newborn hearing screening test. Her parents were referred to an audiologist, who performed a diagnostic evaluation and confirmed that Mary had a profound hearing loss in both ears. Her parents were taken by surprise, because their two other children had normal hearing; however, Mary's mother had both a sister and an aunt who were deaf from birth. The deafness appeared to be a hereditary form of hearing loss affecting the development and function of an inner-ear structure, the cochlea. The audiologist fitted Mary with hearing aids on both ears and referred the family to an otolaryngologist to consider a cochlear implant, which would provide electrical stimulation to the auditory nerve. The Kims learned that Mary was a good candidate for implantation, and when she reached 12 months of age, surgery was performed. Six weeks later, when the implant was activated, Mary heard sound for the first time. She reacted initially by crying, but then became alert to sound, widening her eyes and turning her head in response. The family received speech-language therapy for the next several years to enhance Mary's communication development. She is now starting kindergarten, and her speech and language development are within the range of typically developing children. The Kims informed the classroom teacher that Mary has difficulty hearing in noisy environments so that accommodations could be made to maximize Mary's opportunity for success.

These cases represent the diverse challenges encountered by professionals in the field of communication disorders. Each case demonstrates how difficulty with just one aspect of communication can affect daily life. Ms. Feldman's vocal nodules had a direct impact on her effectiveness as a teacher. Mr. Murrich's stroke forever altered both his and his wife's plans for retired life. Devon's difficulty with language had a significant effect on his school success.

Classification of Communication Disorders

Communication requires the transmission of information from one person to another. Breakdown in communication may be understood by examining the components of this process. Information can be conveyed through tone of voice, facial expression, posture, and gestures. Language, however, is the medium of choice when we wish to communicate specific ideas and speech is the modality that most of us use to transmit these ideas.

The ways in which sounds are combined into words and words into sentences is arbitrarily determined across languages. For example, in English, words may begin with an "st" combination, as in *stairs,* but not with a "ts" combination. However, Navajo includes words that start with the "ts" combination (e.g., *tseí,* meaning "rock"). These conventions within each language are completely arbitrary; English speakers are capable of producing the "ts" combination (e.g., "its") but do not use it at the beginning of words. Other rules govern how words are combined into sentences. These rules of grammar also vary among languages, and do not follow a standard pattern. For example, English requires the use of nouns or pronouns to specify the subject of a sentence (e.g., "I am hungry"). In Spanish, however, the pronoun can be dropped from the sentence without any resulting confusion (e.g., "Tengo hambre"). We will explore the nature of language in more detail in Chapter 7.

For most individuals, language is communicated from speaker to listener through an oral-to-auditory pathway. The larynx, tongue, lips, and other oral structures are used to produce the individual sounds of language that we recognized as **speech**. Mere changes in tongue placement result in different speech sounds, such as "k" versus "t." The addition of vocal fold vibrations changes the "t" to a "d." In some languages, additional manipulations of sound contribute to speech. For example, Chinese is considered a tonal language because changes in the pitch of the voice distinguish specific speech sounds. Our vocal mechanism also allows us to vary the pitch and loudness of speech to convey emotion and emphasis. For the average person, these aspects come together seamlessly to produce a smooth flow of words. We introduce the physical structures that support speech in Chapter 2 and follow with a discussion of the sounds of speech in Chapter 3.

Language is a symbol system used to represent ideas.

Because of their knowledge of the anatomy and physiology of the oral structures, speech-language pathologists have become involved with treatment of certain disorders that do not strictly involve communication, such as swallowing and feeding. Swallowing disorders often result from the same types of disease processes and acquired damage that can affect communication. Evaluation and treatment of swallowing have become prominent components of many speech-language pathologists' work in health-related settings. Swallowing disorders are discussed in Chapter 6.

Spoken language is received by the listener through the aural modality. This requires an intact auditory system. **Hearing** involves the awareness of sound, the ability to distinguish among sounds, and the ability to process sounds that occur at a rapid rate. These abilities are essential for decoding speech. By hearing spoken language, we learn the rules of our native language, the sounds of speech, and even the accent and intonation patterns that characterize our regional dialect. When we speak, we monitor our own production and modify or correct our speech as we talk. The mechanisms of hearing, on which all these skills rely, are addressed in Chapter 10.

> Speech refers to sound production achieved by movements of the vocal mechanism.

Impairments of Speech

When impairments of communication occur, they typically involve a breakdown in one or more of the elements involved in speech, language, or hearing. Impairments of speech may include aspects of **articulation**, or the way the sounds of words are produced. Some disorders of sound production are caused by structural abnormality, as in the case of a child born with a cleft palate. For Rodolfo, his cleft palate altered the oral structures needed for speech articulation. If left unrepaired, he would have little chance to develop normal speech. In other children, developmental articulation disorders may appear without a known cause. Children may also exhibit phonological disorders, in which they are able to produce all speech sounds but combine them incorrectly in words. In many instances, children simply are slow to develop speech. All of these developmental speech sound disorders may appear without an apparent cause. In other cases, the disorder may be associated with a more generalized delay in development, such as occurs with mental retardation. Speech sound disorders also may be acquired following accident or disease. Disorders of speech sounds are reviewed in Chapter 4.

Some speech disorders reflect problems with the voice. **Voice** disorders may alter the pitch, quality, or loudness of the voice, as discussed in Chapter 6. We saw in the case of Ms. Feldman that poor speaking practices may lead to physical changes in the vocal mechanism that interfere with speech over time. In her case, the voice disorder affected her professional life. In other cases, an overly breathy or harsh vocal quality or a loss of voicing may signal a health concern that requires immediate medical intervention.

Finally, a disorder of speech may involve the fluency of speech production. Fluency disorders occur when the normal, smooth flow of speech becomes interrupted, as in the case of stuttering. The individual may struggle to produce words or sentences that come effortlessly for others. For most individuals, stuttering begins during childhood, and many of those who stutter eventually overcome this difficulty. Those

> Some common impairments of speech include:
> - articulation errors
> - voice disorders
> - stuttering

with persistent stuttering have to monitor their fluency indefinitely. Stuttering and other fluency disorders are reviewed in Chapter 5.

Impairments of Language

Some impairments
of language include:
- delayed language
  development
- autism
- aphasia

Language impairments may include conditions that emerge as a child develops. These *developmental* language disorders may first appear during childhood but can persist into adulthood. This was the case with Devon, who had difficulties throughout his school years. In contrast to developmental language disorders, acquired language disorders occur when an individual suffers an injury or disease that causes a loss of language skills. Mr. Murrich experienced one type of *acquired* language disorder called aphasia. Although acquired language disorders can occur at any time during life, the majority of individuals with acquired language disorders are adults. Disorders involving language skills in children and adults are discussed in Chapters 8 and 9, respectively.

Impairments of Hearing

Impairments of
hearing can be
associated with:
- genetically linked
  deafness at birth
- conductive hearing
  loss due to middle
  ear infection
- noise-induced
  hearing loss

Disorders of hearing may arise from factors that block the conduction of sound into and through the hearing mechanism. These are referred to as **conductive hearing loss**. A common cause of conductive hearing loss in young children is the presence of fluid in the middle ear due to infection, which is called otitis media. In contrast to conductive hearing loss, **sensorineural hearing loss** refers to a hearing loss caused by disease of the inner ear or the neural transmission of sound. In Mr. Fields's case, exposure to loud sound over time produced a sensorineural hearing loss. In other cases, an individual may be born with a sensorineural hearing loss, as in the case of Mary. Although we classify hearing disorders as conductive or sensorineural, in some instances, hearing loss may involve a mix of both types. We will discuss disorders of hearing in Chapters 11 and Chapter 12.

Personal Stories about Communication Disorders

The cases described above provide a brief look at the way in which speech, language, and hearing might be impaired at various times throughout the lifespan. It is evident that some communication impairments can have a dramatic impact on the lives of affected individuals and their families. In fact, quite a few people have written personal accounts of living with a disease or disability that affected their ability to communicate. Such stories are part of a relatively new literary genre called *pathography*. Pathography refers to literature that recounts personal stories about living with illness or disability. Such accounts include autobiographies and biographies written by the affected individual, family members, friends, physicians, or other involved parties. Although most pathographies are written as first- or third-person accounts of true events, a few are fictionalized stories. As various communication disorders are introduced in this book, we will list relevant pathographies at the end of the chapter under the heading "Readings from the Popular Literature." These books often capture the true impact of communication disorders, whether they are present from birth or acquired later in life. Although the impairment may not be the primary focus of the story, considerable insight is offered in the context of these personal stories. For example, Mitch Albom's best-seller *Tuesdays with Morrie* recounts the lessons that he learned from his former college professor, whose health was declining due to the progressive neurological disease known as amyotrophic lateral sclerosis (ALS, or Lou Gehrig's disease). In the midst of this poignant story about appreciating life, the reader gains insight into the consequences of reduced motor control for the production of speech and for swallowing. We agree with the observation made by our colleague Raymond Kent, who wrote, "What often emerges in the best of these accounts is not preoccupation with a bad turn of life, but rather lessons in endurance, resourcefulness, and overcoming" (Kent, 1998, p. 22). Professionals in the field of communication disorders have the privilege of sharing in these life lessons with their clients or patients, and they often find it one of the most rewarding aspects of their work.

> Pathography refers to a literary genre that recounts the story of an illness or disability. Can you think of some examples in books that you have read or movies you have seen?

As you read this book, you will learn about the biological foundations for speech, language, and hearing, and will gain an understanding of how these critical human functions can be disrupted. The individual case descriptions interspersed in the subsequent chapters provide some context for understanding the nature and treatment of communication disorders, and how the impairments may affect individuals in real life. Greater understanding of the true impact of communication disorders can be gained by reading books from the popular literature listed at the end of each chapter, or by simply getting to know individuals with speech, language, or hearing impairments. Of course, you may already have knowledge from your own experiences or those of close family or friends. Individual life stories provide insight into the social aspects of disability that are unique to each person. This personalized view of disability was clearly articulated by the World Health Organization (WHO) in a document that provided a framework to consider the impact of health and disability in the context of personal and environmental factors (WHO, 2002). The WHO, which is a specialized agency of the United Nations, promotes the view that all individuals experience some degree of disability over the course of their lives, and that various health conditions can lead to altered physical or cognitive functioning that limits activities or participation in life situations. Professionals who work with individuals with communication disorders typically appreciate this "whole person" perspective, and often express great satisfaction in work that that is devoted to minimizing the negative impact of speech, language, or hearing impairments on their client's daily lives.

Careers in Communication Disorders

As described in the cases at the beginning of this chapter, most individuals with speech, language, or hearing disorders can improve their communication. The professionals who provide services for the remediation of communication disorders are **speech-language pathologists** and **audiologists**. These clinical professionals rely on the information provided by research conducted by speech scientists, language scientists, and hearing scientists, as well as researchers in related fields. The professional organization for speech-language pathologists, audiologists, and scientists in the field of communication disorders is the American Speech-Language-Hearing Association (ASHA). This organization has been certifying professionals in communication disorders since 1952, but the beginnings of modern occupations in "speech correction" and sound amplification for the hearing impaired can be traced back to the early 1800s in Europe. In fact, interest and concern regarding disorders of the ability to communicate were evident in the writings of ancient Greece and Rome philosophers (Wollock, 1997).

In the United States, academic programs specific to communication disorders began to emerge in the 1940s, after World War II, as the need for rehabilitation services was evident for the large numbers of returning soldiers with head injuries and acquired hearing loss. Educational programs for **audiology** and **speech-language pathology** developed in tandem, but in 1989, ASHA passed a resolution that specified these as separate professions. Because of the common concern for human communication impairments and the historical association of these two professions, most individuals in either field have some knowledge and training in areas served primarily by the other. At the present time, for example, the undergraduate curriculum in most training institutions does not divide the two fields. Instead, students specialize in one or the other profession as part of their graduate school training. Although there are some job opportunities for individuals with less training (see Chapter 13 for a discussion of support personnel), a graduate degree is required for certification as an audiologist or speech-language pathologist.

An aspiring speech-language pathologist must complete all graduate courses (typically thirty-six credit hours) for a master's degree (or its equivalent) awarded from an accredited program. In addition, ASHA requires a minimum of 400 hours of supervised clinical practicum (see Figure 1.2). Upon completion of the degree, a clinical fellowship year is completed under the supervision of a certified speech-language pathologist (ASHA, 2005; rev. 2009). In the field of audiology, the entry-level degree for clinical practice is now a doctorate. The Doctorate of Audiology (AuD) has become the most common degree earned by audiologists since about 2004. This degree requires a minimum of seventy-five credit hours of post-baccalaureate study, with supervised clinical training included in the degree program. In addition to academic and clinical training, both audiologists and speech-language pathologists must pass a national certification examination before becoming certified to work independently in any of a wide variety of clinical settings.

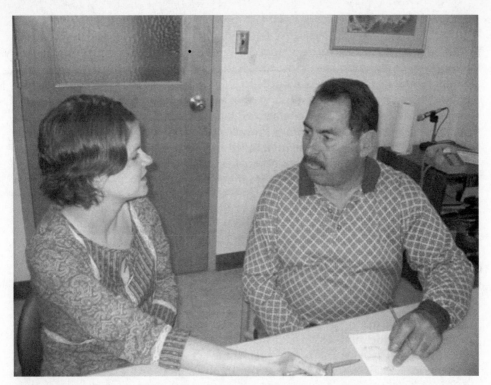

FIGURE 1.2   In addition to academic preparation, students training to be speech-language pathologists or audiologists conduct a supervised clinical practicum with individuals with communication disorders.

Those who are interested in pursuing a research career or an academic position in a college or university typically obtain training for a Doctor of Philosophy (PhD) or a Doctor of Science (ScD) degree. A primary goal of doctoral-level training is to prepare individuals to conduct independent research. Such research may focus on normal aspects of speech, language, and hearing or on the nature and/or treatment of communication disorders. Many of the scientists in this field obtained research training after completing their clinical training, but some researchers pursued a research track from the outset and did not obtain clinical training.

There are over 145,000 professionals with careers in communication disorders and sciences. This includes over 126,000 speech-language pathologists, close to 13,000 audiologists, and about 1,000 individuals with dual certification in speech-language pathology and audiology (ASHA, 2010; Bureau of Labor Statistics, 2011). In addition, there are about 3,600 individuals whose primary employment involves research and/or teaching at the college or university level regarding the nature and treatment of communication disorders. Like the U.S. population, these professionals represent all major racial and ethnic groups: White, African

American, Hispanic, Asian/Pacific Islander, and Native American. A survey of the ASHA membership indicated that most audiologists and speech-language pathologists (73 percent) are employed full-time. For audiologists, the most common place of employment is in a health-care facility (65–75 percent), which includes hospitals, clinics, private practices, and as part of a physician's practice. Other employment settings for audiologists include educational settings (10–15 percent), industrial facilities, or state and local government agencies. In contrast, 50 percent of the speech-language pathologists report working in a school system. Other common employment settings for speech-language pathologists are health-care facilities, colleges or universities, and private practice offices.

The results of the annual ASHA membership survey provide an overview of those who work in the field of communication disorders. To get a more personal view, we asked audiologists and speech-language pathologists from around the country to share their perceptions about their careers. Our informants included individuals who represent nearly all segments of the demographic groups that comprise the professions.

Clinical Careers

A number of years ago, we began interviewing our colleagues and former students in the profession, and asked why they chose a career path in communication disorders. As one might imagine, some were first introduced to the field because they knew someone with a communication disorder. That was the case for Nancy, who lives in Arizona and was a relative newcomer to the field when we interviewed her. Nancy wrote, "I worked for a gentleman who had Parkinson disease, and he piqued my interest in the rehabilitation fields. He persuaded me to 'lose interest in the law' [a previous pursuit] and to become involved in a 'helping profession.' After doing some research, I found speech-language pathology to be the most interesting." A few colleagues had received clinical services themselves or knew someone who was working in the field. Kim, a speech-language pathologist from Colorado, reported that she had received articulation therapy as a young child. She wrote, "I decided one day on my way to my daughter's day care to be a 'speech therapist.' At the time, I only knew the 'r,' 'l,' and 's' part of the field." In her six years in the profession, Kim gained extensive experience working in both school and hospital settings. Donna is an audiologist with thirty-five years' experience who is employed as the director of a university clinic. She reported that a relative was a teacher of the deaf and that this sparked her interest in deafness. As an undergraduate, she was in the enviable position of having three fellowship offers—in theater, linguistics, and audiology—to choose among. She chose audiology and said, "I have *never* regretted this decision."

Those with direct exposure to the professions were in the minority. Many of our colleagues noted a desire to enter a field where they could "make people's lives better." This sentiment was echoed by Jennifer, who wrote, "I always knew I wanted to work with children, but I wasn't sure how until I saw some speech pathologists work with language-impaired preschoolers at a local hospital. Watching them, I realized how much impact a person could have in a child's life." Jennifer has had many opportunities to rediscover this impact in her own hospital-based position as a pediatric speech-language pathologist. Others were attracted because of a specific interest area that was encompassed by the field. Paula reported that she had an initial interest in languages and language development. "Then I took an audiology course and became fascinated with the process of hearing and what can happen when people—especially children—are unable to hear." She has combined these interests for fifteen years as an audiologist. Many who come to the field of speech-language pathology have a background in psychology or linguistics. Celia chose to become a speech-language pathologist after obtaining a PhD in linguistics. Although the two fields are similar in many ways, Celia realized that she wanted more of a clinical focus, which she now enjoys in her work with adults with acquired language disorders.

Increasingly, individuals come into the profession after having worked in another field. Zarina was a bilingual second-grade teacher before deciding to go back to school. In her years of teaching, Zarina said, "I noticed that there were a lot of Spanish-speaking kids with language difficulties. I decided to go into speech-language pathology to help bilingual children. I also wanted the option of working in other settings in addition to schools." Erin was a public relations accounts executive before returning to school for a master's degree in speech-language pathology. "What it all came down to was more meaningful work. I wanted a job helping people instead of just helping a company make money." She picked speech-language pathology because it allowed her to combine her interests in languages (she speaks English and French) and health. Bret wrote, "I've had a long-standing interest in how we communicate; my BA was in speech communication. I was advised by a family friend to investigate speech-language pathology . . . and I learned just how varied the field is and that it could provide a lifelong, stable career." He now works as a speech-language pathologist in a rehabilitation center. Sue discovered speech-language pathology after a diverse career path that included water-quality testing, small business ownership, creative writing, and publishing. She told us, "I wanted to work more closely with people, and my background in language is directly relevant to my work with clients who have reading and writing impairments."

There is also what we like to think of as the "luck factor" that led people to discover the field. Consider Anne, who is a speech-language pathologist in Missouri. "I didn't really know what I wanted to do," wrote Anne. "I had several friends who talked me into taking a speech-language pathology course, and I decided then and there that I was in the right field." Carol, an audiologist of ten years in California, had a similar reaction to her initial academic exposure. "I found the coursework interesting and challenging. There didn't seem to be a single course in the program I wasn't interested in taking." For Ellen, who has now been practicing for eleven years in Tennessee, a problem with her own voice led to a career in speech-language pathology. "I wanted to work with voice disorders, as I was a voice major in music and experiencing problems. I took a class in phonetics and loved the content."

We were impressed by the variety of reasons that led our colleagues to enter the field. This may be because the professions accommodate a wide range of personality traits and backgrounds. We saw this when we asked people to tell us about the traits they considered important in their job. Here are a few of the recurring themes they expressed: Lane's experience in hospitals and skilled nursing facilities in Arizona taught him that "a speech-language pathologist needs to be flexible, adaptable, a team player, a good communicator, and very clear about personal and professional integrity. These characteristics are crucial for survival in a rapidly changing health-care system." Another trait identified by our colleagues was an orientation toward solving problems. Ellen commented, "Task analysis is at the center of what we do: identify problems, then determine the best method of improving function." Not surprisingly, she feels that traits such as analytical skill, inquisitiveness, enthusiasm, and an action-oriented nature apply to her. Rebecca, a speech-language pathologist of twenty-one years and the director of a hospital-based center for communication disorders in New York, adds qualities such as persistence, self-confidence, maturity, and generosity to the list.

Among the most frequently mentioned traits was independence. Angie, a speech-language pathologist from Tennessee, commented, "I believe you must be assertive in this field. People's quality of life is at stake, and you must do whatever you can to help." Independence characterized clinicians in private practice, university clinics, schools, hospitals, rehabilitation centers, and skilled nursing facilities. This is not surprising, in that clinicians in most settings have a great deal of autonomy in how they manage their caseload, develop programs, and provide quality service. Mike, a Colorado resident with twenty-three years' experience, expressed the complementary position: "I think patience may be the key to my success as an audiologist, especially when working with families with young hearing-impaired infants. They need the gift of *time* to accept their child's impairments and to implement the many recommendations we make." In fact, patience was mentioned as an important trait by almost all our respondents. Regardless of clinical setting or clientele, the field demands individuals with the motivation to identify areas of need and seek out information in this ever-advancing field.

We were also curious about what keeps these professionals in the field year after year. Some cited specific aspects of their jobs, such as the experience of developing a new program for service delivery or working with cutting-edge technology. Donna works with new advances such as programmable hearing aids and cochlear implants (see Figure 1.3). She wrote, "Patients who are realizing dramatic functional gains keep me going!" "I love the diagnostic process," writes Shara, a speech-language pathologist of eleven years. "To be able to identify strengths and weaknesses and provide explanations for behavior is very challenging. Also to be able to change those behaviors, to see them 'get it,' is exciting." Shannon, a Michigan-based speech-language pathologist, echoed several common themes: "It's the versatility of being able to work with children or adults. I also like having a solid base of knowledge in a variety of disorders. And there's also the advantage of always being able to find a job!" Angie expressed the sentiments of many of our colleagues. She wrote, "It's a fast-paced field. I am always encountering new situations that allow me to learn." Lou,

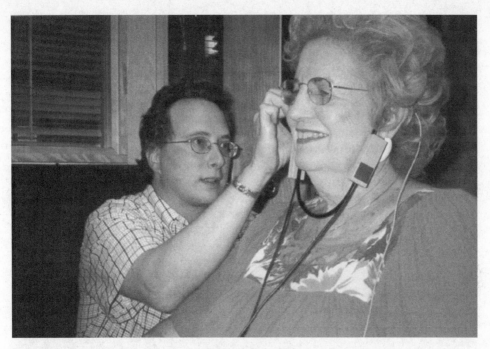

FIGURE 1.3   Audiologists are responsible for the selection and fitting of hearing aids. Hearing aids are programmed using specialized equipment to suit the hearing loss of each individual.

a speech-language pathologist of three years, wrote, "The most exciting thing for me to experience is children's first words—the look in their eyes when they realize they are able to impact their environment using words." All clinicians have stories about particular clients who stand out, punctuating their careers like exclamation points along the way. This was the case for Angie, who wrote about a difficult case involving a man who had had a stroke. The patient recalled that Angie had high expectations for him, and made him work hard, always "cracking the whip." He told Angie, "I never could have done it without you." Ellen writes that one of her staff was able to identify an important medical issue for a patient that had been previously missed by several other professionals. "This speech-language pathologist referred the patient back to the ear, nose, and throat physician and highlighted her findings. The ENT diagnosed the actual cause of the swallowing disorder and was able to surgically repair it. The patient resumed a regular diet." Sometimes the smallest gains are the most important to the clinician. Susan, a speech-language pathologist in Minnesota, wrote of a severely autistic child who, for the first time, communicated a specific desire by selecting a picture of an activity. "We were so excited for him and what this skill will do for him in the future." She is now working to expand that child's first step toward building the skills to communicate with others through the use of pictures. The impact of these cases is captured by Lane, who commented that "the emotional rewards and the opportunity to powerfully impact and connect with people during a difficult time in their lives" are primary advantages to a career in the field of communication disorders.

Research Careers

Audiologists and speech-language pathologists impact lives through direct clinical services. But this is not the only avenue to effect change within the professions. The desire to advance the field beyond its current boundaries inspires professionals to incorporate research into their career. Whereas direct clinical intervention improves lives, one person at a time, research has the potential to improve the lives of many, as new discoveries further the understanding, diagnosis, and treatment of communication disorders for the entire profession. Although opportunities for research exist in almost all job settings, fewer than 1 percent of the professionals see themselves primarily as researchers. Another 3 percent are college or university professors, for whom research is a typical component of their careers (ASHA, 2010). Researchers include not only those with a clinical interest but also those who focus on the scientific aspects of the human communication system (see Figure 1.4). Most of these individuals received doctoral

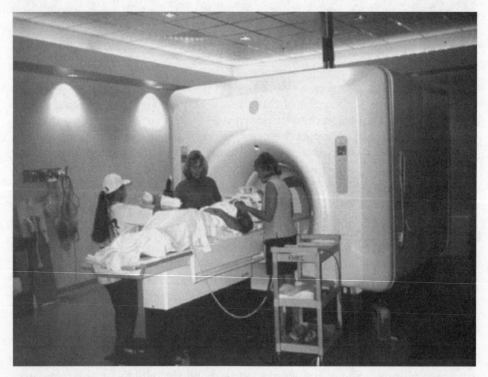

FIGURE 1.4   Research careers in communication disorders involve the study of normal and disordered communication processes. Functional magnetic resonance imaging provides a means to examine how the brain supports speech and language.

education that provided core training in research methods. The majority of these researchers work in university settings. We asked some of these individuals to tell us why they selected this career path and what it is like to be a researcher in the field of communication disorders.

Amy Skinder had just begun her doctoral studies at the University of Washington when we first talked with her. Prior to her enrollment, she had worked as a speech-language pathologist for four years, part of that time as a traveling clinician in a variety of settings around the country. "My goal when I finished my master's was to be able to work with a broad range of disorders. After a while, I decided that instead of knowing a little about a lot, it would be nice to focus on one area. At the same time, I was working with a client in the public school system who had severe developmental apraxia of speech, as well as attention deficit disorder and other learning disabilities. I went to a seminar . . . and asked lots of questions. I found out there weren't a lot of answers. After talking with the speaker [a noted researcher], I felt encouraged to go on for my doctorate. Doctoral studies are an opportunity to indulge in trying to answer all your burning questions."

When we next caught up with Amy Skinder, she had obtained her doctorate, married, and taken a faculty position at the University of Minnesota–Duluth. Dr. Skinder-Meredith filled us in on what it is like to start an academic and research career. "I enjoy my faculty position very much. It's good to be teaching. I work with wonderful people who value my work as a colleague, a teacher, and a researcher." She emphasized the importance of her clinical experience to her teaching and research endeavors. Besides conducting research in childhood apraxia, a communication disorder she encountered as a clinician, Dr. Skinder-Meredith draws on her clinical background to supplement her teaching. In addition to continuing her own research, she forged relationships with others who work in her area of interest in order to foster collaborative research.

This motivation has been echoed by many researchers. Anne Cordes Bothe, PhD, is on the faculty at the University of Georgia, where she conducts research in the area of stuttering. She realized during her master's program that she wanted to go on for a doctorate. "The things that were catching my interest during my coursework and with my practicum clients were the things that we as a field didn't know or didn't yet understand. It wasn't the answers that I thought were interesting, it was the *questions*! And the PhD is a research degree, which is about questions, so it became pretty obvious that this is where I belonged."

Nancy Helm-Estabrooks, ScD, wrote, "In many ways I think I was always an informal researcher—trying new approaches, developing new materials, regarding every individual as a case study—even before my doctoral studies, which I pursued in my thirties. I decided to get a doctorate to further my knowledge and to write grant proposals as a Principal Investigator so I could explore and test some ideas I had for new treatment approaches."

Steven Camarata, PhD, works as faculty at Vanderbilt University. He wrote, "I wanted to teach at a university and was interested in clinical research. Being able to follow my curiosity for research [is an exciting component of the job].

This freedom is a very precious gift. I knew that research would involve a lot of mundane work, but the discovery is worth it. Plus, I want to help children with speech and language problems and realized early on that I could best do this not only by seeing patients (which I still do) but also by developing better treatments."

For our colleagues, the commitment it takes to get a doctorate was definitely worth the time and effort. Barbara Lewis, PhD, of Rainbow Babies and Children's Hospital and Case Western Reserve University, has been conducting research for two decades. Her work on the genetic basis of phonological disorders has drawn her into collaborations with psychologists, pediatricians, epidemiologists, and geneticists. She wrote to us, "I like the challenge of asking difficult research questions and finding results that do not always correspond to my prediction."

This was also apparent to Dr. Skinder-Meredith when she was just beginning her research career. "It is not easy to answer those big, burning questions. It's surprising how small you have to start out with your research. It's a lot more complicated than you anticipate." In the long term, the discoveries made by scientists who systematically follow a line of research, advance the knowledge base of the entire profession. Audiologist and hearing scientist Theodore Glattke, PhD, expressed the importance of researchers within the profession when he said, "If we fail to develop new knowledge, we will face extinction as service providers." Leslie Gonzalez Rothi, PhD, added, "We are the professionals best suited to perform this applied research—a bridge between basic research and clinical application."

Many active researchers in our field hold academic positions. This brings with it the opportunity to interact with students. Dr. Cordes Bothe related some of her favorite aspects of teaching. "I like being able to sit with one student and figure out where she is and what her needs are and be able to point her in the right direction. I get a kick out of phrasing something just right in class so that I can see twenty light bulbs come on over the students' heads. And every so often, I get a kick out of the sudden realization that I *do* know how to solve some problem after all." Dr. Glattke, now an emeritus faculty member at the University of Arizona, held an academic position for over forty years and has extensive experience mentoring students in research experiences. "It is a pleasure to witness the genuine excitement that the students express when they share their work. Sometimes they discover something about themselves as a result of the effort they put into writing about their research or synthesizing the literature base." He also had this to say about working in an academic environment: "Contributing to the development of new knowledge, integrating the new knowledge into the curriculum, and adapting mentoring styles to respond to the needs of the students are invigorating activities. It is a privilege to be allowed to teach in a university setting."

Others conduct research within health-care settings. Among the leading non-university research sites are some of the Veteran's Administration (VA) Medical Centers. Dr. Gonzalez Rothi served as program director of the Brain Rehabilitation Research Center at the Veteran's Administration Medical Center in Gainesville, Florida, where she combined clinical practice with cutting-edge research.

She wrote, "My research background offers me a willingness to open doors that are not yet available to most. Second, no day is ever the same. Each time I come into the hospital, I find that new challenges are facing me, testing the limits of my abilities, and always inspiring me to know more." Dr. Helm-Estabrooks has also worked in the VA system as well as university settings and has extensive experience conducting research in clinical settings. "Research appeals to my detective instincts, developing new assessment and treatment methods appeals to my creative instincts, and clinical research allows me to work directly with patients. Also, there are many aspects to my work—patient evaluations and therapy sessions, writing, teaching, mentoring, etc.—so that I'm always challenged and never bored."

Research careers present their own unique challenges. "One of the main challenges has been to remain focused on my primary interest: genetics of speech and language disorders," Dr. Lewis expressed. "There are many temptations to digress into related but very interesting areas. You have to realize that you can't do it all." Dr. Cordes Bothe agrees. "Balance and organization [are challenges]. My job gives me at least twice as many options as any one human being could reasonably keep track of. . . . An academic position is described as 'teaching, research, and service,' but what that really means is that the challenge is to find time for good teaching, good research, and a reasonable amount of service. It often seems that each day has about two days' worth of little stuff that has to get done. The challenge is to keep track of what's really important for the long term."

What advice do these individuals have for a new generation of potential researchers? Dr. Lewis advises, "a student interested in research should learn as much as possible about research methodology and statistics while keeping a strong tie to the clinic. Most important is to identify an area of interest and explore related disciplines." Other research colleagues emphasize the value of interdisciplinary collaboration. Dr. Gonzalez Rothi urges students to "look for a program where you have an opportunity to see a wide variety of perspectives. Set up an advisory committee that reflects this diversity. Take courses outside of your [major area of focus] that might be able to contribute to your knowledge base." Finally, Dr. Camarata provides this advice: "Look into your heart and mind to determine whether satisfying your curiosity will sustain you. The key requirement for research is not 'intelligence' per se, but an interest in problem solving (with a large dose of persistence thrown in). If you like asking questions, a research career might be the most satisfying option."

Clinical Problem Solving

We have introduced some of types of communication disorders that concern the professions of audiology and speech-language pathology and have heard from some practicing professionals regarding their insights about the field. The ensuing chapters lay the groundwork necessary to understand normal and disordered communication processes in children and adults. We will consistently introduce the reader to clinical cases that bring to life the realities of the communication disorders. These individuals will help the reader appreciate the diagnostic and treatment processes that are at the heart of the professions.

Audiology and speech-language pathology are, by nature, fields in which memorization of facts is not enough for success. They require the application of knowledge to real-life problems. For this reason, we will end each chapter with a section in clinical problem solving. This is an opportunity to take the information covered in a chapter and apply it to a case. We saw in this chapter how individual components of communication can break down in cases of disorder. Many communication disorders involve a combination of difficulties within the areas of speech, language, and hearing. Consider the following case:

> *Bonnie*, age 8, was born with a severe hearing loss in both ears that was detected in the hospital when her hearing was screened as an infant. She could hear some low-frequency sounds in the environment and detect when someone was talking, but she could not perceive the differences in speech sounds. Bonnie was fitted with hearing aids to help her capitalize on the little hearing that was preserved, and she was placed in a preschool program that combined the use of hearing aid amplification with sign language and speech. Despite this early help, her spoken language skills were two years behind other children her age, and most people could not understand her speech when she entered first grade. She has made gains in speech and language but still struggles with spoken and written grammar. Her use of sign language has far outpaced her spoken and written language abilities. Bonnie's speech is still difficult to understand because she makes many articulation errors involving sounds that are outside of her hearing range. Her voice has an effortful quality and sounds like she is speaking from the back of her throat. Bonnie continues to receive academic tutoring and speech therapy.

> 1. What aspects of speech, language, and hearing are affected in Bonnie's case?
> 2. Would Bonnie's communication disorder be classified as developmental or acquired?
> 3. Which professionals are likely to be involved with Bonnie to maximize her communication potential?

REFERENCES

American Speech-Language-Hearing Association. (2005). Standards and implementation procedures for the certificate of clinical competence in speech-language pathology (revised March 2009). Available at www.asha.org/certification/slp_standards.htm

American Speech-Language-Hearing Association. (2011). *Standards and Implementation Procedures for the Certificate of Clinical Competence in Audiology.* Available at www.asha.org/Certification/Aud2011Standards

American Speech-Language-Hearing Association. (2010). *Highlights and trends: ASHA counts for Year End 2010*. Retrieved October 1, 2011, from www.asha.org/uploadedFiles/2010-Member-Counts.pdf#search=%222011%22

Bureau of Labor Statistics. (2011). *Occupational outlook handbook*. Retrieved October 1, 2011, from www.bls.gov/oco/ocos099.htm

Kent, R. (1998, Summer). Renewal and rediscovery: Insights from memoirs of illness and disability. *ASHA* magazine, p. 22.

Wollock, J. (1997). The noblest animate motion: Speech, physiology and medicine in pre-Cartesian linguistic thought. *Studies in the History of the Language Sciences, Volume 83*. Amsterdam: John Benjamins Publishing Company.

World Health Organization (2002). *Towards a common language for functioning, disability and health*. Geneva: Author.

The Biological Foundations of Speech and Language

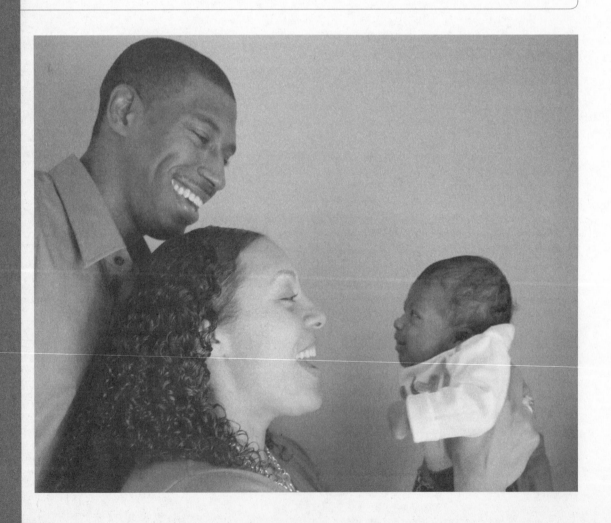

Knowledge of the biological underpinnings of normal speech, language, and hearing is central to understanding the many ways in which communication can be disrupted. In this chapter, we will first examine respiration and the vocal mechanism, which provide the power source and voicing for speech. The position and movement of lips, tongue, jaw, and other articulators transform the sound into individual consonants and vowels that form words. The resulting sounds are perceived by the listener through the auditory system. Finally, they are processed by the language system in the brain, where the information is comprehended, and a response may be formulated. These physical mechanisms work together to support communication. When communication is limited or disrupted by developmental disorder or acquired pathology, the breakdown can often be traced to one or more of the basic biological systems.

PREVIEW

Speech-language pathologists and audiologists are confronted daily with clinical cases that require an understanding of the physical and neurological underpinnings of communication and how impairments to these systems lead to communication disorders. Consider the following child:

> *Alicia*, age 3, was born with Down syndrome. This developmental disorder can be traced to a genetic abnormality that results in an extra copy of chromosome 21. The resulting alteration in brain development causes some degree of mental retardation and is likely to affect the capacity for normal language development. For this engaging 3-year-old girl, the occurrence of this genetic abnormality could impact her communication skills in several additional ways. Low muscle tone associated with the disorder might restrict her ability to move and explore her world, and abnormalities of her oral-facial structure could interfere with speech articulation. Her hearing might be affected because structural characteristics of the ear in children with Down syndrome make them prone to hearing loss. A multidisciplinary assessment team, consisting of a speech-language pathologist, an audiologist, a special educator, a psychologist, a physical therapist, and an occupational therapist, will work together to determine how the effects of Down syndrome manifest in this child. The team will then devise a plan intended to maximize her overall development, including communication skills. In the following sections, we will explore the biological systems that support normal communication and consider how they might be affected in clinical cases such as Alicia's.

The Vocal Mechanism

It is said that speech is an "overlaid function" that makes use of structures that have other primary functions. The same muscles and organs that allow us to breathe also provide the driving force behind sound production for speech. The larynx, which keeps us from choking food or liquid that might otherwise be misdirected into the airway, also provides the sound source for our voice. The structures of the mouth and throat that allow us to eat and drink also permit us to rapidly change the shape of the vocal tract to produce the various sound sequences that make up words and sentences.

The Respiratory System

The main function of the respiratory system is to sustain life through the continuous exchange of gases, primarily the exchange of carbon dioxide for oxygen. The human body requires a continuous renewal of its oxygen supply, usually accomplished by twelve to eighteen breaths (inspiration-expiration cycles) per minute. For the majority of people without respiratory disease, breathing occurs with little conscious effort.

Breathing is achieved by movements of the rib cage and the **diaphragm**. The rib cage can be raised slightly by contraction of skeletal muscles. The diaphragm, a large muscle that separates the chest from the abdomen, is shaped like an inverted bowl. When it contracts, it flattens and descends toward the abdomen, as shown in Figure 2.1. Because the lungs adhere to the inside of the rib cage and diaphragm, the lungs are stretched when the muscles of inspiration contract and cause the rib cage to elevate and the diaphragm to descend. This increase in lung size results in a decrease in pulmonary pressure relative to air pressure outside the body. With the airway open, air flows into the lungs through the mouth or nose (or both) in order to balance the air pressure, and we inhale. Exhalation simply results from relaxation of the muscles of inhalation. The rib cage falls back to its resting state and the diaphragm ascends as it returns to its inverted-bowl shape. The lungs then decrease in size, causing an increase in pulmonary pressure relative to the atmosphere, and air rushes out. This cycle, shown in Figure 2.1, repeats itself continuously as we breathe in and out.

The natural recoil forces of the lungs and muscular contraction function in a natural, synergistic way as we breathe at rest and during sleep. Our "in" breath is about as long as our "out" breath. When breathing at rest, an adult typically moves about a half of a liter of air in and out during each breath cycle. This is about ten percent of the full volume of air that an adult can voluntarily move in and out of their lungs (i.e., their vital capacity). Of course, on average, men have larger torsos (and lungs) than women, and their vital capacity and total lung volumes are typically greater (Hixon, Weismer, & Hoit, 2008). When we talk or sing, we engage muscular forces that enable us to take a quick inspiration and draw in more air than at rest, and then prolong the expiration as we phonate. So, the breathing pattern for speech (or singing) is quite different than breathing at rest. We typically talk at a lung volume that requires the least amount of effort, which is in the mid-range (40–60 percent) of our vital capacity.

> Breathe quietly for a minute. What movements of your torso do you detect? How many breaths do you take in a minute? Find out by counting them.

> Take in a deep breath. What movements do you detect? Now count from one to fifty, noting each breath that you take. How was your breathing pattern different when you were talking compared to breathing at rest?

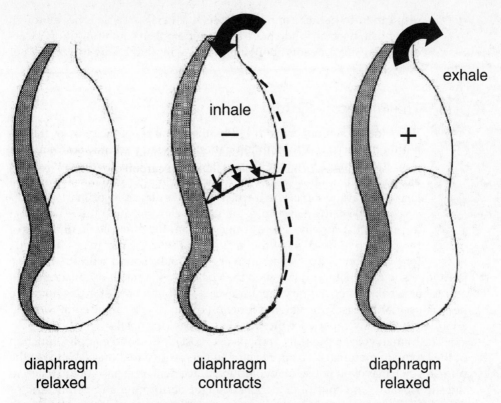

inhale
−

exhale
+

diaphragm
relaxed

diaphragm
contracts

diaphragm
relaxed

FIGURE 2.1   Schematic drawing of the torso during quiet breathing. Note that, for inhalation, the diaphragm moves downward and the rib cage lifts up and forward so that the lung volume increases and a negative pressure is created. For exhalation, the diaphragm relaxes and returns to its dome shape and the chest wall falls back to its resting state so that the air in the lungs is compressed, causing a positive pressure.

Based on Hixon (1973).

The muscles of the torso that support respiration serve another function important to the support of speech breathing—that of postural control. These muscles support the body so that the lungs have room to expand. A person who lacks control of these muscles may have difficulty maintaining a stable posture for efficient speech breathing.

Many disorders can disrupt the musculoskeletal system that underlies control of speech breathing. Let us refer back to Alicia's case from the perspective of the respiratory system. When the evaluation team works with Alicia, several professionals will look at her musculoskeletal system. The physical therapist will examine postural support and gross motor movements. The occupational therapist will examine fine motor control, particularly in relation to age-appropriate play activities. The speech-language pathologist's primary concern will be whether Alicia has sufficient control over the muscles that support posture and

- Adult men have a vital capacity of about 5 liters and a total lung volume of about 6 liters.
- Adult women have a vital capacity of about 3 liters and a total lung volume of about 4 liters.

respiration to permit connected speech. Alicia's muscle tone, although lower than normal, is adequate to support spoken communication. However, there are concerns about her motor skills and ability to support her body.

The Phonatory System

Voice (or phonation) is produced by the vibration of the two vocal folds within the larynx. Although phonation is a vital part of speech production, the primary function of the larynx is to guard the airway against **aspiration**, the inhalation of fluids or other matter into the airway. The larynx sits at the top of the trachea, where it plays this primary "watchdog" role. When we swallow, the larynx elevates and muscles contract to protect the airway. The average person, for example, is unaware of the protective function of the larynx, and when asked what the larynx (or "voice box") does, may answer, "We make sound with it." In some individuals with structural damage to the vocal folds (a result of cancer, for example) or weakness of the laryngeal muscles (perhaps part of a degenerative neuromuscular disease), the valving function of the larynx can be compromised and the patient may experience life-threatening choking spells.

The human voice represents perhaps the most elegant and complex function of the larynx in mammals. To appreciate the perspective that the elegance of the human voice may well not be an evolutionary accident, one has only to listen to the sheer beauty and control of a trained singer performing an operatic aria or melodic ballad. The communicative and artistic functions of the larynx take it well beyond its basic valving responsibilities.

The back (posterior) and front (anterior) views of the larynx can be seen in Figure 2.2. A ring-shaped **cricoid cartilage** forms the base of this structure and the **thyroid cartilage** sits above the cricoid. The thyroid cartilage is shaped like a shield and forms the anterior wall of the larynx. In many individuals (especially young men), we can see the prominent thyroid cartilage, which is often referred to as the Adam's apple. You can feel your thyroid cartilage by placing your fingertips on your throat, and feeling for the V-shaped notch in the front, which is called the thyroid notch (see Figure 2.2). If you are not sure whether you are touching the thyroid cartilage, it will become evident if you prolong an "ah" while you warble the pitch high and low. You will feel the thyroid cartilage move up and down with the changes in pitch.

Place your hand on your neck as you swallow. What is the movement of the larynx during the swallow?

The vocal folds lie in a horizontal orientation and are attached in the front to the thyroid cartilage just below the thyroid notch. The vocal folds extend posteriorly from the thyroid cartilage to the base of two pyramid-shaped cartilages called the **arytenoid cartilages**. In order to see the vocal folds, it is necessary to view the larynx from above, as shown in Figure 2.3. In this figure, we can see the left and right vocal folds and the arytenoid cartilages in a typical position for taking in a breath. The area between the vocal folds is known as the **glottis**, which has a V shape because the vocal

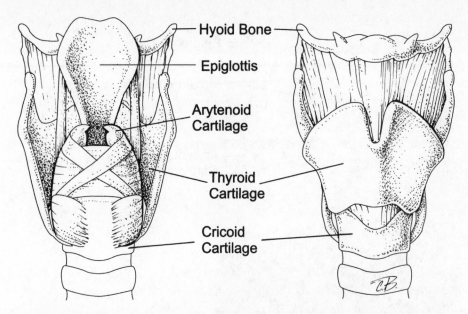

FIGURE 2.2 Structures of the larynx shown from the back (posterior) view on the left and front (anterior) view on the right. Note that the larynx is suspended from the hyoid bone (at the top). The V-shaped "thyroid notch" is evident in the anterior view of the thyroid cartilage.

folds are attached at a common point in the front of the larynx and they diverge in the posterior aspect by the action of the arytenoids. During voicing, the arytenoids move to the midline, closing the glottal opening. In Figure 2.3 the view of the thyroid cartilage is blocked by another structure within the larynx called the **epiglottis**.

As shown in Figure 2.2, the arytenoid cartilages sit on top of the posterior cricoid cartilage. The arytenoid cartilages move and rotate atop the cricoid cartilage, controlled by the action of several muscles within the larynx. For example, when certain muscles contract, they move the arytenoid cartilages in such a way that they pull the vocal folds away from the midline. The muscles that accomplish this movement are known as laryngeal *ab*ductors (they separate the folds). Laryngeal *ad*ductor muscles rotate the arytenoids in such a way that the folds come together. This muscle action is extremely quick, permitting a speaker to produce the rapid changes in voicing needed for continuous speech.

When the vocal folds are brought together (adduction), they are in the position for phonation. The outgoing air from the lungs builds up below the vocal folds, causing increased air pressure, referred to as **subglottal air pressure**. When this pressure is greater than the pressure holding the vocal folds together at the midline, it blows them apart (away from the midline). A puff of air is released between the open folds, and then they

The glottis is the area between the vocal folds. What does the word *subglottal* mean? What does the word *epiglottis* mean?

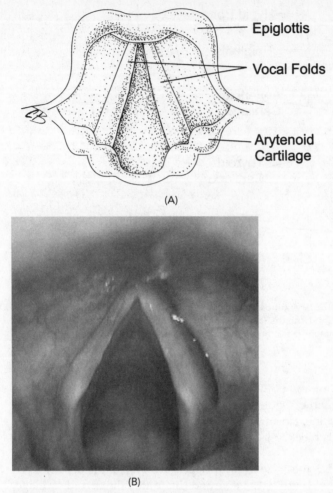

Epiglottis

Vocal Folds

Arytenoid
Cartilage

(A)

(B)

FIGURE 2.3   A drawing (A) and photograph (B) of the vocal folds viewed from above.
The front of the larynx is at the top of each figure, and the back of the larynx is at the bottom.
The vocal folds are apart in a V-shape as is typical during inspiration.

return to the midline. The closure results from the elastic recoil of the vocal fold
tissue and is assisted by the movement of air across the surface of the folds. This
opening and closing produces one cycle of phonation. Repeated cycles produce
sound, or phonation.

What we hear as the pitch of the voice relates directly to the rate, or frequency,
at which the vocal folds open and close. The normal pitch of the speaking voice is
primarily determined by the size and mass of the vocal folds. The tiny vocal folds
in babies produce high-pitched voices because their vocal folds vibrate quickly.
Nine-year-old children typically produce speaking voices just above middle C
on the musical scale. We can describe this in terms of the number of vibrations

per second, or cycles per second (**hertz**). The speaking voice of an adult male, whose vocal folds have increased in size since puberty, is about an octave lower than it was when he was 9 years old. The adult female, whose larynx is usually half again as large as it was when she was 9, typically speaks at a pitch that falls between that of a male adult and a child.

Because outgoing airflow causes the vocal folds to vibrate, changes in intensity, or loudness, of the voice are produced by changes in subglottal air pressure. This pressure can be raised by increasing the muscular force that holds the vocal folds together or by increasing the air pressure from the lungs (i.e., the respiratory drive). When the airflow finally breaks through the vocal folds, they are blown apart with greater force than when a less intense sound is produced. This, in turn, produces greater lateral excursion of the vocal folds, resulting in greater air displacement. In this way, a speaker can increase the intensity, and the perceived loudness, of the voice.

Just as we can regulate the loudness of our voice, we can also change the pitch by making adjustments to the vocal folds. Contraction of certain laryngeal muscles serves to lengthen the folds by stretching and tensing them, or shortens the folds by relaxing and thickening them. When stretched, the vocal folds become thinner, and they vibrate more quickly, producing higher frequencies (perceived as higher pitches). Likewise, when muscle action causes the vocal folds to become shorter and thicker, they vibrate more slowly and produce lower frequencies. Speech scientists study these dynamics of vocal fold function as well as the physical characteristics of the vocal mechanism (see for example, Kent, 1997; Hixon, Weismer, & Hoit, 2008; and Zemlin, 1998).

The Resonance System

Although the source of the voice is the larynx, sound waves are modified by the other structures within the throat, mouth, and nasal cavities. This is analogous to the way the hollow body of a guitar modifies the sound produced by plucking a string. The sound waves that we recognize as the human voice result from both the sound produced by the larynx and the filtering of that sound by the resonance system.

The first area of the vocal tract through which the sound waves travel lies immediately above the larynx. This tubelike cavity is called the **pharynx** (see Figure 2.4). The pharynx can be studied with **videoendoscopy**, which uses an illuminated lens to look down the back of the throat toward the larynx. The structures and their movements can then viewed on a video monitor. Videoendoscopy reveals that the pharynx is constantly changing shape during speech as the tongue moves forward and backward and the pharyngeal walls move inward. The length of the pharynx also changes as the larynx rises (shortening the pharynx) or lowers (lengthening the pharynx). A fascinating videoendoscopic tape distributed by the Voice Foundation (1985) of two famous impersonators, Rich Little and Mel Blanc, revealed that much of the muscle action used to produce different voice impersonations takes place in the pharyngeal cavities. While the

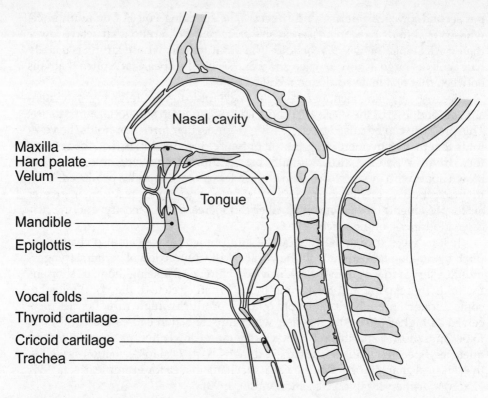

FIGURE 2.4 Sound produced at the larynx is modified by the resonance characteristics of the vocal tract, which consists of the pharynx and the oral and nasal cavities. At rest, the velum allows air to flow into the nasal cavity.

pharynx plays an important role in shaping vocal resonance, it obviously plays another vital role as a conduit for the passage of air and food.

In addition to the pharynx, the oral cavity also shapes the resonance characteristics of the voice. This air-filled cavity within the mouth constantly changes size and shape during speech. The overall size of the oral opening is primarily determined by the position of the **mandible**, or lower jaw, which is continually lowering and elevating during speech. As the jaw drops when saying a low vowel, such as "ah," the tongue drops with it. In contrast, the tongue rides high in the mouth when producing the long "e" vowel. The tongue itself has the greatest flexibility of any muscle group in the body, constantly changing its shape and position during articulation, thus altering the overall shape and size of the oral cavity. Together, the continuous oral and pharyngeal cavities determine the shape of the vocal tract. Speech scientists can study the vocal tract shape using magnetic resonance imaging (MRI) while a person holds a vowel position, as shown in Figure 2.5 (Story, Titze, & Hoffman, 1996, 1998).

The roof of the oral cavity is formed anteriorly by the bony hard palate and posteriorly by the soft palate (also known as **velum**). The velum is a muscular structure,

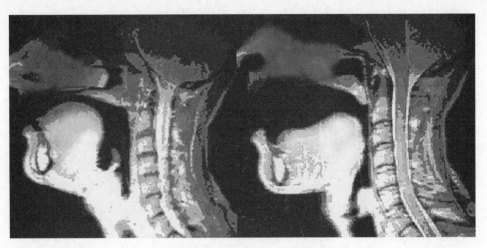

FIGURE 2.5 A side view of the articulators showing the differences in tongue and jaw position during the production of the vowels "ee"(/i/) on the left and "ah"(/a/) on the right. Note that the tongue and jaw are elevated for "ee" (/i/), whereas they are lowered for "ah" (/a/).

noticeable for its dangling appendage, the uvula. The velum hangs down during normal breathing so that air can flow between the nasal cavity and the oral cavity. When eating or drinking, the opening between these two cavities is closed as the velum raises and the pharyngeal wall constricts around it. During the production of most speech sounds, the velum is raised to close off the nasal cavity from the oral cavity. This allows for oral resonance of all the vowels and consonants in the English language except for the sounds "m," "n," and "ng." When these three nasal sounds are produced, the velopharyngeal port is open, allowing sound waves to enter the nasal cavity from the oral cavity, known as nasal-oral coupling. During normal speech production, the velum raises and lowers quickly as you produce oral and nasal sounds. For example, if you say the word *banana*, the initial "ba" requires a raised velum, the following "n" requires a rapid drop of the velum, and the next vowel, "a," requires closure again, only to be followed by another rapid drop for the next "n," ending with an elevated velum again for the vowel "a."

Failure to move the velum rapidly enough to match the demands of the particular utterance can result in excessively nasal speech, called **hypernasality**. Many problems that involve hypernasality are caused by faulty velophryngeal closure, which could be related to a number of factors, such as cleft palate, short velum, injured palate, or paralysis or weakness of the velopharyngeal muscles (disorders that are discussed in subsequent chapters). A less common resonance disorder is *hyponasality*, which is insufficient nasal resonance often due to excessive velopharyngeal closure. Hyponasality also occurs when the nasal cavity is affected by swollen tissues due to allergies or colds that dampen sound waves, and block airflow through the nasal cavities so that you have to breathe through your mouth. Excessive tonsil and adenoid tissue will sometimes create enough obstruction to give the voice a **denasal** vocal quality that has a marked lack of nasal resonance.

The resonance system gives each voice its distinctive quality. Changes in the quality of the voice can signal vocal pathology, as we will see in Chapter 6. Let us consider the resonance system in the case of Alicia, the child with Down syndrome.

> Down syndrome can involve congenital malformations of the pharynx (specifically the naso- and oropharynx), which can result in altered voice quality. In the case of Alicia, the speech-language pathologist noted some instances of hypernasality. This might result from poor control of the velopharyngeal mechanism or from a defect in the articulatory mechanism, explained below. To differentiate between these two possible causes, the speech-language pathologist evaluates both the oral structures and velopharyngeal functioning.

The Articulatory Mechanism

The Tongue

It may be surprising to realize that the tongue occupies most of the space of the oral cavity, as is evident in Figure 2.4. The tongue body is composed of a number of intrinsic muscles that run both the length and width of the structure. These muscles enable us to change its shape easily (curled, pointed, and so on). Other muscles of the tongue originate from various sites outside the tongue, such as the hyoid bone (shown in Figure 2.2). These extrinsic muscles allow the tongue to be elevated, lowered, protruded, and retracted. The way in which the tongue is postured influences the overall sound and resonance of the voice and is critical for the production of individual speech sounds. Vowels are produced primarily through changes in the shape and movement of the tongue (and elevation of the jaw). Precise movement and positioning of the tongue is necessary for many of the consonant sounds, which involve vocal tract constriction that affects the flow of air through the oral cavity. Without the precision of tongue movements, there could be no articulate speech.

> Some have said the tongue is the strongest muscle in your body. Do you think that is true?

The Lips

The lips are the most visible structure of the mouth and are easily shaped and altered to produce a range of facial expressions. They are made up primarily of facial muscles that can be variously contracted, to pucker, retract, protrude, or form a circle. They also play a vital role in oral behaviors such as sucking, chewing, smiling, and kissing. The lips form the end of the oral vocal tract, so their position can also contribute to the resonance of the voice. You can demonstrate the effects of the lips on vocal resonance by prolonging phonation for five seconds while you alternately retract and then pucker the lips. The distinct changes in the resonance that occur with each pucker and retraction reflect the lengthening and shortening of the vocal tract. The lips also play a primary function in the production of several consonants. Sounds such as "m," "p," "b," and "w" are produced by movements of the lips, whereas "f" and "v" are produced with the upper teeth on, or against, the lower lip.

The Mandible

The movement of the mandible, or lower jaw, allows for quick opening and closing of the mouth. Some mandibular movement contributes to change in the shape and size of the oral cavity needed for the production of different vowels. The normal speaker moves the mandible in quick synergistic movements that coordinate with the lips and tongue during normal speech production. If, however, a speaker were to talk with a pen clenched between the teeth, the mandible would stay fixed to trap the pen, and immediate compensatory adjustments of the tongue and lips would be made to during speech production. Optimal articulation and vocal resonance require continuous mandibular movement. Occasionally, we see patients with voice problems who speak with a clenched jaw much of the time, requiring the tongue to make all the muscle movements needed for vowel differentiation. Speaking this way is inefficient and often results in a muffled voice and imprecise articulation.

The Palate

The bony hard palate and the muscular soft palate make up the structures of the roof of the mouth, or **palate**. The underlying bone of the hard palate is the maxilla. It is an arched structure with a vaulted ceiling that contributes greatly to oral resonance. The portion of the palate just behind the front teeth is the alveolar ridge, which is a point of contact for the articulation of several speech sounds, such as "t" and "d." Attached to the posterior hard palate just beyond the last molars is the muscular soft palate, called the velum. As discussed earlier, when the velum makes contact with the pharynx it separates the oral cavity from the nasal cavity, allowing for oral resonance of sounds.

The Teeth

The teeth play a primary role in chewing food, while their contribution to speech articulation is somewhat secondary. However, a few English sounds, such as "f" and "v," are made with the lower lip tucked under the upper central incisors. This placement is referred to as labiodental (lip-to-teeth) contact. The teeth are also the contact point for "th" sounds, which are produced by placing the tongue to the upper teeth (linguadental sounds). The alveolar ridge behind the base of the upper front teeth is an important contact point for the tongue for the production of such sounds as "n," "s," "z," "t," and "d."

When speech is slow to develop or is difficult to understand, it is important to rule out possible problems with the oral and facial structures. In Alicia's case, the speech-language pathologist performed what is known as an **oral mechanism examination**. This is an evaluation of the structure and function of the articulatory mechanisms.

Alicia's oral-peripheral exam revealed several factors that could negatively affect communication. Some of her front teeth are quite crooked, which may interfere with sounds made against the teeth, such as "th" or "s." Her hard palate is highly arched, but does not contain any clefts or holes that would allow air to flow into the nasal cavity to produce hypernasality. Although her tongue appears large for her mouth and tends to protrude a bit, it is not actually too large. Rather, it lacks the muscle tone to rest within the mouth. Alicia's face has a soft, rounded appearance, which also suggests low tone of the facial muscles. Low tone of the oral and facial muscles can interfere with the movements needed to produce the sounds of speech. All these factors may account for the perception that Alicia's words sound "thick" and imprecise.

The Nervous System

The remarkable ability of human beings to communicate efficiently is related primarily to a complex nervous system that permits meaningful interaction between a person and the environment, other people, and other creatures. The nervous systems of other animals may have features that allow them to perform a particular behavior "better" than human beings. For example, predator birds have more acute eyesight than humans, and the porpoise has a more advanced auditory system. However, it is our complex brain that allows humans to master the complexities and subtleties of human language. The brain is part of the **central nervous system** (CNS). It works in concert with the **peripheral nervous system** (PNS), which allows information to travel to and from the body. We will consider each separately.

Central Nervous System

The brain and the spinal cord, seen in Figure 2.6, are considered the two primary CNS structures. The brain enables humans to engage in high-level functions, such as synthesizing information gathered from the environment, making inferences, drawing conclusions, making plans for the future, and communicating about all of these things. Because of its critical role in such functions, factors that alter brain development or damage the brain underlie many types of communication disorders. Between the brain and spinal cord is the **brainstem**. The brainstem and spinal cord comprise the primary pathway for sensory information that comes from the body and travels to the brain. Conversely, the brain sends motor commands through the brainstem to the spinal cord that result in our ability to support and move our bodies. Therefore, damage to the brainstem or spinal cord, with the resulting loss of muscle control, can disrupt the biological support necessary for speech.

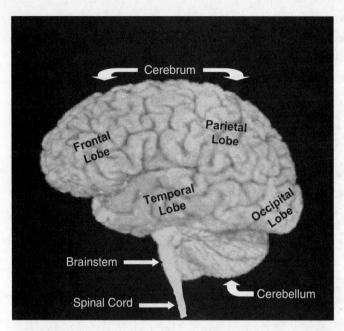

FIGURE 2.6 Components of the central nervous system: the cerebrum, cerebellum, brainstem, and spinal cord. The left cerebral hemisphere is divided into four lobes: frontal, parietal, temporal, and occipital.

The brain consists of the **cerebrum** and the **cerebellum** (see Figure 2.6). The cerebrum occupies the majority of the brain cavity within the head. The cerebellum sits below the cerebrum and behind the brainstem. Both the cerebrum and the cerebellum can be further divided into right and left **hemispheres**. The hemispheres of the cerebrum are joined at the midline by a large band of fibers called the **corpus callosum**, which carries information between the cerebral hemispheres (see Figure 2.7). The surface of the brain appears as a series of ridges, called *gyri,* and grooves, called *sulci.* Large sulci are referred to as *fissures.* The gyri and sulci can be individually identified by name, so that the location of both normal and pathological features of the cortex can be described in specific terms.

The cerebral hemispheres are further divided into four lobes (see Figure 2.6), each of which contains regions that are associated with particular functions. The **frontal lobes** contain the primary motor cortex, which sends neural commands, including those needed for speech, to specific parts of the body. They also contain regions that are involved with attention, impulse control, and judgment. The **parietal lobes** contain the primary sensory cortex, which receives sensory information from the body, as well as other regions that support a number of cognitive functions. The **occipital lobes**, at the back of the brain, receive and process visual information. The **temporal lobes** contain the primary auditory cortex as well as regions important for language comprehension and memory.

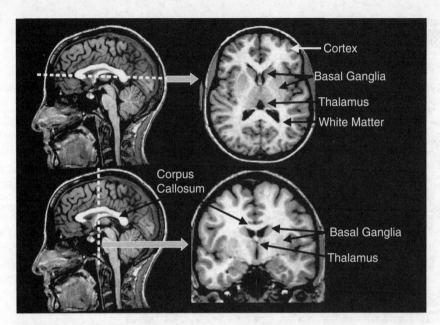

FIGURE 2.7 A midline view of the brain (on the left), a horizontal cross section of the brain (on the upper right), and a vertical cross section (i.e., coronal) of the brain (on the lower right). The cross sections allow you to see the gray and white matter distinctions and the deep subcortical structures called the basal ganglia and the thalamus. On each view, the corpus callosum can be seen bridging the right and left hemispheres.

The specialized functions of specific regions of the brain are attributed to differences in cells found within these regions. If we examine a cross-section of the cerebrum (see Figure 2.7), we can see the surface layer, or cortex. The cortex contains layers of **neurons**, which are cells that support different types of brain activity. Because the bodies of these neurons appear gray, the cortex is also called *gray matter*. The layers of the cortex within the primary motor area of the frontal lobe, for example, contain many neurons that send signals to the body for the control of movement, whereas the primary sensory cortex contains many cells that receive incoming signals from the body. If we look at the cross-section of the cerebrum (Figure 2.7), the lighter gray tissues beneath the cortex consist of nerve fibers that originate in the gray matter. These fibers connect regions of the brain, receive sensory information from the body, and send impulses to move the muscles of the body. Such fibers are collectively referred to as *white matter*.

The brain also includes a collection of subcortical (i.e., beneath the cortex) bodies known as the **basal ganglia** (see Figure 2.7). These neural bodies are connected to the cerebellum and to cortical regions involved in movement. Disorders of the basal ganglia, such as Parkinson disease, often result in impaired movements. Near the midline of the brain, just behind and below the basal ganglia, is another collection of subcortical

Much of what we know about the brain was first discovered by studying individuals who acquired communication impairments after damage to specific regions of the brain.

neurons known as the **thalamus**. This highly complex region receives and processes sensory and other types of information that is relayed to other areas of the brain.

Several regions of the brain are particularly important for communication and may be involved when communication disorders occur. Neural impulses from the ear, that occur in response to sound, travel to a region of the brain called the *primary auditory cortex*. This cortex is located on the superior surface of the temporal lobe (inside the Sylvian fissure) and is sometimes called *Heschl's gyrus* (see Figure 2.8). Within the left hemisphere, the primary auditory cortex is surrounded by cortical tissue that supports higher-level auditory function, including the comprehension of spoken language. Areas particularly important to this skill occupy the posterior regions of the superior temporal lobe and parts of the parietal lobe. Portions of the left inferior frontal lobe, on the other hand, are particularly important to aspects of language expression. Finally, the motor movements of speech are supported by the *primary motor cortex,* which is located in the frontal lobe of each hemisphere. This area works in conjunction with sub-cortical structures and the cerebellum to produce the movements needed for speech.

In a normal, healthy brain, these various regions work in concert to support communication in all its complexity. However, when a brain is compromised during development or due to disease or injury, communication breakdowns can occur.

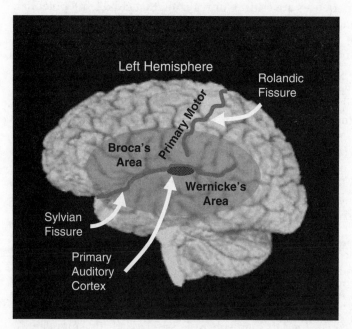

FIGURE 2.8   Important anatomical areas of the left hemisphere. The left perisylvian region that is important for language is shaded in light gray.

For Alicia, the effects that brought her to the developmental center began long before the day of her birth. The genetic anomaly that leads to Down syndrome affects the development of the brain. Research with this population has revealed certain brain characteristics that co-occur with this disorder. In Down syndrome, changes in fetal brain development can be detected by ultrasound between 16 and 21 weeks gestation (Bahado-Singh et al., 1992). These changes reflect neurobiologic features such as reduced brain size (particularly in the frontal lobes), fewer cells within specific layers of the cortex, and smaller cerebellar size (see Schmidt-Sidor, Wisniewski, Shepard, & Seren, 1990, for a review of the brain correlates of Down syndrome). After birth, these neuroanatomic differences can have functional correlates of concern for communication. For example, neuroimaging research has demonstrated reduced metabolic activity in the language areas of the brain associated with Down syndrome (Azari et al., 1994), as well as weaker interactions among the important language regions (Horowitz et al., 2000).

Normal prenatal brain development is characterized by overproduction of neurons and the connections between cells. After birth, the brain begins a lifetime of refining itself by pruning back excess cells and connections, and strengthening those connections that are most functional. What determines which cells and connections are most functional? A large determinant of functionality is the experience the young child receives. In other words, all babies' brains are shaped by what they see, hear, and explore. Even for a baby like Alicia, brain development is not complete at birth. Experience continues to shape the brain throughout life, and a child's early experiences are critical for realizing that child's full potential. This is one reason that professionals advocate for early intervention with children who have, or are at risk for, communication disorders.

In some individuals, the brain may have developed normally, only to be damaged later by illness or injury. In fact, much of what we know about the brain's organization was learned by observing the behavior of people who suffered damage to localized regions of the brain. This work began in the 1800s with two landmark medical cases. Paul Broca described a case of a man who lost his ability to express himself through spoken language, but retained much of his general cognitive functioning and his ability to understand language. When this man died, Broca examined his brain and found damage to the left inferior frontal lobe, a region that has come to be known as Broca's area. This area has been closely associated with processes important for expressive language. Conversely, Carl Wernicke described a man who lost the ability to comprehend spoken language and whose brain lesion was in the posterior part of the left temporal lobe. This general area, associated with language comprehension, has come to be called Wernicke's area.

The work begun by Broca and Wernicke gave rise to the **cerebral localization** perspective on brain functioning. The premise of a localizationist approach is that certain regions within the brain appear necessary for a particular skill or function. For most people, the left hemisphere is specialized for language. In particular, the regions of the left hemisphere that surround the **sylvian fissure** are critical language areas. This so-called **perisylvian region** includes the primary auditory cortex and the primary sensory and motor regions for the face that are located on either bank of the **Rolandic fissure**, which is roughly at right angles to the Sylvian fissure (see Figure 2.8). It also includes both Broca's and Wernicke's areas and additional cortex in the region. Damage within this broadly defined perisylvian region can lead to various types of language disorders, as we will see in Chapters 8 and 9.

The localization perspective focuses on brain regions that contribute to particular functions. However, we have become increasingly aware that brain areas do not act in isolation. Rather, systems composed of various brain structures, and the connections among them, act together to support behavior. This insight has given rise to a *connectionist* perspective, which emphasizes the interconnectedness of functionally related brain regions. Current connectionist models of language are implemented with computer programs intended to simulate how the brain works (Plaut, McClelland, Seidenberg, & Patterson, 1996; Rumelhart & McClelland, 1986). Information from these computational models provides understanding that complements that learned from the study of the effects of damage to critical brain regions. Another important means of understanding how the brain supports language and other cognitive processes comes from neuroimaging research, including functional magnetic resonance imaging (fMRI). As shown in Figure 2.9, fMRI provides evidence regarding what regions of the brain are involved in specific language processes in healthy individuals. This information provides a means to test hypotheses that emerged from studies of language impairment following brain damage and to refine our understanding of the language networks in the brain.

For most individuals, language is a left hemisphere function; however, effective communication relies on many regions within both hemispheres of the brain. For example, listening to a lecture can involve all lobes simultaneously. As each person in attendance concentrates on the speaker, he or she tries to ignore other

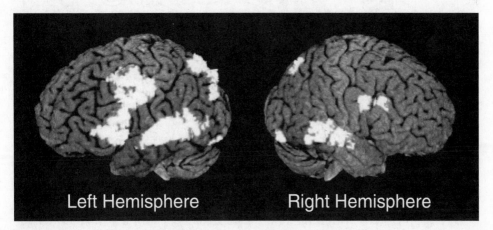

FIGURE 2.9   A functional magnetic resonance image illustrates the principle of language dominance. Note that brain activation associated with language processing (areas in white) is more widespread in the left hemisphere than in the right.

Data based on Plante, Ramage, & Maglöire (2006).

distractions (using frontal and parietal lobes), take in the auditory and visual speech signal (temporal and occipital lobes), interpret its content (left temporal lobe), and visually monitor the facial expressions and affect of the speaker (occipital and right parietal lobes). It is the integrated function of all these brain regions that allows the listener to receive the verbal and nonverbal information and to comprehend its meaning.

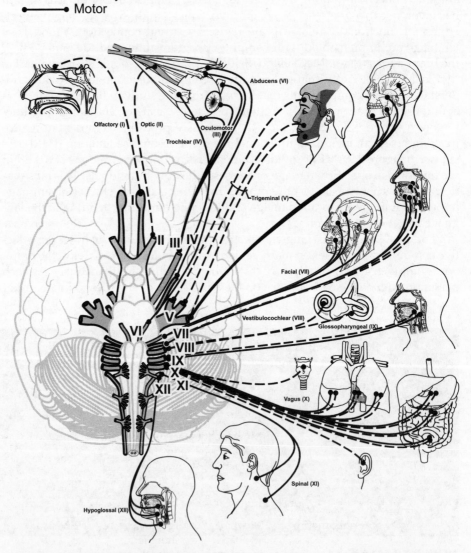

FIGURE 2.10 Twelve pairs of cranial nerves connect the brainstem to regions of the head and neck. Of particular interest are those cranial nerves that provide motor control for speech (the lips, tongue, jaw, velum, and larynx), and sensory input from the face, tongue, and ear.

Peripheral Nervous System

To be functional, the brain must be connected to the body and the outside world. This connection is made through the peripheral nervous system. The upper portion of the peripheral nervous system includes twelve pairs of nerves that enter or exit the CNS within the cranial space occupied by the brain and brainstem (see Figure 2.10). These are known as the **cranial nerves** (see Table 2.1).

TABLE 2.1   The Cranial Nerves

Cranial Nerve	Name	Primary Function	Role in Communication
I	Olfactory	Sense of smell	—
II	Optic	Vision	Face-to-face communication Reading and writing Sign language
III	Oculomotor	Eye movement	Reading and writing Sign language
IV	Trochlear	Eye movement	Reading and writing Sign language
V	Trigeminal	Movement of jaw Sensation from face	Speaking
VI	Abducens	Eye movement	Reading and writing
VII	Facial	Movement of facial muscles Sensation from tongue, velum	Speaking
VIII	Auditory	Hearing and balance	Listening
IX	Glossopharyngeal	Movement of pharynx Sensation from posterior tongue, pharynx	Speaking
X	Vagus	Movement of larynx, pharynx, velum, diaphragm, heart, abdominal viscera Sensation from larynx, pharynx, inner ear, other body organs	Speaking
XI	Accessory motor	Movement of large muscles of the head, neck, shoulders	Speaking
XII	Hypoglossal	Movement of tongue, supralaryngeal muscles	Speaking

As one can see from Table 2.1, most of the cranial nerves play some role in communication. Therefore, injury or disease that affects individual nerves may also impair specific aspects of communication. It is not surprising, then, that speech-language pathologists and audiologists consider cranial nerve function when evaluating individuals with communication disorders.

Below the level of the cranial nerves are thirty-one pairs of nerves that enter or exit the spinal cord, referred to as the **spinal nerves**. The **spinal cord** is made up of ascending and descending nerve tracts. There are anterior and posterior nuclei (clusters of cell bodies) at thirty-one levels of the spinal cord. The motor nerves that innervate the muscles of the chest, the abdomen, and the limbs exit the anterior (front) portion of the spinal cord, and sensory information from the body is received in the posterior portion of the spinal cord. Sensory nerves come into the posterior spinal nuclei from various peripheral sites, such as glands, tissues, joints, and muscles. Some of the peripheral sensory information is processed directly at the spinal level, where various sensorimotor reflexes may occur. In other cases, the sensory information travels to the central nervous system through the brainstem and cerebellum, where sensorimotor adjustments may be made. The sensory information may also travel to the thalamus, where it is processed and relayed further. Some sensory impulses from the spinal nerves probably project directly (with some filtering or adjustment along the way) to the sensory cortex.

Clinical Problem Solving

Consider the following clinical case:

Mr. Blades, age 71. In an acute-care hospital, a speech-language pathologist is asked to evaluate the speech and language of a right-handed, 71-year-old man named Mr. Blades. He had been admitted to the hospital the day before, following a car accident in which he was a passenger. He had several broken bones and had hit the left side of his head. Although alert on the following day, he seemed to have difficulty understanding what was said to him. The clinician was concerned that the blow to the head damaged regions of his brain that support language, but also needed to consider other reasons for his language comprehension difficulty.

1. Why would the clinician suspect that the car accident may have produced the language comprehension problem?
2. What other biological system(s) could also be the source of poor comprehension?

REFERENCES

Azari, N. P., Horowitz, B., Pettigrew, K. D., Grady, C. L., Haxby, J. V., Giacometti, K. R., & Schapiro, M. B. (1994). Abnormal pattern of cerebral glucose metabolic rates involving language areas in young adults with Down syndrome. *Brain and Language, 46,* 1–20.

Bahado-Singh, R. O., Wyse, L., Dorr, M. A., Copel, J. A., O'Connor, T., & Hobbins, J. C. (1992). Fetuses with Down syndrome have disproportionately shortened frontal lobe dimensions on ultrasonographic examination. *American Journal of Obstetrics and Gynecology, 167,* 1009–1014.

Hixon, T. J. (1973). Respiratory function in speech. In F. D. Minifie, T. J. Hixon, & F. Williams (Eds.), *Normal aspects of speech, hearing, and language* (pp. 73–126). Englewood Cliffs, NJ: Prentice Hall.

Hixon, T., Weismer, G., and Hoit, J. (2008). *Preclinical speech science: Anatomy, Physiology, Acoustics, Perception.* San Diego, CA: Plural Publishing.

Horowitz, B., Schapiro, M. B., Grady, C. L., & Rapoport, S. I. (2000). Cerebral metabolic pattern in young adult Down's syndrome subjects: altered intercorrelations between regional rates of glucose utilization. *Journal of Intellectual Disability Research, 34,* 237–252

Kent, R. D. (1997). *The speech sciences.* San Diego: Singular Publishing.

Plante, E., Ramage, A., & Maglöire, J. (2006). Processing narratives for verbatim and gist information by adults with language learning disabilities: A functional neuroimaging study. *Learning Disabilitites Research and Practice, 21,* 61–76.

Plaut, D. C., McClelland, J. L., Seidenberg, M. S., & Patterson, K. (1996). Understanding normal and impaired word reading: Computational principles in quasi-regular domains. *Psychological Review, 103,* 56–115.

Rumelhart, D. F., McClelland, J. L., & PDP Research Group (Eds.). (1986). *Parallel distributed processing: Explorations in the microstructure of cognition: Volume 1. Foundations.* Cambridge, MA: MIT Press.

Schmidt-Sidor, B., Wisniewski, K. E., Shepard, T. H., & Seren, E. A. (1990). Brain growth in Down syndrome subjects 15–22 weeks gestational age and birth to 60 months. *Clinical Neuropathology, 9,* 181–190.

Story, B. H., Titze, I. R., & Hoffman, E.A. (1996). Vocal tract area functions from magnetic resonance imaging. *Journal of the Acoustical Society of America, 100*(1), 537–554.

Story, B. H., Titze, I. R., & Hoffman, E. A. (1998). Vocal tract area functions for an adult female speaker based on volumetric imaging. *Journal of the Acoustical Society of America, 104*(1), 471–487.

Voice Foundation. (1985). *The voice of the impersonator.* (Videocassette developed by R. Feder.) New York: Author.

Zemlin, W. R. (1998). *Speech and hearing science: Anatomy and physiology* (4th ed.). Boston: Allyn and Bacon.

Sounds in Communication

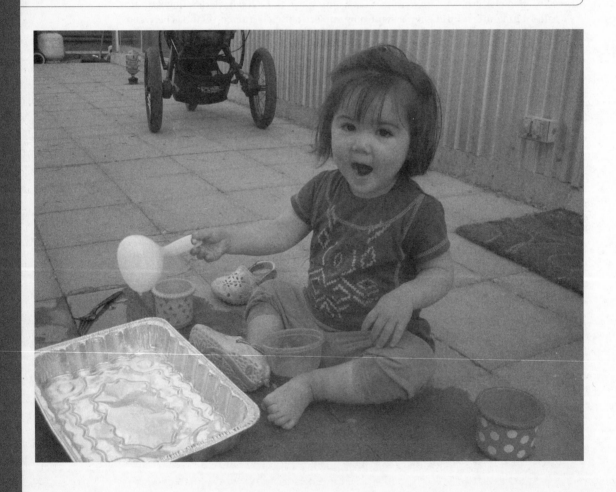

Sounds are the currency of auditory-oral communication. Speech-language pathologists and audiologists, as well as speech and hearing scientists, are concerned with the acoustic elements of sound. This includes an understanding of the basic physical nature of sound, how speech sounds are produced, and how such sounds can be measured and described. Given the complexity of the sounds of language, it is amazing that young children master the language of their environment with such ease. We will examine this process in a young child who is acquiring English as his native language.

PREVIEW

Auditory functioning supports communication at many levels. A short bark at the back door lets us know that the dog wants to come inside. The telephone's ring or cell phone buzz tells us someone is trying to reach us. With speech, humans are able to use sound to express an infinite variety of ideas, moods, and attitudes. We will examine sound first at its most basic level, as an acoustic signal, and then in the form of human speech.

Acoustic Aspects of Sound

The essence of sound is motion. When someone talks to you from across the room, the vibrations created by his or her voice and articulation are carried through the air to your ears. Sound energy "travels" because air molecules that are adjacent to a source of vibration bump up against neighboring molecules and push them a bit. Those molecules likewise displace their neighbors, and so on, so that the vibration is propagated. The individual molecules do not move far before they rebound back in place, but they set off a chain reaction of motion that radiates from the source. As depicted in Figure 3.1, the disturbed molecules alternately bunch close together (causing areas of *compression*) and spread apart as they return to their original locations (causing regions of *rarefaction*). This vibratory motion produces a sound wave that travels through the air but can also be carried through other media, including liquids, such as water, and solid structures, such as dormitory walls. One way to represent the transmission of sound is to graph the moment-to-moment position of the sound source (or a molecule that is moving in response to the force applied by the source). Such a graph is a **waveform**, as shown in the lowest panel of Figure 3.1. The horizontal axis indicates time, and the vertical axis reflects displacement from a resting point.

Frequency

The rate of vibration of the sound source is the **frequency** of the sound. It is the number of complete cycles of to-and-fro motion that occur in one second. The units of measurement for frequency are named Hertz to honor a scientist who

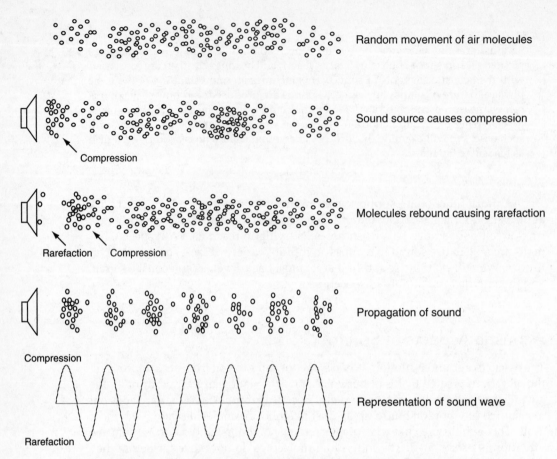

Random movement of air molecules

Sound source causes compression

Compression

Molecules rebound causing rarefaction

Rarefaction   Compression

Propagation of sound

Compression

Representation of sound wave

Rarefaction

FIGURE 3.1 Illustrations of compressions and rarefactions of air molecules, which serve to propagate sound. The waveform at the bottom of the figure depicts the sound.

made important contributions to the development of the radio. The waveform in Figure 3.2 (A) shows a pattern of vibration with three complete cycles during three-hundredths of a second (or three milliseconds). Over the course of a full second, the vibratory cycle would repeat one hundred times, so that it is a 100 Hertz (Hz) tone. Because the vibration is at only one frequency, it is called a **pure tone**. A pure tone is also called a *sine wave*. Pure tones do not occur naturally but can be produced in the laboratory and are used to test hearing at specific frequencies. Sounds in the environment are not pure tones but rather are produced by energy located at more than one frequency.

Children and young adults with normal hearing are able to hear sounds that range in frequency from about 20 to 20,000 Hz. Sounds at different frequencies are each perceived as having a different **pitch**. In other words, frequency refers to that actual number of vibrations per second (an acoustic property of the sound), whereas pitch reflects how those frequencies sound to us.

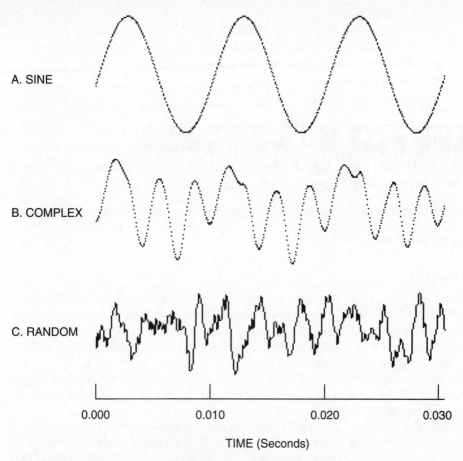

FIGURE 3.2 Examples of simple and complex waveforms. The sine wave (A) is a pure tone from an audiometer; the complex wave (B) reflects speech; the random wave (C) is noise.

The notes on a piano keyboard span a frequency range of about 20 to 4000 Hz. As shown in Figure 3.3, this frequency range includes much of the energy produced by people's voices and speech sounds. Middle C on the piano corresponds to a frequency of 256 Hz, which means that, when the piano string is struck, it vibrates 256 times in one second (see Figure 3.3). This frequency is typical of the fundamental frequency of the voice of an adult woman. The average male voice has a fundamental frequency of 128 Hz, or half the frequency of a typical woman's voice. When the frequency of sound is doubled, it increases by one octave, so a woman's voice is about one octave higher than a man's voice. Additional information in a speaker's voice is carried at higher frequencies. The most important frequencies for speech sounds range from about 500 to 4000 Hz.

Do you know the pitch of your speaking voice? There are computer and smart phone applications that allow you to measure it.

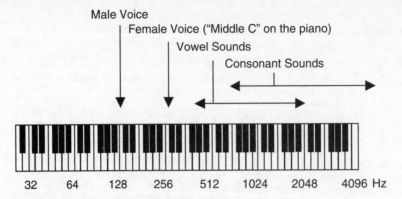

FIGURE 3.3 Frequency of sound in Hertz represented on a piano keyboard. Note that the frequencies that allow us to distinguish between specific vowels or consonants are higher than those that distinguish between male and female voices.

Intensity

What we perceive as the loudness of a sound is determined primarily by its **intensity**, or the pressure produced by the vibrating motion. Sound pressure level (SPL) is typically measured using a **decibel** (dB) scale. The decibel was named to honor Alexander G. Bell, the inventor of the telephone. The scale is based on logarithms of the ratio between an arbitrary reference point and the pressure, or intensity, of a sound. The reference point for hearing, denoted as 0 dB SPL, is approximately the smallest pressure that can be detected by a person with no hearing loss. In other words, 0 dB SPL can be considered the threshold for "perfect hearing." The actual range of sound pressure from the threshold of hearing to a sound that is so loud that it causes discomfort is about a million to one (Kelly, 1985), but on the logarithmic scale the difference between these two levels is only about 120 dB. The sound pressure levels for some common sounds are shown in Table 3.1. If you compare the loudness of the human voice to various environmental sounds, you see that conversational speech falls in the middle range of intensities. It is obvious that it is easier to hear speech when we are not also confronted with louder environmental sounds.

Complex Sounds

Most sounds in the world are not pure tones with energy restricted to one frequency; they are complex sounds with energy at more than one frequency. For example, the waveform in Figure 3.2 (B) was generated by an adult male producing the vowel "ah." It is an example of a *complex waveform*, which means that more than one frequency is produced by the source. The motion pattern is complicated, with several peaks and troughs. Nonetheless, it is possible to see that the overall pattern is repeated three times within the time frame illustrated in Figure 3.2. In other words, the repetition rate of the complex pattern is the same as that of the

TABLE 3.1   Possible Sound Pressur e Levels of Common
Environmental Sounds

10–20 dB	Whispering heard from over five feet away
40 dB	The ambient noise in a quiet room
50 dB	The hum of a refrigerator
57 dB	The dial tone of a phone
60–70 dB	Conversational speech
74 dB	A door closing
79 dB	A dog barking
89 dB	A door slamming
100 dB	A household fire alarm
120 dB	A police siren
140 dB	An airplane taking off

100 Hz pure tone shown in the figure. The lowest of the frequencies that make up this complex tone is 100 Hz. This is called the *fundamental frequency*.

The waveform illustrated in Figure 3.2 (C) is also complex, but it does not reveal any regular or repeated pattern of motion. This type of motion pattern represents *noise,* such as that produced by a waterfall or jet engine or simply the sound made by producing "sssss" or "shhhh." When noise is produced by motion that is completely random, it is called *white noise* because it contains all frequencies. This is analogous to white light, which contains all colors. We hear white noise on the television when we try to tune in a channel that is not broadcasting or that is not available through the cable company. Noise can be produced also by abrupt or brief sounds, such as consonants produced without voice (e.g., /p/, /t/, /k/).

Speech sounds can also be displayed in terms of the intensity of their energy at various frequencies over the period of time that they are spoken. This display is known as a **spectrogram**. The spectrogram in Figure 3.4 shows the differences among the words *bit, bat,* and *bait* that are readily apparent to the listener. These words differ in the two parameters of sound that we have already discussed: frequency and intensity. For each of these words, we can see the distribution of sound energy (intensity) at different frequencies. The energy appears as horizontal bands on the spectrogram with greater intensities shown as darker bands at particular frequencies. The lowest dark band of energy is the fundamental frequency of the speaker's voice.

For each of the words in Figure 3.4, we see differences in the relative intensity and duration of each sound that makes up the word. The portion of speech corresponding to vowel sounds contains regions of strong acoustic energy. When we listen to words, we pick up information about the speaker's voice primarily

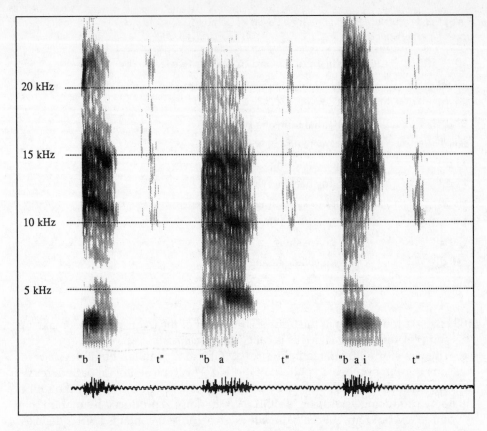

20 kHz

15 kHz

10 kHz

5 kHz

"b i   t"   "b a   t"   "b a i   t"

FIGURE 3.4 Complex speech sounds can be analyzed to show the component frequencies that we hear as different speech sounds. The words shown in this spectrogram are *bit*, *bat*, and *bait*.

from vowels because of the relatively long duration of voiced sound production. In contrast to the vowels, the unvoiced consonant "t" produces a short and relatively weak burst of energy, which is represented by a much lighter shade of gray on the spectrogram. These differences in the frequency and intensity of speech sounds may seem subtle when examined visually. However, they are adequate to distinguish between words, for those with normal hearing.

> A spectrogram is your "voice print." It reflects the unique characteristics of your voice and your vocal tract, but it is not as identifiable as your fingerprint.

The spectrogram also reveals a third parameter that differentiates the sounds of speech: time. It is the combination of the distribution of sound energy over certain frequencies and the particular timing patterns that lead to the perception of three different vowels and, thus, three different words, in the case of *bit*, *bat*, and *bait*. Changes in the spectral energy and timing also help differentiate consonants, as in the words *pot*, *got*, and *not*.

The Spoken Sounds of Communication

Vocalization

As we learned in Chapter 2, the production of speech sounds relies on the co-ordinated action of many physical elements, including muscles of the larynx, throat, face, and oral structures. **Vocalization** requires a sound generator—the larynx—and a force to drive this generator—air. During normal breathing, the vocal folds of the larynx are "open" (i.e., away from the midline), allowing air to flow in and out unobstructed. For speech, the vocal folds are apart during the production of voiceless sounds and are closed to produce voiced sounds. When exhaled air hits the closed (or closing) vocal folds with sufficient force, the folds blow apart and the exhaled air pushes against the stationary air above the folds, setting in motion a sound wave.

The frequency of the sound created by the vibrating vocal folds depends on the mass and length of the folds. Larger vocal folds tend to vibrate fewer times per second and therefore produce sounds at a lower frequency. Thus, men's voices tend to be lower than women's, and women's voices are lower than children's. Table 3.2 shows some frequencies of different voices for comparison. The fundamental frequency of the voice is carried by the vowel sounds in speech. The frequency of consonant sounds is much higher than the fundamental frequency of the voice.

Speech Sounds

As clinicians, we need a precise system for differentiating among the sounds that people produce. The written word, as produced with the English alphabet, is inadequate for this task because one letter can correspond to more than one sound. Consider the "o" in *off* versus in *over*, or the "c" in *cat* versus in *certain*. For

TABLE 3.2   The Fundamental Frequency of the Human Voice and Some Consonant Sounds

Source	Frequency Level of the Voice
An infant cooing	380 Hz
Boys or girls, age 9, talking	260 Hz
An adult woman talking	256 Hz
An adult man talking	128 Hz
Consonant Sounds	
s or z	4000–8000 Hz
t or v	6000–7000 Hz
th (as in "thick")	7000–8000 Hz

other consonants, two or three letters represent the sound (e.g., "th," "sh," "ng," "tch"), and the same sound can be represented in more than one way (e.g., "f" and "ph"). Further complicating matters is the occurrence of "silent letters" (e.g., "p" in *ptomaine*, "gh" in *weight*) in English orthography. For these reasons, those who study speech use the *International Phonetic Alphabet* (IPA). The IPA symbols for consonants appear in Table 3.3, along with their corresponding sounds in words, and the IPA symbols for English vowels are depicted in Figure 3.5. Some additional symbols are used for specific vowel sounds; in all, more than forty different symbols are needed to specify the sounds of English, compared with the twenty-six letters of our alphabet. These symbols allow us to specify the individual sounds, or **phonemes**, of the English language. A unique IPA symbol is associated with each phoneme in a manner that avoids the confusion caused by a single letter having more than one pronunciation (e.g., the letter "c" can be produced like a "k" or an "s"). The actual production of a sound by a speaker is referred to as a **phone**. The term **allophone** refers to the variations in phones that are still categorized as the same phoneme. For example, we say the "t" in *tap* slightly differently than in *setting*, although both are considered versions of "t." By convention, phonetic symbols are written between two forward slash marks to indicate a phoneme with all its various acceptable allophones (e.g., /t/).

TABLE 3.3   The Consonants in English

Manner of Articulation	Place of Production						
	Bilabial	Labiodental	Interdental	Alveolar	Palatal	Velar	Glottal
Stop or Plosive	p (*pat*)			t (*toe*)		k (*kick*)	
	b* (*bat*)			d* (*doe*)		g* (*gap*)	
Fricative		f (*fat*)	θ (*thin*)	s (*sip*)	ʃ (*shoe*)		h (*hip*)
		v* (*vat*)	ð* (*that*)	z* (*zip*)	ʒ* (*measure*)		
Affricate				tʃ (*chop*)			
				dʒ* (*job*)			
Nasal	m* (*mom*)			n* (*num*)		ŋ* (*sing*)	
Lateral				l* (*lap*)			
				r* (*rare*)			
Glide	w* (*wall*)				j* (*yes*)		

* Consonant is voiced.

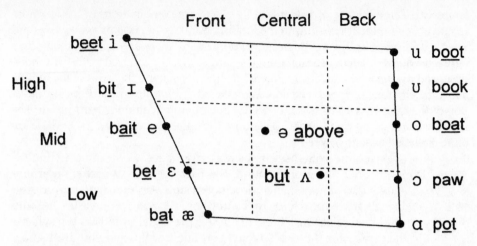

FIGURE 3.5 The vowel quadrilateral showing twelve vowels used in English, their place of articulation in the oral cavity (front, central, back), and the relative height of the highest part of the tongue (high, mid, low).

Consonants

Consonant sounds are the result of precise placement and movement of the articulators. They can be characterized by three general parameters: the *place* of articulation, the *manner* in which the sound is produced, and whether the consonant is voiced. This place-manner-voicing system can be used for describing the production of specific sounds. Table 3.3 includes the consonants used in English and shows how each phoneme is distinguished by its place, manner, and voicing characteristics. The anatomical *place of production* is named for the articulator(s) involved or the contact point for the tongue. These are shown across the top of Table 3.3, ordered from front to back in the vocal tract: *bilabial* (lips), *labiodental* (lips and teeth), *interdental* (between the teeth), *alveolar* (ridge behind upper teeth), *palatal* (hard palate), *velar* (velum, or soft palate), and *glottal* (glottis). The glottis is not strictly an articulator but functions to produce the unvoiced /h/ sound, as in "hip." We see the *manner of production* on the left-hand margin. There are six consonants (/p/, /b/, /t/, /d/, /k/, /g/) classified as *stops* or **plosives**, produced by briefly obstructing the airflow and then releasing it. The consonants that are paired in Table 3.3 (e.g., /p/ and /b/; /t/ and /d/) are called **cognates**. Each pair has the same manner and place of production, differing only on the dimension of voicing in that some sounds are accompanied by voice and others are not. For example, /b/ is a voiced stop, whereas /p/ is the voiceless cognate for /b/. In Table 3.3, voiced sounds are marked with an asterisk. The **fricative** consonants (/f/, /v/, / θ / as in thin, /ð/ as in that, /s/, /ʃ/ as in shoe, /ʒ/ as in measure, and /h/) are created by articulators forming a constriction of the airway that produces some audible noise as air flows through. All of the nine fricatives are also **continuants**, because they can be continued as long as the airflow is present. The **affricate** consonants (/tʃ/, /dʒ/) are combinations of a stop and a fricative. Only three consonants in the English language are **nasals** (/m/, /n/, and /ŋ/), produced with the velopharyngeal port open. There are two commonly recognized liquid, or *lateral,* consonants. The lateral /l/ is produced with the tongue tip raised to contact the alveolar ridge while openings along the sides of the tongue allow the air stream to pass. The liquid consonant /r/ requires retraction and elevation of the tongue, with the sides of the tongue often touching the hard palate. The last consonant grouping in Table 3.3 includes the glide sounds (/w/, /j/), which are often classified as semivowels.

Consonant systems vary across languages. For example, English contains only one glottal sound, the fricative /h/, whereas other languages, such as Navajo, include a glottal stop. A glottal stop is produced by bringing the vocal folds to the midline, allowing air pressure to build up, and then releasing a burst of air. It is the initial sound of each syllable in the expression, "uh-oh," which you might say when you drop something. When using the International Phonetic Alphabet, a glottal stop is coded with the symbol /ʔ/, but of course this sound is not coded in English orthography. In languages like Navajo that mark the glottal stop, it is coded with an apostrophe, as in *ts'in* (meaning "bone"); the traditional pronunciation and spelling of *Hawa'ii* also marks the glottal stop.

English contains some consonant distinctions that are not found in some other languages. For example, Japanese does not make the distinction between /l/ and /r/ that is made in English, but rather, has one lingua-alveolar, liquid consonant. As a result, it is often quite difficult for a native speaker of Japanese who learns English as a second language to clearly articulate these two sounds; sometimes an /l/ sounds more like an /r/, or vice versa. What we perceive as the "accent" of a non-native speaker of English relates to the replacement of some sounds with those from the native language, or simply our perception of subtle alterations in the place, manner, or voicing of the consonant sounds.

Correct production of speech sounds requires specific positioning and movement of the articulators to achieve the ideal place of contact, shape of the oral cavity, force, airflow, and pattern of movement. These movements must be accomplished quickly in running speech, which requires a steady stream of air and continuous sequencing of articulatory movements. The sounds that precede or follow a particular phoneme influence the production of that sound, a process often called sound **assimilation**. For example, when you say "hot rod," you probably do not actually produce the /t/ sound. Contrast that with your production of "hot afternoon." The dropping of the /t/ in "hot rod" or "hot potato" reflects assimilation processes that help you speak rapidly with ease. If you were paying close attention, you may have noticed that you actually substituted a glottal stop for the /t/ in "hot rod." A similar characteristic of connected speech is the tendency to simultaneously produce adjacent sounds. For example, the last two sounds of the word "tenth" are typically produced at the same time, a process known as **coarticulation**. It would certainly sound odd if you first produced

> Place your hand on your throat and produce a "p" sound; now produce a "b" sound. Can you feel a difference? Which one has voicing?

> The glottal stop is essential for a good Cockney accent: "Wo' ya like a liʔl biʔ o buʔer wiv your toast?"

the /n/ and then the "th." These processes of assimilation and coarticulation provide evidence that planning for speech production involves units larger than the single phone.

Vowels

Like consonants, vowels are also coded using IPA symbols, as shown in Figure 3.5. Vowels are produced with the mouth relatively open, and voicing is generated by vocal fold vibration. The sound generated by the vocal fold vibration is then modified by positioning of the pharynx, soft palate, tongue, jaw, and lips to create a distinct configuration of the vocal tract. The unique sound for each vowel is dependent on the position and height of the tongue in the oral cavity as well as the configuration of the lips. For example, as shown in Figure 3.5, in the production of the /i/ ("ee" as in *beet*) vowel, the tongue is positioned high and forward in the mouth. In addition, the jaw is elevated, and the lips are slightly withdrawn. Conversely, we see that the /a/ ("a" as in *father*) vowel is produced with the jaw dropped and the back of the tongue held low in the oral cavity. In addition to single vowel sounds, we also produce sounds called **diphthongs** that contain a combination of two vowels. Diphthongs, such as /ai/ in *buy* or /oi/ in *boy*, are assimilated blends of separate vowels that produce a two-vowel glide. Production of a diphthong requires a quick sequence of vocal tract adjustments, usually involving rapid movements of the tongue from low to high (or vice versa) and back to front (or vice versa).

Each vowel found in a particular language has its own distinctive production characteristics. For example, listening to an Australian speaker and an American speaker, one will perceive the same English language with the same consonants embedded within markedly different vowels and diphthongs. These differences may cause difficulties for the listeners as they try to understand each other. As mentioned earlier in this chapter, vowels allow us to hear the voice of the speaker. Although consonants play a primary role in how well speech is understood, or its *intelligibility*, the vowels we utter also contribute to how well someone can understand us.

> Say the sentence "Tom wants tea, too." What are the differences in the lip and tongue positions for each of the four instances of /t/?

Prosody

So far, we have discussed the constituents of speech that make up the individual sounds within words (i.e., the consonants and vowels). However, additional aspects of sound are critical in conveying meaning in conversation. These aspects include the tempo, rhythm, and intonation with which the sounds and words are spoken. These elements make up the **prosody** of speech.

Prosody conveys information about the grammatical structure of a spoken sentence. For example, the speaker uses short pauses to set off a phrase embedded within the sentence (separated by commas in written text), as in "The report, which appeared to be composed by monkeys typing at random, received a failing grade." Variations in intonation also allow us to discriminate between statements and questions. For example, the words "You liked rhubarb pie" can be expressed as a statement (meaning, "You had it before, and you liked it") or as a question (meaning "Did you really like it?"). The difference between a statement and a question is conveyed in English by the steady or falling intonation in the statement form and the rising intonation on the question form. These types of prosodic cues are referred to as *linguistic prosody*, because they provide information about the sentence structure and type.

Prosody can also convey information about the feelings or emotions of the speaker. This *emotional prosody* is how others detect, from the tones of our voices, whether we are upset, or secretly pleased, or simply neutral. In other cases, we purposefully mismatch the content of our words with the emotional tone of our speech to express sarcasm or irony. Most individuals are exquisitely sensitive to the myriad of overtones that can be added to speech via emotional prosody. In fact, when there is a mismatch between what we say (i.e., the words used) and how we say it (i.e., the emotional prosody), our listener is likely to assume that the prosodic information conveys our true meaning. That is why we hear comments such as, "She said it was OK, but she didn't seem too happy about it." The additional information conveyed through emotional prosody may be intentional or unintentional, which is why we sometimes say, "Your voice is telling on you."

Speech Sound Development

A child who is born with a normally functioning hearing mechanism and raised in a speaking environment will systematically acquire the perceptual capabilities needed to understand the language he or she hears. As the baby develops, we see a corresponding development of the baby's knowledge and use of the sound system (see Table 3.4). In order to understand the development of the child's auditory and early sound production capabilities, let us look at the experiences of a single child.

Birth

Abraham was born in the early morning of May 15. He was the first child in his family. On his second day of life, Abraham's hearing was screened as he slept beside his mother's hospital bed. Newborn hearing screening using electrophysiological measures can detect possible hearing loss in the first few days of a baby's life. In Abraham's case, the results confirmed normal hearing.

The development of Abraham's sound system actually began while he was still in the womb. A developing fetus responds to sound by the third trimester of gestation (Birnholz & Benacerraf, 1983; Kisilevsky et al., 2003). The fetus will change positions and increase heart rate in response to sound. If the sound persists, these behavioral signs of hearing will wane, only to return if the characteristics of the sounds change (Leader, Baillie, Martin, & Vermeulen, 1982).

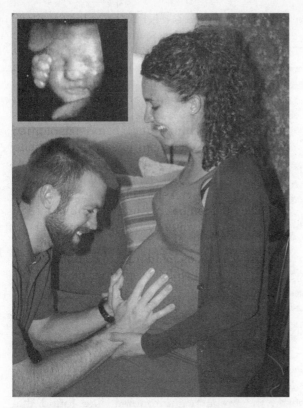

FIGURE 3.6   Not only does the third trimester fetus respond to sound from outside the womb, there is evidence that newborn babies recognize the voices of their parents. Inset photo: 3-D sonogram of 33-week fetus.

However, the sounds that reached Abraham *in utero* were probably more limited in scope than what he can now hear. First of all, his mother's body tissues attenuated, or reduced, the sounds (Walker, Grimwade, & Wood, 1971). Because the voice of Abraham's father had to travel from the air through his wife's body to reach his developing child (as in Figure 3.6), Abraham probably heard only a muffled version of his father's voice in the womb. The lower frequencies carried by vowel sounds and the pitch, rhythm, and intonation of the father's voice were probably heard more clearly than the higher frequency sounds that distinguished the consonants of his speech. In contrast, the mother's voice had a direct route to her fetus via internal sound vibrations that traveled through her body to the womb. This advantage makes maternal speech recorded within the womb more intelligible than the speech of others (Armitage, Baldwin, & Vince, 1980; Bench, 1968).

The influence of prenatal auditory experience can be measured in babies soon after birth. Researchers use techniques such as "high-amplitude sucking," in which infants suck on a pacifier that is wired to data-recording instruments. Infant abilities are explored by conditioning babies to change their rate of sucking

TABLE 3.4 Approximate Ages for Milestones in the Comprehension and Production of Sound

Age	Milestone
0 weeks	Startles at loud sound Prefers mother's voice to strangers' Produces reflexive, vegetative sounds
4 months	Responds to household sounds Can discriminate among many speech sounds Produces differentiated cries Produces vowel-like sounds
7 months	Produces canonical babbling Uses sound with communicative intent
10 months	Produces "protowords" Repeats sounds made by others Produces jargon Understands some words
12 months	Produces first words with simplified forms

in response to what they hear. DeCasper and colleagues examined infant responses to sounds available in the prenatal environment and found that the infants showed preferences for recordings of an intrauterine heartbeat (DeCasper & Sigafoos, 1983) and the voices of their own mothers (DeCasper & Fifer, 1980). Therefore, it is no surprise that Abraham is comforted by being held against his mother's body as she speaks gently to him. The warmth of her body and the sound of her heartbeat and voice are already familiar to him.

At home, Abraham is already a beginning communicator. However, much of this is unintentional on his part. As his uncle holds him, Abraham makes a series of lip smacks. In response, his uncle responds playfully as if the baby just related a shocking secret. Later, as his mother gives him a sponge bath, Abraham is fussy and emits a series of cries. His mother "explains" to him that she is bathing him and that she is trying to do this as fast as she can. She then picks him up in a towel to rock him, telling him he is okay. While dressing him, she "trades" sounds with him by repeating his short cries and other vocalizations. Soon, his parents begin to recognize the different types of cries he makes. For example, Abraham's father recognizes a cry of protest as he removes a bottle of formula from Abraham's mouth in order to reposition him. These early interactions provide the infant with important information about communication. The infant learns that vocalizations have the positive effect of parental attention and response. The close proximity of the parent's face allows the infant to see his or her parent's facial expressions. The give-and-take interchanges lay the groundwork for conversational turn-taking.

6 Weeks

Abraham awakens from his nap. His legs and arms stretch and move about as he makes a series of sounds. His mouth is open, and he emits a series of short, vowel-like sounds as well as lip and tongue smacks. Sometimes these sound like exclamations, comments, or complaints. Early on, infants' cries and other vocalizations often occur with the velopharyngeal port open, giving sounds a nasal quality (Oller, 1980). Infants may produce sounds on both expirations and inspirations. Each infant is quite variable in how he or she produces sounds from one time to the next. It may be that the infant is "trying out" the many combinations of positions and movements that can be used to produce grunts, cries, and other vocalizations (Boliek, Hixon, Watson, & Morgan, 1996).

Abraham's father enters the nursery and gets down to eye level with his son. When he calls his son's name, the infant turns his head and looks at his father's face. His father asks, "Are you waking up? Are you waking up now?" Abraham gives his father a big smile. These types of interactions demonstrate the infant's early response to, and preference for, familiar faces and voices. In return, Abraham's interest in his father's voice is rewarded by more verbal attention from his father. In fact, Abraham's parents speak to him quite a lot. They name his body parts as they wash him. They tell him about his fashion options while dressing him for the day. They recite nursery rhymes while changing his diaper. Although all this language stimulation may seem beyond his level of comprehension, it provides him with an ongoing stream of information from which he is already beginning to gain knowledge about his native language.

Like parents around the world, Abraham's parents talk to him with exaggerated stress and pitch variations, slower rate, and liberal use of repetitions. This type of speech is often called *child-directed speech* or, sometimes, *motherese*. Adults and older children often use child-directed speech when speaking to infants and toddlers, and babies seem to prefer this type of speech. Researchers feel that the exaggerations of child-directed speech may also play an important role in helping the young child segment the ongoing stream of speech into units of phrases, words, and individual sounds (Jusczyk, 1997; Kuhl & Iverson, 1995).

4 to 6 Months

At 4 months, Abraham's major activity for the day is putting things into his mouth, with a secondary emphasis on drooling. He tries putting his hands, his feet, his toys, and even dry leaves into his mouth, then makes a grab for his grandmother's earrings. This is a typical mode for exploring the world at this age. Regardless of whether his mouth is full, he makes a variety of vowel sounds. Sometimes, they are abrupt exclamations (e.g., "eh!"). These sounds are not necessarily directed toward anyone, although they stop when his mother approaches. His mother gets down on the ground with him and exclaims, "How's my big boy?! How's my big boy?!" He looks at her intently and then squeals in response. Although Abraham does not yet understand just what is said to him, he is learning about the give-and-take of "conversation" and sounds that comprise his native language (see Figure 3.7).

We know that infants have perceptual capabilities from very early on that allow them to begin to recognize the individual sounds of speech. As we discussed earlier, the production of individual sounds varies from one word to the next due to coarticulatory effects. Nonetheless, we perceive all the variations of the sound "b" as the phoneme /b/, and all the variations of "p" as the phoneme /p/. This trait, common to mammals including humans, is known as *categorical perception* because acoustic signals that lie on a physical continuum between sound pairs such as /b/ or /p/ are perceived as one sound or the other. A complementary situation exists for vowels, wherein a large variety of acoustic representations are perceived as one of a much smaller set of vowel sounds. This is known as the *perceptual magnet effect* (Kuhl, 1994; Kuhl & Iverson, 1995) because, when we hear an acoustic signal that is vowel-like, our perception of that signal is drawn, like a magnet, toward the prototypical vowel that is closest to the sound heard.

These early perceptual capabilities are shaped by the listener's experience with the language or languages heard. An early study by Eimas, Siqueland, Jusczyk, and Vigorito (1971) showed that infants could distinguish between language-relevant acoustic contrasts at four weeks after birth. Subsequent work

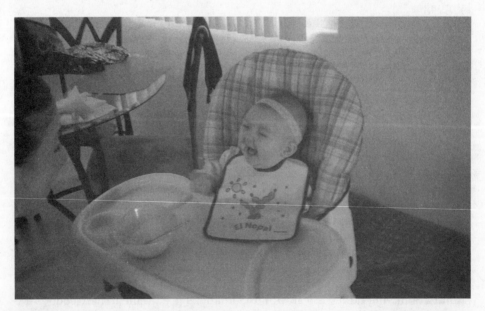

FIGURE 3.7 Even before the first words are spoken, babies use a range of vocalizations to communicate.

(e.g., Burnham, Earnshaw, & Clark, 1991; Kuhl, Williams, Lacerda, Stevens, & Lindblom, 1992; Streeter, 1976; Werker & LaLonde, 1988) has shown that infants initially perceive contrasts that include sounds not found in their native language but later lose the ability to discriminate between non-native speech sounds. This suggests that the perceptual change reflects a developmental milestone that requires exposure to spoken language to be achieved.

7 to 9 Months

At 7 months of age, Abraham celebrated this first Christmas. Wearing his pajamas and a red Santa's hat, he sat on the couch and reached for the small gift that fell out of his Christmas stocking. His parents began to unwrap the gifts for him, but, once they were started, he was able to tear the remaining paper off them. He mouthed each piece of torn wrapping paper before tossing it aside. He patted an unwrapped box with his open hand and watched his parents as they held up each gift, naming and commenting about each one. This "joint reference" between parent and child provided Abraham with the opportunity to observe objects and actions at the same time that he heard the words that related to them. His breathing was rapid and loud, and he waved his arms with excitement.

During this period, Abraham reached a new milestone in the development of the speech sound system. His production of sounds no longer consisted solely of vowels. The first consonants were added to his repertoire. Abraham exclaimed "Da!" as he reached for an as-of-yet untasted piece of wrapping paper. These first consonant-vowel (CV) and consonant-vowel-consonant-vowel (CVCV) utterances are referred to as **canonical babbling**. This type of babbling is nonspecific, in that babies Abraham's age do not use these CV or CVCV combinations to refer to specific objects or intentions. However, Abraham, like other babies, produced these sound combinations with the prosody of speech, so that it seemed as though he was speaking even though no true words were produced.

Abraham's initial production of canonical babbling at 7 months was about average for developing infants. Eilers and Oller (1994) reported that normally hearing infants may enter the stage of canonical babbling as early as 3 months or as late as 10 months. Auditory experience seems critical for the development of this milestone. Hearing-impaired infants are delayed in canonical babbling, with the onset occurring after 11 months of age. In contrast, infants with other developmental problems but no hearing loss may show little or no delay in reaching this milestone (Eilers & Oller, 1994).

At 6 and 7 months of age, babies continue to make vowel-like sounds, and they also produce consonant-vowel (CV) combinations. They make these sounds regardless of whether another person is interacting with them. However, there are qualitative changes in sound production at this stage as well. For example, Abraham often seemed fascinated with his own babbling. He seemed to play with variations of his own babbling, producing a string of sounds and then repeating them with a slight change in the overall pattern. For example, while playing, he produced "di da . . . di da . . . daaaaaah . . . da." As at earlier ages, these sounds appeared to be a form of vocal play, without reference to any object in particular.

Another change is the emergence of communicative intent motivating Abraham's use of sound. This preverbal use of sound is typical among babies at this age. Parents recognize their baby's use of sounds to direct their attention to an object, to request actions ("give me"), or just as a social interaction. At this age, Abraham used sounds to signal refusal, for example. His mother offered him a spoonful of strained peas, which appeared to be out of favor at the time. He exclaimed his disgust and turned his face away from the offending food. These first intentional vocalizations are quite probably precursors of linguistic behaviors yet to come. In fact, babies at this stage begin to comprehend a few spoken words, signaling the onset of the first true linguistic stage of development.

10 to 14 Months

Abraham learned to walk before his first birthday. Initially, he used a coffee table or the couch to lift himself up and then "cruised" around the room, holding on to the edges of the furniture. Then he walked without support. But often, he was able to take only a few steps before landing on his seat. His most efficient mode of locomotion was still crawling.

Abraham also expanded his sound repertoire. In addition to the single syllables that were heard at 7 to 9 months, he learned to produce consonants in combination. As he stood ready to walk to his mother's outstretched arms, we heard "yee yeah adee di hee." Then Abraham's father, holding a video camera, caught his attention. His mother asked, "Do you want to walk to Daddy?" Abraham piped in with an enthusiastic "da! dee!" Although this approximated the word "daddy," it was not yet a true word for Abraham. In fact, a few minutes later, we heard Abraham utter a chorus of "da dees" when attempting to walk toward his mother and also when attending to neither parent. In this particular case, "da dee" reflected a different milestone in the development of speech sounds: the ability to repeat sound strings produced by others. We saw this new ability to repeat more explicitly when Abraham's mother was encouraging him to show off for the camera. She told him, "Wave to the camera. Wave! Wave!" He echoed back "ey . . . ey" as a shortened form of "wave." Then he waved his hands, first one hand and then both. Next, his mother told him, "Say 'Hey!' You know how to say 'Hey!' Say 'Hey!'" And he repeated "Hey!"

At this stage, we often hear a chain of syllables with sentence-like inflectional patterns, such as "ba to aa aa na?" We refer to these speech-like sound strings as *jargon.* Such an utterance is directed toward a listener, with the baby often searching to make eye contact, causing the listener to feel almost obligated to answer the jargon question with "yes" or "no." Abraham appeared to demand an object from the listener, give it back, and then demand it again. He changed his role within the communicative exchange, alternating between asker and giver. The sound of his voice carried as much of the message as the reaching gestures or looking at the object.

Jargon includes many combinations of consonants and vowels, and there does not appear to be a one-to-one representation between a particular object or desire and the sounds produced. That is, the baby is not using the same combination of sounds to represent particular words. At this stage, we hear front, middle, and back vowels sandwiched between many different consonant-like sounds. Although many of the consonant-vowel combinations are repeated, others are unique. The intention of the utterance is carried more in the inflection and prosody than in the consonant-vowel combination. When they use vocalized jargon as intentional communication, babies begin to use the inflectional patterns that have been heard in their native language that represent particular needs and wants. For example, a rising intonation may accompany a jargon "request."

Around the age of 11 months, Abraham entered a stage characterized by "variegated babbling" (Schwartz, 1984), meaning the jargon sounds were individualized and not frequently repeated. At this stage, the infant begins to show real control over the stress and intonation of vocalization, with the jargon pattern closely resembling the language that the baby has been hearing. Ingram (1976) presented a number of diary studies that described particular babies at 11 to 12 months who were beginning to repeat the same vocalization patterns for a given situational context. There was still enough phonetic variability to preclude the utterance from being classified as true words. Many of the utterances at this age sound more like phrases than single words.

A baby this age produces phonetically consistent forms that are the immediate precursors to true words. Schwartz (1984) describes these precursors as **protowords** (primitive, early forms of an actual word). Whereas jargon vocalization appears to be more related to the affective, emotional state of the infant and is therefore rather free-flowing, protowords have much greater specificity and appear to be more object- or action-specific. Sometimes, babies this age embed a protoword in the prosodic jargon. At other times, we observe a combination of jargon, then a slight pause, followed by the production of a protoword. It would seem that the first true words that often appear at 12 to 13 months do not come suddenly but have developed gradually, from babble to jargon to protowords and then finally to a true word with relative phonetic stability.

Despite the arrival of the first few words, typical 1-year-olds seem to attempt most of their communication by continuing differentiated jargon. The first words are not said very often. The jargon pattern becomes longer, sounding more like real language and occasionally containing a real word. Although a wide variety of sounds may be heard in the jargon of children, relatively few sounds are heard in the first few words. Much of the intended message, when understood by the listener, is communicated not by the occasional word but by the general intonation pattern of the utterance, gestures, and by the situational context.

When imitating the sounds of others, there is some selectivity regarding the kinds of sounds chosen for play. We also see this pattern as babies begin to produce their first words (Ferguson, 1978). Babies imitate the sounds they can physiologically produce. If a sound is too complex to make, babies will usually simplify the utterance, perhaps changing the consonant to one they can produce and preserving the vowel that was in the model. Abraham was heard doing just this when he looked at a tiger in a picture book and said, "tita." As the first words are produced, there is similar selectivity, such that the first words require less complex motor control. Many of the first words may involve sounds with a similar place of production, often voiced consonants produced at the front of the mouth, such as /m/ and /b/. Babies often use the same consonant-vowel combination for several different words. For example, /ba/ may be used for words as different as *ball* and *car*. Over time, as children add to their repertoire of speech sounds, the pronunciation of these two words becomes distinct (see Figure 3.8).

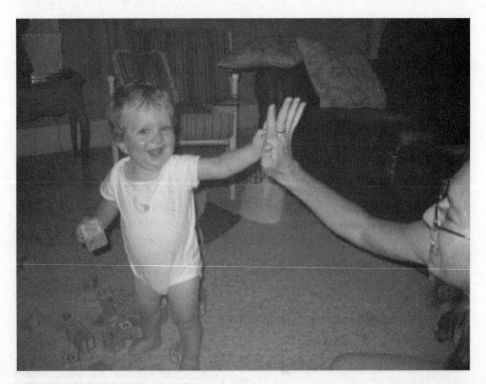

FIGURE 3.8   Babies begin to produce their first words around 12 months of age, around the time that they begin walking.

15 Months and Older

At this age, Abraham has entered the true verbal stage of communication development. We will look in some detail at his development from single words to sentences in Chapter 7. However, Abraham will continue to add to his sound system as well during this time (see Figure 3.9). As he grows, he will add sounds in a fairly predictable way. Irwin and Wong (1983) described the sequence in which typically developing children like Abraham add sounds to their repertoire between 1½ and 3 years of age. Their work shows that most children at 18 months have one or two distinct vowels and a few consonants that they use to produce approximations of their first words. By 24 months, many of the vowels are produced distinctly, and a few new consonants are added. As depicted in Figure 3.9, by the age of 3, children have expanded their consonant repertoire, which greatly aids the overall intelligibility of their speech. Over time, children learn to use their acquired sounds in different positions within words (Dyson, 1988). The job of learning the sounds of speech and using them correctly in connected

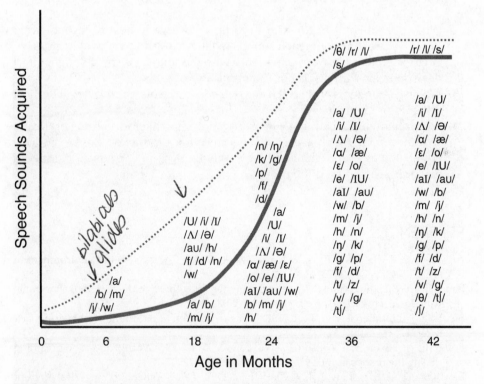

FIGURE 3.9 A depiction of speech sound acquisition. The solid line indicates the increase of the number of speech sounds that children acquire with age. The dotted line represents additional sounds that are in the process of being acquired; that is, they are mastered by some but not all children at a given age.

Based on Sander (1972) and Irwin & Wong (1983).

speech takes years to complete. Some normal 5-year-olds, for example, may still be mastering some of the latest acquired sounds, such as /r/ and /l/ (Kenney & Prather, 1986), although these sounds begin to emerge much earlier. Likewise, normally developing children may make sound errors in some words and not in others. This is because the production of a particular sound is influenced by all other sounds contained in the word. As children mature, their speech is less affected by these coarticulatory effects (Nittrouer, Studdert-Kennedy, & McGowan, 1989). By age 4, most children can be readily understood, even by those who do not know them well.

Clinical Problem Solving

Kim was born with a severe hearing loss affecting both of his ears. He responded reliably to sounds of 500 and 1000 Hz at 40 dB HL; sounds at 2000 to 4000 Hz were heard at 50 to 60 dB HL, and sounds above 4000 Hz required even greater intensities (up to 80 dB HL).

1. What does this mean for Kim in terms of everyday hearing experiences? What types of environmental sounds will he hear, and what will he miss?
2. Give examples of how his experience with the sounds of speech might affect development of this aspect of communication.
3. Which components of speech (i.e., vowels, consonants, prosody) will be most difficult for him to hear?
4. Some children (and adults) who experience a hearing loss become proficient speechreaders. Which aspects of speech sound production can be best discriminated by this method and why? What aspects of conversational speech make speechreading difficult?

REFERENCES

Armitage, S. E., Baldwin, B. A., & Vince, M. A. (1980). The fetal sound environment of sheep. *Science, 206*, 1173–1174.

Bench, J. (1968). Sound transmission to the human fetus through the maternal abdominal wall. *Journal of Genetic Psychology, 113*, 85–87.

Birnholz, J. C., & Benacerraf, B. R. (1983). The development of human fetal hearing. *Science, 222*, 516–518.

Boliek, C. A., Hixon, T. J., Watson, P. J., & Morgan, W. J. (1996). Vocalization and breathing during the first year of life. *Journal of Voice, 10*, 1–22.

Burnham, D. K., Earnshaw, L. J., & Clark, J. E. (1991). Development of categorical identification of native and non-native bilabial stops: Infants, children, and adults. *Journal of Child Language, 18*, 321–260.

DeCasper, A. J., & Fifer, W. P. (1980). Of human bonding: Newborns prefer their mother's voices. *Science, 208*(1), 1741–1776.

DeCasper A. J., & Sigafoos, D. (1983). The intrauterine heartbeat: A potential reinforcer for newborns. *Infant Behavior and Development, 6*, 19–25.

Dyson, A. T. (1988). Phonetic inventories of 2- and 3-year old children. *Journal of Speech and Hearing Disorders, 53,* 89–93.

Eilers, R. E., & Oller, D. K. (1994). Infant vocalizations and the early diagnosis of severe hearing impairment. *Journal of Pediatrics, 124,* 199–203.

Eimas, P. D., Siqueland, E. R., Jusczyk, P. W., & Vigorito, J. (1971). Speech perception in infants. *Science, 171,* 303–306.

Ferguson, C. (1978). Learning to pronounce: The earliest stages of phonological development in the child. In F. Minifie & L. Lloyd (Eds.), *Communicative and cognitive abilities: Early behavioral assessment.* Baltimore: University Park Press.

Ingram, D. (1976). *Phonological disability in children.* New York: Elsevier North Holland.

Irwin, J. V., & Wong, S. P. (1983). *Phonological development in children 18 to 72 months.* Carbondale: Southern Illinois University Press.

Jusczyk, P. W. (1997). *The discovery of spoken language.* Cambridge, MA: MIT Press/ Bradford Books.

Kelly, J. P. (1985). Auditory system. In E. R. Kandel & J. H. Schwartz (Eds.), *Principles of neural science.* New York: Elsevier.

Kenney, K. W., & Prather, E. M. (1986). Articulation development in preschool children: Consistency of production. *Journal of Speech and Hearing Research, 29,* 29–36.

Kisilevsky, B. S., Hains, S.M.J, Lee, K., Xie, X., Huang, H., Ye, H. H., Zhang, K. & Wang, Z. (2003). Effects of experience on fetal Voice recognition, *Psychological Science, 14,* 220–224.

Kuhl, P. K. (1994). Learning and representation in speech and language. *Current Opinion in Neurobiology, 4,* 812–822.

Kuhl, P. K., & Iverson, P. (1995). Linguistic experience and the perceptual magnet effect. In W. Strange (Ed.), *Speech perception and linguistic experience.* Baltimore: York Press.

Kuhl, P. K., Williams, K. A., Lacerda, F., Stevens, K. N., & Lindblom, B. (1992). Linguistic experience alters phonetic perception in infants by 6 months of age. *Science, 255,* 606–608.

Leader, L. R., Baillie, P., Martin, B., & Vermeulen, E. (1982). The assessment and significance of habituation to a repeated stimulus by the human fetus. *Early Human Development, 7,* 211–219.

Nittrouer, S., Studdert-Kennedy, Y. M., & McGowan, R. S. (1989). The emergence of phonetic segments: Evidence from the spectral structure fricative-vowel syllables spoken by children and adults. *Journal of Speech and Hearing Research, 32,* 120–132.

Oller, D. (1980). The emergence of speech sounds in infancy. In G. Yeni-Kamshian, J. Kavanaugh, & C. Ferguson (Eds.), *Child phonology. Vol. 1: Production.* New York: Academic Press.

Sander, E. K. (1972). When are speech sounds learned? *Journal of Speech and Hearing Disorders, 37*(1), 55–63.

Schwartz, R. (1984). The phonologic system: Normal acquisition. In J. Costello (Ed.), *Speech disorders in children.* San Diego: College-Hill Press.

Streeter, L. A. (1976). Language perception of two-month-old infants shows effects of both innate mechanisms and experience. *Nature, 259,* 39–40.

Walker, D., Grimwade, J., & Wood, C. (1971). Intrauterine noise: A component of the fetal environment. *American Journal of Obstetrics and Gynecology, 109,* 91–95.

Werker, J. F., & LaLonde, C. E. (1988). Cross-language speech perception: Initial capabilities and developmental change. *Developmental Psychology, 24,* 672–683.

Disorders of Speech Sound Production

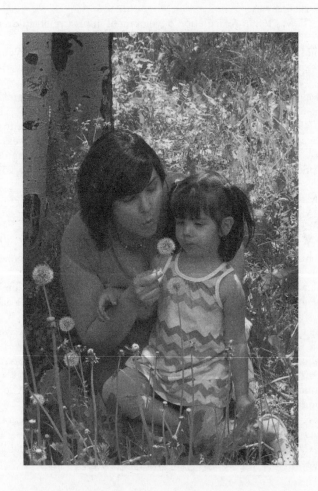

PREVIEW

Disorders of articulation affect both children and adults. Speech sound errors may range from a mild lisp to nearly unintelligible speech that results from many sound substitutions, omissions, and distortions. Childhood speech sound problems may be caused by structural anomalies, such as cleft palate, but are more frequently related to faulty or incomplete learning of the sound system. Some adults show the residual signs of a childhood speech disorder. In others, speech sound errors result from damage to the central nervous system. Brain damage may produce the slurred or labored speech of dysarthria or the unpredictable errors of apraxia of speech. In evaluating the wide range of speech sound disorders, the speech-language pathologist must recognize the factors that cause and maintain the disorder. Intervention may include medical procedures, behavioral therapy, or the application of technology to improve communication.

The emergence of spoken words is one of the most important milestones in a toddler's life. We commonly hear from excited parents who report hearing "dada" or "mama" in their child's babblings, well before these sounds are used as true words. As long as the baby's word attempt contains sufficient phonemes to be recognized, the listener accepts it as the target word. In the first three years of life, parents pay more attention to the emergence of new words and overall communication, rather than to the precision of articulation. If the young child's speech can be understood, there is usually little concern. During the preschool years, children's articulation improves and approximates adult sound production. However, some children persist in using immature patterns of speech, often interfering with their ability to make themselves understood. In the case of acquired articulation disorders, an adult may begin to make speech errors following an illness or injury. Persistent speech sound errors in either adults or children may warrant a referral to a speech-language pathologist.

> From 2 to 4 years of age, the intelligibility of a young child's speech increases from about 50 percent to nearly 100 percent

Types of Speech Sound Errors

In Chapter 2 we studied the speech mechanisms required for the production of normal speech, and in Chapter 3 we considered the consonants, vowels, and diphthongs used in English. We also learned that sounds are strung together to form words in connected speech. We say these sounds very rapidly. It is often in the rapid production of sounds required for normal speech that speech sound errors become most noticeable. Whether heard in a single syllable, a word, a phrase, or sentences, such errors are known as **misarticulations**. There are four forms of misarticulation: **substitution errors** (*fith* for *fish*), **omission errors** (*fi'* for *fish*), **distortion errors** (a lisped "sh" in *fish*), and **addition errors** (*fisha* for *fish*).

Substitutions

Substitutions are a common type of speech sound error in young children. Pre-school children often substitute one phoneme for the target phoneme, with a certain logic or predictability. In many cases, the incorrect sound is similar to the target sound in terms of the place and manner of articulation and voicing characteristics of the sound (see also Chapter 3). For example, the child who says, *I tee the wabbit* has used two common substitutions heard in the speech of young children. Like the /s/ in *see*, the substituted /t/ is a voiceless sound that is made near the same spot in the front of the mouth; the /w/ has many production similarities to the target sound /r/ that it replaces. In other cases, the incorrect sound shares similarities with other sounds found within the word. For example, when a child says *bate* for *bake*, the /t/ replaces /k/ because /t/ is produced forward in the mouth, closer to where /b/ is produced.

> Four types of speech sound errors can be remembered by the acronym SODA.
> S = substitution
> O = omission
> D = distortion
> A = addition

Until children acquire a particular sound of the adult phoneme system, they often replace it with a sound they have some success in making. Many of the substituted sounds are ones that are acquired by children at earlier ages than the target sound. For example, if 4-year-olds cannot say an /s/, they might substitute a sound that they can say, such as /t/. Substitution is perhaps the most common articulatory error in the child who is learning to talk. However, these errors may persist or be far more frequent in a child with a speech disorder.

Omissions

When speakers omit sounds from words, their speech is difficult to understand. Consider the following exchange between a 28-month-old boy and his father:

> **Dad:** Look at all that stuff!
> **Child:** I bri a boo. A bir boo. [I bring a book. A bird book.]
> **Dad:** (Looks at book.) Is it a bird book?
> **Child:** I ge thi un, you ge tha un. [I get this one, you get that one.]
> **Dad:** Oh. Ok, I get this book about shells.
> **Child:** I a pi un. [It's a pink one.]
> **Dad:** It's a pretty pink shell.

As we can see, it is difficult to tell what this child is saying from his words alone. If not for the father, who provides a running translation, we might not know what this child was actually saying.

The omission of consonants, known as a syllable-simplification process, is a natural part of phonological development. One particular sound or a whole class of sounds may be omitted. Occasionally, a young child will leave all endings off words. For some children, the simplification processes can lead to omission of an entire syllable, which is what occurs when the young child says *nana* for *banana* or *amblance* for *ambulance*. In each case an unstressed syllable has been omitted from the word. These omissions of sounds or syllables occur frequently in the speech of toddlers and become less common as the child grows older. However, when a 4-year-old child persists in omitting sounds, or an adult begins to produce them after years of normal speech, the omissions signal an articulation disorder.

Distortions

As we saw in Chapter 3, the production of a sound must be relatively close to the target to be perceived by listeners as correct. Slight variations that still sound like the target sound are considered acceptable **allophones**, but when the sound is markedly different from the target, it is classified as a distortion. With a distortion error, the target sound is produced with some change of the sound, although not enough to be classified as a sound substitution or an addition. One of the most common distortions is the lateral lisp, in which the target /s/ or /z/ phonemes sound slushy, as if an unvoiced /l/ is part of the sound. Such errors may be developmental, wherein the child has not learned the precise articulation for the sound, or may emerge in the speech of an adult if they acquire a neurological condition that affects their speech.

Additions

A fourth type of articulatory error involves an addition of a sound where it does not belong. For example, we might hear an individual with an addition error saying *boata* for *boat*. In other cases, an extra vowel may be inserted between the two sounds of a consonant blend (e.g., *galass* for *glass*). As in these examples, the addition error is often an unstressed vowel. Unlike other types of articulation errors, addition errors are not typically seen as a part of normal development. We sometimes hear speakers with foreign accents make sound editions. Additions may also occur when an individual has difficulty with the timing and coordination of articulatory movements, so that vowel-like intrusions emerge within or at the ends of words. This type of error may occur in individuals with impaired motor control, such as cerebral palsy or progressive neurological disease.

Speech Sound Disorders in Children

Disorders affecting the speech sound system affect approximately 3.8 percent of 6-year-old children (Shriberg, Tomblin, & McSweeny, 1999). Boys are identified as having difficulty with speech sound production slightly more frequently than are girls. Some children experience difficulty because of structural abnormalities that affect the speech system. Others seem to make speech sound errors despite the lack of any obvious cause. We will consider both types of speech sound disorders in this chapter.

Structural Impairments in Children

In Chapter 2, we saw that sound production relies on a number of physical systems. If one or more of these systems are compromised, due to genetic disorders, birth defects, or injury, the ability to produce speech sounds may also become impaired. For children, there may be a collection of structural anomalies that fit a broader pattern of anomalies known collectively as a **syndrome**. A syndrome is identified when a certain number of features co-occur across individuals. For example, a child may be classified as having the Treacher Collins syndrome, characterized by a lack of mandibular growth, downward-slanting eyes, notched lower eyelid, and microtia (a lack of external ear development). This syndrome is genetic in origin and may often be observed in several members of the same family. A syndrome is often named after the physician(s) or other professional who first described the group of signs that co-occurred in their patients. Other syndromes, such as fetal alcohol syndrome, are named for the factors that cause the condition. In addition to abnormalities of orofacial structures, the signs of fetal alchohol syndrome may include hearing loss, language delay, mental retardation, or problems with speech sound production.

Occasionally, the structure of the tongue may contribute to articulation difficulty. The tongue may appear to be too large (macroglossia) or too small (microglossia). Macroglossia occurs with certain developmental syndromes, and appears to contribute to poor articulation. At one time, tongue reduction surgery was recommended for these children, but follow-up studies failed to document improved articulation (Lynch, 1990). Sometimes the tongue appears to be too large because it is riding forward in the mouth and protruding, possibly because of abnormalities in the back of the oral cavity, such as enlarged tonsils. In other cases, a forward tongue carriage may be the result of muscle weakness and inadequate neural innervation of the tongue muscles, so the problem is not related to the structure of the tongue, but to other factors.

Another structural problem related to the tongue, which seems to get undue attention, is what is referred to as being "tongue-tied." This is the lay term for a condition in which the small band of tissue that connects the underside of the tongue to the floor of the mouth is too tight, so that forward and upward movement of the tongue tip is restricted. This connective membrane is referred to as the lingual frenulum (or frenum). When the lingual frenulum is tight, it is evident by the heart-shaped appearance of the tongue when it is protruded because the tip is tethered and a bit indented. The condition is evident in some newborns, and raises concerns when there are breastfeeding difficulties (Ballard et al., 2002; Ricke et al., 2005). In such infants, surgery to clip the frenulum has been associated with improved breastfeeding (Buryk, Bloom, & Shope, 2011). With regard to speech development, it appears that some individuals who appear to be "tongue tied" learn to accurately produce speech sounds without difficulty; however, in other instances tongue movement is restricted to the extent that it negatively affects the production of certain lingual sounds, such as /l/. Some research indicates improved articulation following surgical release of the tight frenulum in such children (Messner & Lalakea, 2002), but the value of such surgery remains controversial and a topic of investigation (Suter & Bornstein, 2009).

People say they are "tongue tied" when they have difficulty speaking, but what does the term really mean?

Dental abnormalities have also been blamed for articulation problems. Shelton and colleagues (Shelton, Furr, Johnson, & Arndt, 1975) looked closely at the influence of various dental abnormalities on improvement in articulation therapy, concluding that even children with severe malocclusion could learn to articulate normally. Sometimes orthodontic correction procedures that include the wearing of braces, bands, retainers, and the like will require slight changes in the tongue placement in order to achieve precise articulation. In other words, the contact points for the tongue may be shifted a bit due to the dental appliances, so it may take some time for the wearer (child or adult) to adjust their motor patterns for clear articulation. Such problems are usually temporary but can be challenging, especially for adults who are suddenly confronted with the need to shift their firmly established speech patterns. If the orthodontic device is not temporary (e.g., braces), a consultation with a speech-language pathologist can be helpful to identify the optimal placement of the articulators to achieve the best speech sound production.

Cleft Lip and Palate.   Among the more common structural anomalies that are relevant to speech production are cleft lip and palate. A cleft (or gap) occurs when there is not proper fusion of the tissues that form the upper lip or those that form the roof of the mouth. The disruption occurs early in embryonic development, between the fifth and twelfth weeks of pregnancy. Depending on the timing and extent of the disruption in development, there may be a cleft palate in isolation, a cleft lip alone, or they may co-occur. Clefts may occur on either side of the midline of the upper lip, to the right or left of the bone that holds the upper front teeth (the **alveolar ridge**), or along the midline of the hard or soft palate. These predictable locations for clefts relate directly to the fact that these structures grow as separate segments that must fuse together during embryonic development.

Estimates of the incidence of cleft lip or palate range between 1 in 500 to 1 in 750 babies (Peterson-Falzone, Hardin-Jones, & Karnell, 2001). Clefts vary widely in severity. A small defect may involve a partial division in the uvula and a gap within the soft tissues of the velum. Severe facial clefts may involve both sides of the lip and alveolar ridge (in which the top front teeth are rooted). A cleft may also extend from the velum forward into the hard palate so that the nasopharynx is open to the mouth. For many children, the cleft is part of a syndrome that affects other aspects of development (Shprintzen, Siegal-Sadewitz, Amato, & Goldberg, 1985). For example, a child born with velocardiofacial syndrome may have other facial anomalies and heart defects in addition to cleft palate. These children frequently have problems with language development as well. For other children, the cleft lip or palate is the only problem.

Perhaps we can best appreciate the impact of a cleft on the life of a child by considering the case of Andres.

Andres is an engaging 3-year-old who was born with a left unilateral cleft lip and palate. In the country of his birth, his mother lacked the resources to feed and care for her child, and Andres was brought to an orphanage. When he was adopted at 14 months, he was small for his age, weighing only 14 pounds. In addition, his language skills lagged well behind age expectations. Whereas children of 14 months are typically producing some words, Andres was not yet producing anything that even sounded like the speech sounds of his native language. His adoptive parents were a U.S. couple who brought him to the United States. Andres's adoptive mother was a speech-language pathologist who had special expertise in cleft palate.

Because Andres's parents adopted him knowing he had a cleft palate, they did not experience the initial emotional shock that is common when parents discover their baby has this condition. Moreover, Andres's parents had a much better understanding of the implications of raising a child with a cleft palate from a medical and communication standpoint. For example, they were aware that some of the corrective surgery would need to be scheduled quickly. In fact, many babies born with cleft lips and palates have already had a repair of the lip well before Andres's age. Therefore, Andres's parents arranged for an initial evaluation with an ear, nose, and throat (ENT) doctor and a plastic surgeon soon after arriving home. By 16 months, Andres had his first surgery, during which his lip cleft was closed and preliminary work was begun to close the palate. In addition, tubes were inserted through Andres's eardrums to drain the fluid that accumulated due to his chronic middle ear infections.

Much to his parents' delight, the day after his first surgery, Andres produced his first speech sound, /m/. As his mother related, "His eyes just lit up." He seemed to recognize that this sound was important, and he produced several more in succession. His first word approximations, *more*, *mom*, and *milk* built on this early appearing sound. Subsequently, he added /h/, /n/, /p/ and a nasal-sounding /b/, along with several different vowels. These additional sounds allowed him to expand his repertoire of words to include social routines like *hi* and an approximation of *please*. He also produced some vocalizations that were unidentifiable as English sounds.

Andres made a return trip to the hospital for a second round of surgery at 18 months. This time, surgery targeted repairs of the soft and hard palate. Andres and his parents stayed overnight, which was required by the hospital staff to assure that he was alert and able to drink independently before he was released. After an episode the next day in which he ran down the hall with his mother gamely attempting to keep up with his IV pole and tubing, the staff decided he could go home. Another post-surgery challenge was that Andres was fitted with arm splints to prevent him from reaching his stitches. However, these did not always remain on this active boy. On several occasions, Andres handed the splints to his mother to indicate she should put them back on.

It is safe to say that Andres's cleft lip initially had an impact on every aspect of his life. However, we also see how quickly intervention with these children can improve both their communication skills and the quality of their lives. For Andres, a good home environment and medical and behavioral treatment transformed him from a child with a cleft lip and palate and delayed speech and language development into an active little boy whose cleft was just one more fact of his life.

Andres's case illustrates that treatment of the child with cleft palate typically involves both medical and behavioral interventions. Indeed, Andres's treatment in the early years of his life involved his parents, a plastic surgeon, an ENT, and a speech-language pathologist. The cleft palate team may also include additional members, such as a pediatrician or orthodontist. An audiologist may be called upon to evaluate hearing loss that can occur with structural anomalies involving the auditory system, or bouts with middle ear infection (see Chapter 11). In Andres's case, tubes that allow middle-ear fluid to drain helped him to maintain normal hearing. Hearing loss due to middle-ear infection is common in children with cleft lip and palate (Handzic-Cuk, Cuk, Gluhinic, Risavi, & Stajner-Katusic, 2001). Later in this book, we will learn more about how the various professionals on a cleft palate team function together (Chapter 13).

> By 23 months, Andres was producing two-word utterances, but his spoken vocabulary was still quite limited. In addition, the words he did use were difficult to understand because they only approximated the adult form. For example, he rarely used sounds that required contact of the tongue to the alveolar ridge. He also did not use "back" consonants (i.e., /k/, /g/). His sound preferences probably reflected a combination of factors, some related to his cleft and some that may have reflected his early attempts to compensate for his abnormal oral structures. Children with complete clefts often have difficulty producing the tongue-to-palate contact and movement of the soft palate for back consonants, and thus they may avoid them. In contrast to his difficulties with speech sound production, Andres seemed to understand very well for his age. At 28 months, his parents made the decision to enroll him in language therapy with the goal of expanding his vocabulary and increasing his utterance length. This focus was intended to help him achieve parity with his preschool classmates, whose skills were somewhat more advanced.

A cleft palate often results in hypernasality and nasal escape of air. What consonant sounds are difficult to produce with a cleft palate?

The consequences of a cleft lip are fairly straightforward in that labial (lip) sounds are difficult to produce until the lip repair is accomplished. The effects of the cleft palate are a bit more complicated. The normal speech mechanism includes a structural separation between the oral and nasal cavities (the hard palate), and the muscular actions of the velum (the soft palate) allow complete separation of the two cavities. Closure of the velopharyngeal opening between the oral and nasal cavities is typically accomplished by the elevation of the velum and its firm contact against the pharyngeal wall. In contrast, an unrepaired cleft palate results in a lack of separation between the oral and nasal cavities, so that sound resonates in both cavities. This results in excessive nasal resonance (i.e., hypernasality), but in addition, the cleft also prohibits complete separation of the oral cavity from the nasal cavity, which is necessary to generate adequate air pressure for plosive sounds (e.g., /p/ and /b/) or to maintain the steady air flow necessary to produce fricative sounds (e.g., /f/ and /v/). Attempts to generate adequate air pressure for such consonant sounds may result in an escape of air through the nose that is audible (sounding like a soft snort). Even after the hard and soft palates are surgically repaired, it is not uncommon for there to be some remaining difficulty in achieving complete velopharyngeal closure, so that hypernasality often persists to some extent and may be the focus of treatment with the speech-language pathologist.

> Speech sound disorders that result from neuromotor impairment may have a congenital or an acquired etiology. Give an example of each.

Neuromotor Impairments in Children

Children may develop a motor impairment after injury or disease that affects the nervous system. For example, a child who suffers a head injury in a car accident may have difficulty controlling the oral structures necessary for producing speech sounds with precision. Other children may display motor impairments from the time of birth. Some of these children are diagnosed as having **cerebral palsy**. These children tend to have motor impairments that involve the speech musculature and other body systems. Some children may show delays in the development of speech without the involvement of other motor systems, in other words, such children have motor control impairments that are specific to speech. We will examine each of these forms of neuromotor speech impairments.

Cerebral Palsy.   Cerebral palsy is not a disease *per se*, but rather a term used to refer to a number of conditions that result from damage to, or imperfect development of, the central nervous system. It is estimated that between 2 and 3 infants per 1,000 newborns are classified as having cerebral palsy (Odding, Roebroeck, & Stam, 2006). This neurological impairment may occur before birth, during birth, or during the first three years of life. Therefore, a delay in motor skills including crawling, sitting, standing, walking, chewing/swallowing, self-feeding, and talking may be evident. The finer the motor skill required, such as in talking, the more likely the child will have a problem. In cerebral palsy, motor deficits may be grossly divided into four types:

Spasticity.   **Spasticity** is characterized by severe tightness of the muscles. Speech prosody is often interrupted by respiratory and voice breaks. Articulation is often severely defective.

Athetosis.   **Athetosis** is characterized by a series of involuntary muscle contractions, with flailing of extremities and much facial grimacing. Lack of respiratory control causes a monotonic voice, often lacking sufficient loudness. There are many phonemic distortions.

Mixed.   This type of cerebral palsy, sometimes called tension athetoid, represents a mixture of both tight spasticity and flailing athetosis.

Ataxia.   **Ataxia** is characterized by a lack of balance and severe problems in coordination of movements. Ataxic speech sounds like the slurred, arhythmical speech of someone inebriated.

The motor speech problems of the child with cerebral palsy can be classified as a type of dysarthria. Dysarthria refers to an impairment involving the motor control for speech production that is characterized weakness, slowness, and/or incoordination of the speech musculature that results in imprecise articulation. It can be developmental, as in the case of cerebral palsy, but it also occurs in children or adults who suffer brain damage later in their lives. If the condition is severe, the affected child enjoys few normal developmental experiences and a marked delay in speech. The treatment of the dysarthria for the child with cerebral palsy, therefore, may be quite different from that of one who acquires dysarthria after normal speech patterns have been established.

Often the child with cerebral palsy is so physically active with muscle contractions or unstable head and trunk posture that speaking appears almost impossible. The speech-language pathologist may work closely with other treatment specialists, such as an orthopedic surgeon, a physiatrist (a physician specializing in physical or restorative medicine), a physical therapist, an occupational therapist, and a special educator in order to address speech goals in concert with these other issues. For some children with cerebral palsy, articulate speech is not a realistic goal, and some form of nonvocal communication system must be introduced. A manually or electronically operated communication board can be an effective alternate communication system. Thanks to modern technology, there are assistive communication devices available to meet the basic communication needs of even the most severely handicapped child with cerebral palsy.

Developmental Dysarthria.   Whereas children with cerebral palsy tend to have pervasive impairment of motor control, other children exhibit difficulties that are specific to the motor control for speech. Some of these children are identified as having developmental dysarthria characterized by abnormal tone of the facial muscles, which may be worse on one side than the other. Low muscle tone may result in a soft, somewhat drooping facial expression. Muscle tone that is abnormally high may produce a taut appearance or contribute to facial distortions and grimaces. Some children with dysarthria have trouble eating and controlling saliva, so that they may drool. Affected children typically are late in acquiring their first words. As they grow older, their speech often remains very difficult to understand. When tested, the motor impairment is particularly evident when they are asked to produce rapid speech or nonspeech movements.

Bell's Palsy.   A sudden (acute) onset of facial paralysis occurs when the cranial nerve that innervates the muscles of the face (cranial nerve VII) is damaged or inflamed. The unilateral (one-sided) facial droop of unknown cause is referred to as Bell's palsy. The weakness of the facial muscles makes it difficult to produce sounds that require lip movement (such as lip retraction for a long "ee" sound), or tight lip closure (such as a /p/). In most cases, the symptoms resolve within several weeks; however, the condition persists in some individuals.

> Bell's palsy refers to sudden onset of paralysis of one side of the face. It typically resolves completely, or nearly completely. A quick search on the Internet reveals some surprises regarding people who have had bouts of Bell's palsy.

Childhood Apraxia of Speech.   Another type of motor speech impairment observed in young people is childhood apraxia of speech (also referred to as developmental apraxia of speech). Apraxia refers to the impairment of the ability to program, combine, or sequence the movement for speech. The problem is not related to muscle weakness, as observed in dysarthria. Rather, the problem relates to planning the correct motor movements for speech sound production. A child with a pure apraxia of speech demonstrates relatively normal comprehension of language but a striking inability to imitate even simple spoken words, despite having no muscular weakness or paralysis. A case presentation of a 6-year-old girl with apraxia of speech illustrates the problem:

> *Esme* was a friendly and enthusiastic 6-year-old enrolled in a public school kindergarten. From her first day, it was apparent that her speech skills were well below average. Esme was nearly impossible to understand. Her kindergarten teacher asked the school's speech-language pathologist to observe Esme in the classroom. The speech-language pathologist noted that Esme's language comprehension appeared to be within normal limits, but she was rarely understood by her teacher or classmates and often showed signs of frustration and distress while trying to communicate. Immediate intervention was needed.

> The speech-language pathologist contacted Esme's mother to obtain permission to see Esme for a formal evaluation and for therapy. Esme's mother confided that her child had been evaluated once before. At the age of 2, Esme had been seen at the county's developmental disabilities center because she had not yet started to speak. At that time, based on her poor motor and speech development, the developmental specialist suspected mental retardation. Her mother was so distressed at this diagnosis that she refused all preschool services and refused to release the records of that diagnosis to anyone. She was sure her child was bright and feared Esme would be stigmatized and held back by this diagnosis. Instead, the mother kept Esme at home and spent a great deal of time taking her on field trips and engaging in other creative activities with her. The mother waited until Esme was 6 to enroll her in kindergarten, hoping that the extra year would give her a developmental advantage to compensate for her poor communication. Although still wary of therapists and special education professionals, after some discussion she agreed to allow the speech-language pathologist to see Esme.

> A formal evaluation revealed that Esme rarely pronounced any words correctly, even when speaking only single words. She often made errors on initial sounds in words and omitted endings altogether. Her sentences tended to be short, with an average of three words per sentence. A battery of language tests indicated that her receptive language skills were slightly above average and her expressive language skills were poor. She did not have mental retardation.

> During subsequent therapy sessions, Esme made slow and inconsistent progress. The speech-language pathologist noted that she sometimes showed facial tension while speaking. Once, when trying to imitate a /d/sound, she used her fingers to move her tongue into position. These behaviors suggested problems with planning and sequencing speech movements. The speech-language pathologist confirmed the diagnosis of childhood apraxia of speech.

As noted in Esme's case, childhood apraxia of speech is a motor speech problem, not a language problem; however, the limited ability to express language through speech results in a marked discrepancy between expressive and receptive language performance. Children with apraxia of speech require intensive individual therapy as well as language-based intervention in which efforts are made to encourage the development of a variety of communication skills.

Phonological Disorders

Some children's poor articulation skills are not readily attributable to structural abnormalities or obvious disorders of motor control. They may have persistent difficulty with just a few speech sounds, or their errors may be so numerous that connected speech is nearly impossible to understand. A careful evaluation of speech sound production allows the speech-language pathologist to characterize the individual sound errors and to determine whether there is a consistent error pattern that affects numerous sounds. The results of the assessment are evaluated relative to the typical age at which children demonstrate consistent correct production for certain sounds.

When a 4-year-old preschool child mispronounces only a few sounds, such as /r/, /l/, or /s/, the speech-language pathologist may recommend a "wait and watch" approach because not all typically developing children produce those sounds correctly. In other words, intervention may be limited or deferred while the child is given a chance to self-correct articulation through normal maturation. For school-age children, however, even a few sounds produced in error is unusual. A 10-year-old boy's lisped /s/ rarely interferes with his ability to communicate his ideas. It can, however, negatively affect the way other children view him (Hall, 1990). Such children are typically candidates for therapy and may be quite motivated to correct their speech.

A phonological approach to speech sound disorders recognizes that the child has difficulty mastering the adult phonology, or speech sound system, of the child's native language. All children, in their early attempts to use spoken language, make simplifications of speech sound patterns. As Dunn (1982) wrote, "The term phonological process . . . is frequently used as a way to describe the systematic simplifications observed in child speech" (p. 147). Children with phonological disorders, however, continue to use these simplification processes long after their peers have ceased using them (Grunwell, 1980). Some common **phonological processes** are shown in Table 4.1.

Because phonological processes represent systematic error patterns, treatment is directed toward correcting the processes to a greater extent than treating individual sound errors. Robbie is one such child.

At age 4, Robbie was brought to a university speech-language clinic by his concerned parents. Robbie's parents, most other family members (including three older siblings), and neighbors had difficulty understanding him. He had normal hearing, normal cognitive ability, and a normal speech mechanism at the time of

TABLE 4.1 Phonological Processes

Phonological Processes	Examples	
	Adult Word	Child Word
Simplification of syllables		
Final consonant deletion	bat	"ba–"
Unstressed syllable deletion	above	"–bove"
Cluster reduction	step	"–tep"
Assimilation		
Regressive (backward) assimilation	dig	"gig"
Progressive (forward) assimilation	goat	"toat"
Substitution		
Stopping—stop sounds are substituted for fricative	sheep	"teep"
Fronting—alveolar sounds are substituted for palatal and velar sounds	came	"tame"

the speech evaluation. His articulation errors were abundant. He could correctly say all vowel sounds, and /m/, /p/, /b/, /t/, /d/, /n/, when these were the initial sounds in a word. He correctly said /m/, /p/, /b/ when they occurred in the middle of words. However, he routinely dropped the final consonants from the end of words. Most of his consonant errors were omissions, although he made a few consonant substitutions: t for k, d for g, t for f, b for v, t for Θ. His overall attempts at conversation were restricted to two- or three-word utterances, many of which were not intelligible. He appeared to limit his mean length of response to two or three words as a conscious gesture to accommodate his listeners; he apparently had learned that if he said more than that, no one would understand him.

Because Robbie could say six consonants correctly in the initial position, a phonological approach to his problem focused on making him aware that many words had consonant endings that he could say. At the start of therapy, the stop consonants that he could produce correctly (/p/, /b/, /t/, /d/) were presented at the beginning and the end of a word, and he was cued to say these sounds in both word positions. In treatment, he was soon able to produce most of the six target sounds (the ones he could say at the evaluation) at both the beginning and the end of a word, such as *pop, top, mop, Bob, tub, mom, Pam* (his sister), and so forth. Later sessions included working on phonetic sounds that Robbie should have been making correctly by focusing on the processes that characterized his sound substitutions.

Studies of children with phonological disorders reveal that they frequently have features in common, including impairments in other domains (Ruscello, St. Louis, & Mason, 1991; Ruscello, 2008; Shriberg, Kwiatkowski, Best, Hengst, & Terselic-Weber, 1986). About two-thirds of children with disordered phonology are boys. Frequently, there are signs of general neuromotor problems, including mild muscle weakness and incoordination. A phonological disorder is often accompanied by a developmental language disorder (see Chapter 8). Half of all children with speech sound disorders also have difficulty learning to read. Problems with academic skills may persist long into the school years, even after speech is no longer obviously impaired (Shriberg & Kwiatkowski, 1988). Sometimes a family history of phonological as well as other speech or language disorders can be documented for these children (Lewis, 1990).

Tongue Thrust

Several generations of Americans have been evaluated and treated for **tongue thrust** as part of an orthodontic management program. Children with tongue thrust use an unusual sequence of oral movements when swallowing. The tongue pushes forward against the anterior teeth (particularly the upper incisors). This forward tongue movement while swallowing has led some to refer to tongue thrust as reverse swallowing. The forward tongue movement is accompanied by high tension in the muscles controlling lip movement, which is needed to prevent the tongue from protruding as it pushes forward during swallowing. This abnormal and inefficient pattern of swallowing tends to make children with tongue thrust messy eaters. In addition, the frequent forward pressure of the tongue forces the teeth out of alignment. For this reason, many orthodontists are reluctant to fit a child with braces until the tongue thrust habit has been overcome. This problem frequently requires direct intervention with special procedures known as **myofunctional therapy** to develop optimal intraoral tongue postures for swallowing (Barrett & Hanson, 1978).

Some children with identified tongue thrust also have an associated articulation disorder, most commonly heard by others as a lisp because the anterior sibilants (particularly /s/ and /z/) are mispronounced. Speech-language pathologists who have been trained in myofunctional therapy techniques may choose to treat the articulation disorder and tongue thrust simultaneously. When there is tongue thrust but no articulation disorder, the speech-language pathologist may elect to administer myofunctional therapy to correct abnormal tongue and lip postures and movements (ASHA, 1991; 2004).

> Are you aware of some characteristic features of the speech of individuals with very limited hearing? What are they?

Hearing Loss

In Chapters 10 and 11, we will see the importance of the hearing mechanism in the development of normal communication. Human communication is primarily an oral-aural interaction. The loss of auditory information can seriously impair aural reception of language. Hearing loss is a frequent cause of a developmental communication problem, affecting speech sound production as well as language. Some children simply cannot hear certain phonemes, which clearly makes it difficult to learn to produce them. Common causes of hearing loss and its effect on speech sound development are described at length in Chapter 11.

Evaluation of Speech Sound Disorders in Children

Many times, children (and adults) are referred for a speech evaluation because others find their speech difficult to understand. Formal evaluation of the speech sound production may involve several steps that are designed to determine whether errors are part of normal development or consistent with a speech disorder that warrants therapy. A complete evaluation may include testing to determine which individual sounds or patterns of sounds are affected and whether there is any physical reason (e.g., an orofacial anomaly, hearing loss) that these speech errors are occurring.

> Sometimes you are listening to a speaker and you know there is something odd about their articulation, but you can't quite determine what it is. How can you focus your attention better to figure out what it is?

Speech Sound Production Screening

A screening measure is not designed to determine whether a disorder exists, but whether additional testing is warranted to make this kind of determination. Screening programs for children are common in the public schools, particularly in kindergarten and the first few elementary grades. Such programs are typically set up in the fall, and all new children in a school district (kindergarten and other grades) meet with the speech-language pathologist or a speech-language assistant (see Chapter 13) for a brief screening. The screening might focus on conversation with the children to observe their articulation and their overall language function, voice quality, and speech fluency. However, many young children are reticent about talking to a stranger, making a natural conversation impossible. Therefore, it is usually necessary to structure the screening so that a maximum amount of information can be obtained from a relatively brief speech sample.

It should be noted that certain speech sounds are stressed in the screening program—usually those that young children typically should be able to pronounce in the early years. Ideally, the screening test should differentiate between those children who will outgrow their problem with maturation and those with articulation problems that need remediation.

Assessing Children with Speech Sound Disorders

Formal evaluation of speech production may begin with simply listening to the child (or adult) in conversation. The conversation may be with other children, between parent and child, or between clinician and child. This may involve discreet observation of a child at home, on the playground, or in the classroom. Other children may be seen in a clinic testing suite (which often looks like a playroom, for young children) that has observation mirrors permitting the clinician to observe the child in as natural a communication setting as possible. A conversation during spontaneous play will often reveal how the child actually talks outside of the testing situation. With an older child, an actual conversation about topics of interest will reveal the communicative ability, offering information about articulation proficiency as well as about voice, language, and fluency.

The well-trained and experienced speech-language pathologist is able to observe the child's productions systematically and make a useful summary statement based on the observations relevant to the articulatory adequacy, the type and place of errors, and so forth. It is possible, however, that observation of play and conversation will not reveal all of the child's speech errors, nor will conversation alone provide the diagnostic information that a more structured evaluation will include. Therefore, the evaluation is likely to include conversational speech and more formal testing.

Assessing children with speech sound disorders will typically include procedures designed to assess whether physical problems are contributing to the speech problem. Two common measures include a hearing screening and an examination of the oral mechanism.

Audiometric Testing. Audiometric testing, or at least a hearing screening measure, should be part of every speech evaluation. As we will see in Chapters 11 and 12; even a mild hearing loss can affect which sounds are heard and produced. The child's ability to perceive the sounds of words is an important part of the evaluation. Therefore, audiometric testing may include evaluation of speech sound reception and discrimination levels.

Oral Mechanism Evaluation. An oral mechanism evaluation provides the speech-language pathologist with information about the adequacy of oral structures and function. As discussed earlier in this chapter, structural defects and incorrect movements of the articulators can all contribute to faulty speech production. An oral mechanism examination form (see Figure 4.1) lists the clinician's observations about various structural areas of the vocal tract and how well they function for speech.

The particular form pictured in Figure 4.1 could be used for either a child or an adult. It allows the clinician to note structural abnormalities (facial and oral) that are relevant for speech. It is important to note that many minor, or even some significant, deviations from normal structure may not impede correct articulation, or may do so only temporarily. A child who has lost his front teeth may lisp temporarily until the permanent teeth grow in, but in general, misalignment of teeth (dental malocclusions) are not a major cause of poor speech.

The oral mechanism form also requires the clinician to note whether specific speech gestures are being made with precision (e.g., lip closure to produce /pa/; lifting the tongue during production of /ta/). In addition to simple speech gestures, the ability to produce rapid alternating speech sounds (e.g., /pʌ pʌ pʌ/) is tested. Individuals who have normal control over speech articulation are able to produce these repeating or alternating syllables (i.e., /pʌ tʌ kʌ/) rapidly, smoothly, and without pauses between syllables. The ability to produce repeated syllable strings is called **diadochokinesis**. Those with neurological impairments or physical deviations of the oral structures may produce these syllables more slowly, struggle to produce them, or produce them with imprecise movements.

ORAL MECHANISM SCREENING FOR SPEECH

Structures	Function
Instructions: Visually inspect structures to complete each item. Note deviations that occur.	**Instructions**: Demonstrate item. For each item, obtain 3 trials. Note deviations that occur.

Structures

Facial Structures
    facial muscle tone
    facial symmetry
    lip symmetry
    Other:_____

Oral Cavity
    tongue
    teeth
    hard palate
    soft palate
    uvula
    faucial pillars
    tonsils
    Other:_____

Function

Lip closure achieved for /pa/
Tongue tip raised for /ta/& /la/
Rounded lips for /wʌ/
Dental-labial position for /vʌ/
Comments:_____
_____

Velum raised for sustained /a/ (three trials)
Comments:_____
_____

Sound quality for sustained /a/
Comments:_____
_____

Diadochokinesis (16 repetitions each)

	accurate		rhythmic		time (secs)
/pʌpʌpʌ.../	Y	N	Y	N	
/tʌtʌtʌ.../	Y	N	Y	N	
/kʌkʌkʌ.../	Y	N	Y	N	
/pʌtʌkʌ.../	Y	N	Y	N	

FIGURE 4.1 Oral mechanism screening for speech.

The advantage to the speech-language pathologist of using a standard form to summarize the data from the oral examination lies in the need to be complete and systematic. The form, in effect, provides a checklist for each part of the oral mechanism in terms of its structural and performance adequacy. For patients with dysarthria or a major structural defect (such as a cleft palate), a more detailed and supplementary examination would be required.

Articulation Inventory.   Many commercially available articulation tests provide the clinician with a ready inventory of speech sounds. Most tests can identify not only the actual sounds produced incorrectly but also the place in the word where the error occurs (initial, medial, or final position) and the type of error (omission, substitution, distortion, or addition). A typical articulation inventory will use words that contain each of the English speech sounds in word initial, medial, and final position. A typical articulation inventory will provide the type of information found in Figure 4.2. This form shows the results of a single-word articulation test given to 5-year-old Katie, who demonstrated a number of speech sound errors. The errors may be described individually as substitutions (e.g., p for f)

ARTICULATION TEST				
Name: Katie	**Age:** 5.0 years			
SOUND ITEM	I	M	F	PHONOLOGICAL PROCESS
p pencils, zipper, cup	✓	✓	-/p	Final consonant deletion
m matches, Christmas, drum	✓	✓	-/m	F.C.D.
n knife, Santa, gun	✓	✓	-/n	F.C.D.
w window	✓			
h house	✓			
b rabbit, bathtub	✓	✓	-/b	F.C.D.
g gun, wagon, flag	✓	✓	-/g	F.C.D.
k cup, chicken, duck	✓	✓	-/k	F.C.D.
f fishing, telephone, knife	P/f	P/f	-/f	F.C.D., Stopping
d duck, window, bed	✓	✓	-/d	F.C.D.
ŋ finger, ring		g/ŋ	-/ŋ	F.C.D., Stopping
j yellow	✓			
t telephone, bathtub, carrot	✓	✓	-/t	F.C.D.
ʃ shovel, fishing, brush	t/ʃ	t/ʃ	-/ʃ	F.C.D., Stopping
tʃ church, matches	t/tʃ	t/tʃ	-/tʃ	F.C.D., Stopping
l lamp, yellow, squirrel	w/l	w/l	-/l	F.C.D., Liquid Simplification
r rabbit, carrot, car	w/r	w/r	-/r	F.C.D., Liquid Simplification
dʒ jumping, pajamas, orange	d/dʒ	g/dʒ	-/dʒ	F.C.D., Stopping
θ thumb, bathtub, bath	t/θ	-/θ	-/θ	F.C.D., Stopping
v vacuum, shovel, stove	b/v	b/v	-/v	F.C.D., Stopping
s scissors, pencils, house	d/s	t/s	-/s	F.C.D., Stopping
z zipper, scissors	d/z	d/z	-/z	F.C.D., Stopping
ð this, feather	d/ð	d/ð		Stopping

FIGURE 4.2 Articulation test results for Katie, age 5 years. Note: F.C.D. = final consonant deletion. Based on the Goldman-Fristoe Test of Articulation-2nd Edition (Goldman & Fristoe, 2000) and the Khan-Lewis Phonological Analysis (Khan & Lewis, 1986).

or omissions (e.g., – for f) in the initial (I), medial (M), or final (F) position in the word. In the column labeled Phonological Process, errors are ascribed to one of three phonological processes demonstrated. Additional testing follows the formal articulation test to see whether incorrect sounds can be produced correctly under special circumstances (e.g., with a model, in a sentence), and to determine the status of specific phonological processes.

Phonological Process Analysis.   For many children, speech sound errors are not limited to a few consistently misarticulated sounds. More often, the speech-language pathologist finds errors on many of the consonant sounds. These errors at first glance may seem inconsistent. Certain consonants may be correctly produced in a few words, whereas in others they are omitted, distorted, or replaced with another consonant. A careful examination of these speech-sound errors almost always reveals a pattern. For example, when a child says *Tuta too my tir* for *Susan took my shirt*, the errors might be classified in the two ways shown in Table 4.2. Substitution errors are shown by writing the error sound followed by a slash (/) and the target sound. Omitted sounds are denoted with a minus (–) sign.

When the sound errors are listed individually in Table 4.2, we notice that the child is inconsistent in the use of the /t/ sound. The child uses it correctly when attempting the word *took* but substitutes it for the /s/ and /z/ in *Susan* and /ʃ/ in *shirt* and omits it altogether at the end of *shirt*. This use would be puzzling if we concentrated only on the individual sound errors. However, all these errors, plus those not involving /t/, can be accounted for by two general patterns, or **phonological processes**. The substitutions of /t/ for /s/, /z/, and /ʃ/ are all examples of a process called *stopping*, in which a stop consonant (e.g., /t/, /d/, or /g/) is substituted for a continuant (e.g., /s/, /f/, or /v/). All the errors of omission occur on the final consonant, indicating a process of final consonant deletion. Many phonological processes are seen in normally developing children, but persist in children with phonological disorders.

Stimulability.   An important part of the articulation evaluation is assessing how well the client can produce omitted or incorrect sounds when provided help to do so. This is known as *stimulability*. After the formal articulation test is

TABLE 4.2   Examples of Sound Errors in Children's Speech

	Individual Errors	Phonological Processes
Attempted Statement		
Susan took my shirt.		
Child's Statement		
Tuta too my tir.	Initial t/s, t/ʃ	Stopping
	Medial t/z	Stopping
	Final –/n, –/k, –/t	Final consonant deletion

completed, the speech-language pathologist selects several incorrect sounds to determine if the child is stimulable for those sounds. Children who can correct their sound errors when given visual, auditory, or tactile cues have a better prognosis for correction than those who cannot.

Stimulability testing can occur at several levels. The higher the level at which the child is able to produce the sound correctly, the easier it is to correct the production of the sound. At the highest level, the clinician may ask the child to say a mispronounced word over again by prompting, "Can you say that better?" If the child does not correct word production, the clinician might ask the child to repeat the word after a model is given. If the child's attempt is incorrect, the clinician might draw attention to visual cues to aid articulation by instructing the child to "watch how I say it." If the addition of visual cues is not effective, the clinician might ask the child to produce the target sound in a consonant-vowel combination, like *la-la-la*. If necessary, visual and tactile cues may be added to help the child. These steps are taken to determine what capacity the child has for producing the sound and how much support and cueing the child needs to do so.

Severity and Intelligibility. Formal testing of the sounds a child (or an adult) can produce does not always reflect the overall severity of the problem. For example, consider the speech of the following two children:

> **MARIA:** He go bi tee [He's got big teeth]. Bu i no a he [But it's not a he]. I a she! [It's a she!]
>
> **JOSEPH:** I see a amblance [I see an ambulance]. Let me see. I see an elphant [I see an elephant].

Both of these children have one phonological process that describes their speech errors. Maria tends to delete final consonants, and Joseph shows a pattern of weak syllable deletion. Although both children's errors can be described with a single process, Maria is much more difficult to understand than Joseph. This illustrates that knowledge of specific error types does not always provide accurate insight concerning overall severity. Kent, Miolo, and Bloedel (1994) reviewed the wide variety of available methods for estimating the overall intelligibility of speech. They noted that these measures tend to emphasize different aspects of speech analysis. A clinician may select among measures that emphasize phonetic contrasts, phonological error patterns, whole-word identification in isolation or in connected speech, or measures that require listeners to rate how well speech can be understood. Some of these measures were developed with the characteristics of a particular type of articulation problem in mind (e.g., speech associated with hearing impairment, dysarthria, phonological disorders). Therefore, the clinician's decision concerning which measure to select may reflect the type of client he or she needs to evaluate and even the types of speech sound errors the client shows (Kent et al., 1994; Shriberg, Austin, Lewis, McSweeny, & Wilson, 1997).

Other Testing.   Speech sound disorders may co-occur with other disorders. For example, children with genetic syndromes or multiple handicaps may have conditions that require coordinated evaluation by multiple professionals. In other cases, a speech sound disorder co-occurs with a language disorder. In these cases, the speech-language pathologist must try to determine the extent to which the sound errors are affecting the ability of the child (or adult) to produce elements of the language. For example, a phonological process such as final consonant deletion will eliminate parts of speech like the past tense -*ed*. Other processes like stridency deletion will eliminate the plural and possessive /s/. Because phonological disorders frequently co-occur with language difficulties, many clinicians routinely include one or more language measures in their assessment. We will consider the evaluation of language skills further in Chapter 8.

Intervention Methods for Children

There are several approaches to treating speech sound errors in children. If a child has physical problems that affect his or her ability to produce speech, a team approach involving several professionals may be involved. For example, treatment may include surgical interventions to repair a cleft palate or coordinated efforts by a speech-language pathologist and physical therapist to provide support for a child whose control of his or her overall posture and muscle tone is too poor to support speech. If hearing loss is contributing to poor articulation, treatment of speech may follow fitting the child with hearing aids.

For a child whose only difficulty involves poor speech sound production, a number of methods are available for treatment. Which method is selected may depend on how many and what types of speech sound errors the child makes, and how stimulable the child is for these sounds. The least effective clinicians may be those who apply the same intervention method to all children. Treatment methods are typically tailored to meet the needs of the individual child. However, two components are important to all forms of intervention: methods to assist the child in acquiring an adult-like speech sound system and methods to assure that newly acquired sounds are used in all words and in all speaking situations.

Acquisition Training

There are many published programs and informal programs that are designed to improve the speech of children. Here we examine general approaches to acquisition training that use different ways of achieving correct sound production. Semantic approaches attempt to make the child realize that his or her current method of speaking is not communicating the meaning intended. This cognitive approach can motivate a child who is capable of producing correct pronunciations but does not do so. Other children may not know how to produce correct sounds and may require more direct instruction. We will consider several approaches that concentrate on correcting sound errors by helping children achieve correct movements of the speech articulators.

A *semantic* approach to articulation therapy emphasizes the changes in meaning that sometimes accompany phonological errors. Let us look at an example of a semantic approach to therapy.

> Brian is a school-based speech-language pathologist who has a group of three first-grade children with phonological disorders. All of these children make systematic substitutions of one class of sounds for another. For example, Amon, one of his students, reduces clusters like /st/ or /bl/ to one sound (/t/ or /b/). Another student, Marta, uses stop consonants in the place of fricatives (see Table 4.1 for example of phonological processes). Brian is able to address each of these children's different patterns of sound errors through a semantic approach. He has selected pairs of picture cards that contrast the error sound with the sound pattern each child needs to master. For example, one card shows a stop sign and its pair shows a toy top. The words *stop* and *top* contrast the cluster /st/ with the word that would be produced if the child reduced the cluster from /st/ to /t/. Other pairs of cards contrast the error patterns of the other children. Brian and the children play a modified game of *go fish*. There are two sets of each picture, so that a child holding one picture can ask another child for that picture in an attempt to obtain matching pairs. Each child has to show the picture he or she requests so that Brian can tell whether each child produces the target sound. Amon is holding the stop sign card, but asks, "Do you have any top signs?" Brian replies, "No, I don't have any tops, but I do have a stop." This highlights for Amon the difference between what he asked for and what he meant to ask for. Likewise, when Marta asks Amon for a "tail" when she meant to say "sail," Amon has the opportunity to model the correct word. This approach works for these children because they are able to produce the sounds they are working on, but don't necessarily do so when they need to. It doesn't take long before the children realize that to get what they want, they have to produce the sound patterns that correspond to the correct word.

Many children need only a few examples of these minimal pairs before they are able to produce the target sounds in additional words (Elbert, Powell, & Swartzlander, 1991). The semantic method serves to alert the children to the fact that there is a difference between what they are saying and what they should be saying and that this difference is important. This method does not require children to think about the sounds themselves, an advantage for young children, who have little awareness of sounds as units smaller than words.

Some children will not benefit from a semantic approach. They may see the differences in meaning between their sound errors and the correct production but are unable to produce the sound correctly without additional assistance. A *cross-modality* approach may provide that assistance. Cross-modality approaches utilize sensory information to facilitate correct articulation. For example, a client and clinician may face a mirror (e.g., Figure 4.3) while the clinician demonstrates the target sound. The client may then attempt to repeat the sound while monitoring his or her movements visually in the mirror. In another case, a clinician may rub a child's alveolar ridge with a mint so that the child can feel and taste where the tongue belongs for /t/ and /d/. Or clients are instructed to put their hand

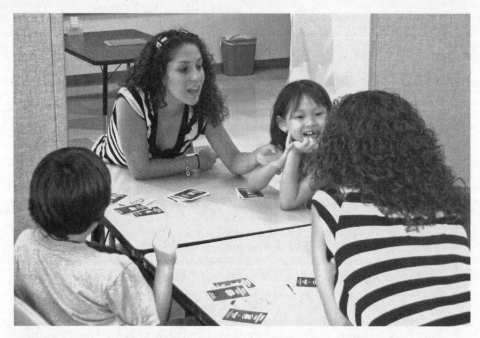

FIGURE 4.3   A graduate student training to be a speech-language pathologist makes use of a mirror to help two children with correct tongue position for the /l/ sound.

over their larynx to feel the difference between /s/ and /z/. This additional sensory input can be an effective way for adults or children to monitor their performance.

For some sounds, there are few available cues that the client can see or feel. Sometimes it is possible to take advantage of the *coarticulatory context* to promote correct sound production. Coarticulatory context refers to the fact that the sounds preceding and following a phoneme will influence the way the target sound is produced. For a phoneme like /r/, for which there are few visual cues, coarticulatory context can help in learning correct production. For example, the /g/ and /k/ in /gr/ or /kr/ blends require a high, back tongue carriage, which carries over to facilitate a correct production of /r/. Once this correct tongue placement is established in blends, it can be used in words with other sound combinations. Let's take a look at an approach that capitalizes on coarticulatory context.

> Makayla has teamed with her school's art teacher to integrate her articulation therapy into her students' classes. The art teacher's lesson plan involved constructing hand puppets in the shape of dragons. Makayla sat at the table with one of her students, Amy, who was working on the production of /r/. A number of other students were seated at the table as well. As Makayla assisted these students with the construction of their puppets, she asked them what sounds dragons might make. Several children offered that they may make a sound like /grrrrr/. Makayla readily agreed that /grrr/ was a strong candidate for dragon speech. She encouraged

each of the children to make their puppets imitate sentences that contained extended /gr/ blends. Soon, the children were pronouncing sentences like "Grrrr, I will grrrrab the grrrreasy grrrrrapes!" or "Grrrr, grrrasshoppers are grrrross!" By saying /grrrr/ at the start of each sentence, Amy had an opportunity to position her tongue for a correct /r/ before it came up in a full word. The use of /gr/ in word blends facilitated tongue position during running speech. Finally, by extending the /gr/ to /grrr/, Amy could slow down production of the blend to increase her chances of correct productions. Through this activity, Amy had an opportunity to work on her speech without missing out on art class. In addition, because many children were engaged in "dragon talk," she didn't feel singled out.

These different techniques can be used in conjunction with behavioral techniques. Many behavior-modification programs are commercially available for use with children with articulation disorders. These programs offer a number of attractive therapy materials designed to make the learning task interesting and fun for the young child. As a first step, the speech-language pathologist establishes a baseline of what the child is able to produce. For example, a particular target sound is selected, and the number of productions the child is able to say correctly, either spontaneously or by prompting, is established as the child's general proficiency for that sound. The treatment program for that sound then begins, following the systematic presentation of a particular protocol. The child is given an occasional prompt (a helping suggestion) to aid in production tasks, and as the typical program progresses, the clinician fades out support by doing less and less.

Generalization

If clients have learned the correct pronunciation of the /r/ sound, it does them little good if they can produce it only in /gr/ blends or only in the therapy setting. The goal of articulation therapy is for clients to be able to use the newly corrected sounds in all words and in all situations. When clients are able to transfer their newly learned articulation skills to untrained words and new settings, we say that they are demonstrating generalization of articulation skills. Generalization does not always occur automatically. The therapist should incorporate activities into the therapy program that promote generalization.

Generalization goals may be broken down into categories, such as generalizations to other sound contexts, to different speaking tasks, and with different speaking partners. Research has shown, for example, that training children on developmentally late-appearing sounds facilitates more generalization to other untrained sounds than when children are trained on earlier-appearing sounds (Gierut, Morrisette, Hughes, & Rowland, 1996). Therefore, through careful consideration of which sounds to train, a clinician can see gains on other sounds "for free." In some cases, the therapist may be able to find a few words in which the client is able to correctly produce the target sound. Generalization then involves transferring this limited skill to greater numbers of words (Prather & Whaley, 1984). For example, the client may lateralize the /s/ (air escapes over the sides of the tongue) in /sl/ blends but produce /st/ blends accurately. In this case, the therapist may present /sl/ blends in conjunction with /st/ blends to facilitate generalization. If the target sound is never produced correctly, the therapist may select a small set of words that begin with the target sounds for initial training. When these are mastered, the therapist may incorporate new words containing the target sounds into the therapy sessions. This set of words is expanded to include words with the target sounds in the medial and final position. The therapist may also include combinations of sounds within words that are more difficult for the client. Different words will be included in each session to promote generalization to new words.

Single-word responses can be expanded into short phrases and sentences. Sometimes a standard carrier phrase can be used initially to facilitate articulation in longer utterances. For example, a group of children might play a game of twenty questions in which each child asks, "Is it a . . . ?" to find out what card the therapist holds. Older children and adults can practice articulation while reading sentences and short passages. The use of carrier phrases or reading tasks allows clients to practice their articulation skills without having to concentrate on the content of the message. As articulation skills become increasingly automatic, the clinician will incorporate conversational tasks into the therapy session.

As therapy progresses, children and adults become increasingly adept at monitoring their articulation during the therapy session. This self-monitoring process appears to relate to the client's ability to generalize articulation skills (Shriberg & Kwiatkowski, 1990). Outside of the therapy session, clients are typically more concerned with the content of their speech than their articulation. To promote generalization to other settings, the therapist may enlist the cooperation of others. For a child, the therapist may provide parents with tips for facilitating correct articulation at home. Teachers may monitor articulation in the classroom. A peer may be enlisted for activities outside the therapy setting. McReynolds (1982) writes that bringing other people into generalization sessions as critical listeners will sometimes accelerate generalization; however, she notes that we must caution others "not to overdo their help, so that the person does not become overly self-conscious about the problem" (p. 136). Individuals should be treated gently when they make mistakes and given realistic positive reinforcement when they produce sounds well.

Acquired Speech Sound Disorders in Adults

Adults who have developed normal speech and language abilities give little attention to how they speak. The motor patterns for speech are well established and relatively automatic under most circumstances; however, adults may acquire structural or neurological impairments that disrupt their ability to produce speech sounds. Treatment of such impairments differs from treating developmental speech sound disorders, because adults may need to change their articulation patterns, and formerly automatic processes may need to become more intentional.

Speech Sound Disorders Due to Structural Impairments

Structural changes of the speech articulators can result from traumatic damage or surgical removal of all or portions of the larynx, tongue, jaw, teeth, or lips. Removal of the larynx results in the dramatic loss of the laryngeal voice and is discussed in Chapter 6. In some cases, portions of the tongue must be surgically removed because of cancer. The procedure is called a **glossectomy**, and it may be either partial or total, depending on the extent of the disease. Articulation is a challenge without the tongue; recall from Chapter 2 that many of the sounds of English are differentiated by movements of the tongue. The goal of treatment following glossectomy is to adjust the placement of the remaining articulators to produce the most intelligible speech possible. There are many subtle adjustments that can be made to approximate speech produced without the tongue. For example, the sound /t/ normally requires the tongue to touch the alveolar ridge, just behind the teeth, but in the absence of the tongue, the patient might touch the lower lip behind the front teeth in a manner that stops and then releases the airflow. Because the manner of production is still a plosive and it is produced at the alveolar ridge, listeners may be tricked into thinking they heard a /t/. In fact, it is typically easier to understand the speech of a glossectomy patient if you do not look at the mouth, where some surprising articulatory placements are being made.

It is rare when the tongue must be surgically removed. When this is medically necessary, the ability of an individual to compensate and produce understandable speech without a tongue reminds us that the role of the articulators is to change the shape of the vocal tract.

In some cases, structural changes of the articulators can be compensated for by specially designed artificial replacements, such as a prosthetic tongue and jaw (Arcuri, Perlman, Philippbar, & Barkmeier, 1991; Leonard & Gillis, 1982, 1983). The artificial tongue does not move but fills the gap resulting from tongue removal. This improves the speaker's ability to use the remaining articulators to overcome the changes in the oral structures. Some speakers adapt to their new anatomy by making appropriate articulatory adjustments. When treatment is needed, the speech-language pathologist works with the patient to come up with the most satisfactory approximation of sounds that are in error due to structural changes. In some cases, the rate of speech must be slowed to allow the necessary time to articulate in a manner that is different from lifelong speech patterns.

Motor Speech Disorders

The most commonly acquired articulation disorders in adults are due to neurological impairments that affect the motor control for speech. They are collectively referred to as motor speech disorders and include the disorders of dysarthria and apraxia of speech. As discussed earlier in this chapter, motor speech disorders can occur in children as well. When they occur in adults, they are typically caused by damage or dysfunction of the motor control centers in the central or peripheral nervous systems, or both. These disturbances may affect any or all aspects of speech production, including respiration, phonation, resonance, and articulation.

> The gradual onset of speech difficulties may be the first sign of a progressive neurological disease, because speech sound production requires rapid and precisely timed movements of the articulators.

Dysarthria.   The dysarthrias are a group of motor speech disorders caused by weakness, paralysis, slowness, incoordination, or sensory loss in the muscle groups responsible for speech. The muscle weakness and poor control typically result in imprecise articulation, so that speech is difficult to understand. The sounds may be distorted or involve the substitution of an incorrect sound. The specific characteristics of dysarthria tend to reflect the location of the damage to the nervous system, so that certain clusters of symptoms have been associated with certain diseases (Duffy, 2005). Some of the causes of dysarthria are stroke, Parkinson disease, Huntington's disease, amyotrophic lateral sclerosis (ALS, or Lou Gehrig's disease), and cerebellar diseases. In addition to imprecise articulation, symptoms include hypernasality because of poor motor control of the soft palate, disturbed voice quality including harshness or breathiness due to poor control of the larynx; and abnormal prosody because of poor control of changes in pitch, loudness, and timing. If motor control is so severely impaired that no understandable speech can be produced, it is called **anarthria**.

Apraxia.   **Apraxia of speech** differs from dysarthria in that there is no muscle weakness, paralysis, or incoordination, but there is impaired ability to plan the movements for speech production. Thus, apraxia of speech has been referred to as an impairment of the motor planning for articulation. Speech is difficult to understand because of substitution errors, sound repetitions, and some inappropriate sound additions. The errors are often inconsistent, so that repeated attempts at the same word come out differently each time. In adults, apraxia of speech often co-occurs with the language impairment of aphasia, and in those cases it is difficult to separate the speech and language disorders. However, apraxia of speech can exist independently of aphasia, so that language formulation, reading, and writing are unimpaired, but speech production is disturbed (Duffy, 2005).

Treatment of Motor Speech Disorders

The goal for the management of motor speech disorders is to improve communication. This can be accomplished through therapy designed to improve the intelligibility, naturalness, and efficiency of speech production, but it may also be achieved by the use of assistive devices. There are excellent resources that provide treatment approaches specific to particular syndromes (Duffy, 2005; Moore, Yorkston, & Beukelman, 1991; Square-Storer, 1989; Yorkston, Beukelman, & Bell, 1988). Treatment may be directed toward the restoration of normal speech production processes or the compensation for impaired motor control. In some cases, adjustments need to be made to overcome the impairment. For example, Parkinson disease often results in a dysarthria characterized by imprecise articulation, decreased loudness, and flat prosody. A treatment approach called the Lee Silverman Voice Treatment trains patients to increase the effort that they exert while speaking by adjusting their loudness. With increased loudness, the Parkinson patients also increase their articulatory precision and thus remarkably improve their speech intelligibility (Ramig, Countryman, Thompson, & Horii, 1995).

Although the symptomatology of apraxia and dysarthria differs, there are similarities in some of the behavioral treatment approaches appropriate for these speech disorders. For both types of disorders, treatment involves in an orderly progression of tasks and intensive drill to re-establish and stabilize the motor movements. For example, a treatment continuum for apraxia of speech might begin with the clinician saying the target word, followed by the patient and clinician producing the target together. If the patient correctly produces the response simultaneously with the clinician, then the clinician reduces support by mouthing the word along with the patient, and ultimately the patient produces the word in response to a question without support from the clinician (Wertz, LaPointe, & Rosenbek, 1984). In cases where speech production is not adequate for everyday communication, augmentative communication devices may be appropriate.

Augmentative and Alternative Communication Systems

Some adults and children have physical limitations so severe that oral speech may not be an attainable goal. For these individuals, alternate methods must be found for communication. These range from a simple signaling device, like the call bell on a bedside nightstand, to sophisticated electronic devices that are tailored to the client's individual needs. Off-the-shelf laptop or tablet computers may be adapted to serve as communication systems with specialized software (see Figure 4.4). The speech-language pathologist's challenge is to find the combination of features in a communication device that best matches the client's needs and abilities. A child who can identify pictures but cannot yet read may start with an electronic touch-screen device that displays and speaks the names of objects and actions common to his or her daily life. Those with moderately impaired intelligibility may need to augment spoken communication with an alphabet or picture board or other form of visual support to achieve successful communication. An adult who can read may do well with a device that can produce both synthetic speech and written output.

Before a device can be selected, an initial assessment of the client's abilities must be obtained, often through the coordinated efforts of a variety of professionals, such as audiologists, vision specialists, psychologists, speech-language pathologists, and physical and occupational therapists. These individuals contribute information concerning the client's sensory, motor, cognitive, and language abilities. This evaluation is designed to determine the client's limitations as well as strengths that might be used for communication. For example, an individual with limited visual acuity may do better with simple line drawings than with glossy photos. An individual with severe cerebral palsy and limited use of the hands may have sufficient control of eye movement, head movement, or even foot movement to use a special switch with an electronic device. Different

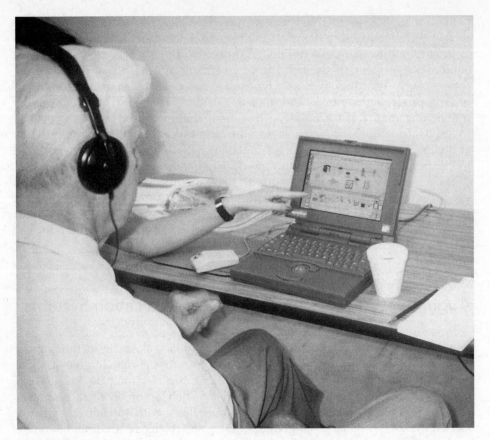

FIGURE 4.4 An adult uses a computer-based communication device to communicate recent events in his life.

devices may be needed to allow the child or adult to communicate from different positions, such as sitting in a wheelchair or lying in bed. The devices selected must be able to accompany the client and be available whenever the client needs to communicate.

The decision about how the child or adult will communicate is closely related to what information will be communicated. Communication involves a code that is passed from sender to receiver. For normal speakers, this code is oral language. For a patient who is recovering from surgery to remove the larynx, the code might be written language. For a child who cannot write, the code might be a symbol system. For a child with more limited language or cognitive abilities, pictures might be used. In selecting the code, both the client's abilities and the people he or she needs to communicate with must be considered. It makes no sense to train clients to expert levels with a symbol system, for instance, if their families, teachers, and classmates prefer not to learn this system as well.

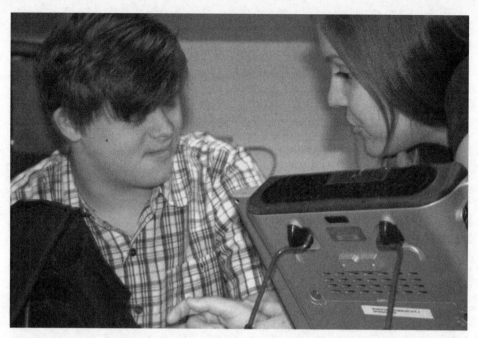

FIGURE 4.5 A teen with Down syndrome learns to use an electronic communication system.

After one or more communication systems are selected, training is vital for developing successful communication (see Figure 4.5). Training is geared toward the client's developmental level and daily needs. For a toddler, it may mean starting with toys and activities that develop turn-taking skills and communicative intent. For a school-aged child, it might include the use of language for academic purposes as well as for interpersonal communication. For the adult, the goal may be to reestablish communication that has been affected by illness or injury. Training often involves trial and error on the part of both the client and the clinician. Imagine the dilemma of the clinician who must try to adapt a communication system to meet the particular needs of the client before the client has the means of communicating those needs. And imagine the frustration of the client who must wait until the clinician figures it out!

A person with the desire and means to transmit a message is still only half of a successful communication exchange. Communication requires other people. Family members often receive direct training on how to use and maintain augmentative devices, but the client is also likely to encounter others who have never seen an augmentative device. Unfortunately, some people may not want to take the considerable time and effort involved in communicating through an alternative system. Communication is inevitably slower and is often less accurate. It can be tiring for both the sender and receiver. However, for many nonverbal individuals, the basic need to interact with other people provides the motivation and reward for the effort involved. This can clearly be seen in the case of Mr. James.

Mr. James had been a medic in the army and then became a nurse in a Veteran's Administration medical center after discharge. At age 57, he began to notice difficulty with his speech. It sounded slurred and was increasingly difficult for others to understand what he was saying. A visit to his primary care physician resulted in a neurology consultation, and ultimately it was determined that he had a progressive neurological disease called amyotrophic lateral sclerosis (ALS), or Lou Gehrig's disease. The neurologist referred Mr. James to a speech-language pathologist to help him address his declining ability to produce intelligible speech. In the context of several treatment sessions, Mr. James learned that he could improve his speech intelligibility by talking more slowly, allowing him to make necessary movements of his articulators. He also began carrying a pad of paper to write down single words or phrases to clarify his message when people could not understand him. At a two-year follow-up visit to the speech-language pathologist, it was evident that his speech was no longer a reasonable means of communication. Although his hand muscles were also weakening, they were still adequate for written communication. In order to expand Mr. James's communication options, the speech-language pathologist showed him several augmentative communication devices with synthesized speech. He liked one of the handheld devices that simply produced synthesized speech from the text that he typed with his index finger. He found this easier than handwriting, and also liked the fact that he could use the device to communicate with his wife over the phone. This device supported Mr. James's communication needs well for three years, until his hands became too weak to make good use of it. Over the course of the years that he had the disease, Mr. James became active in the local ALS support group. He and his speech-language pathologist helped other individuals to adopt strategies to maximize communication success as speech was declining. Ultimately, Mr. James succumbed to pneumonia at the end of his illness as the muscles of respiration were too weak to maintain good ventilation.

Clinical Problem Solving

Kiesha, age 6, was brought into our research lab to participate in a language study. While she was there we taped the following conversation:

Kiesha: Hey, Piget [Piglet]!

Dad: There he is. You found him. There's Piglet.

Kiesha: Shhhhh.

Dad: Oh, is it because he's sleeping?

Kiesha: Kaiet [quiet]!

Dad: Okay, I'll be quiet. Are they all asleep?

Kiesha: We da he seep [Where does he sleep]?

Dad: What are they doing?

Kiesha: Let's make 'em seep [sleep]. He's at home.

Dad: Who's this guy.

Kiesha: Gover [Grover]. And Ernie. Cookie Monser [Monster].

1. Does this speech sample indicate an articulation disorder? Would you feel the same if the child had just turned 3? (To review normal development, consult Chapter 3.)
2. Using Table 4.1, can you identify any phonological processes among the sound errors? Remember that identification of a phonological process requires evidence of a pattern that affects more than one individual sound.
3. What factors would you need to rule out as causes of these speech errors before considering therapy?
4. Which therapy approaches might you consider for remediation in this case? Which would not be appropriate? Why?

REFERENCES

American Speech-Language-Hearing Association. (1991). The role of the speech-language pathologist in management of oral myofunctional disorders. *ASHA, 33* (Suppl. 5), 7.

American Speech-Language-Hearing Association. (2004). Preferred practice patterns for the profession of speech-language pathology. Retrieved August 5, 2011, from www .asha.org/docs/html/PP2004-00191.html

Arcuri, M. R., Perlman, A. L., Philippbar, S. A., & Barkmeier, J. M. (1991). The effects of a maxillary speech-aid prosthesis for the combined tongue and mandibular resection patient. *Journal of Prosthetic Dentistry, 65*(6), 816–22.

Ballard, J. L., Christine E. Auer, C. E., & Khoury, J. C. (2002). Ankyloglossia: Assessment, incidence, and effect of frenuloplasty on the breastfeeding dyad, *Pediatrics, 110*, e63.

Barrett, R. H., & Hanson, M. L. (1978). *Oral myofunctional disorders* (2nd ed.). St. Louis, MO: Mosby.

Buryk, M., Bloom, D., & Shope, T. (2011). Efficacy of neonatal release of ankyloglossia: A randomized trial. *Pediatrics, 128*, 280–288.

Duffy, J. R. (2005). *Motor speech disorders: Substrates, differential diagnosis, and management* (2nd ed.), St. Louis, MO: Mosby-Year Book.

Dunn, C. (1982). Phonological process analysis: Contributions to assessing phonological disorders. *Communicative Disorders, 7*, 147–163.

Elbert, M., Powell, T. W., & Swartzlander, P. (1991). Toward a technology of generalization: How many exemplars are sufficient? *Journal of Speech and Hearing Research, 34*, 84–87.

Gierut, J. A., Morrisette, M. L., Hughes, M. T., & Rowland, S. (1996). Phonological treatment efficacy and developmental norms. *Language, Speech, and Hearing Services in Schools, 27*, 215–230.

Goldman, R., & Fristoe, M. (2000). *Goldman-Fristoe Test of Articulation-Second Edition*. San Antonio, TX: PsychCorp-Pearson.

Grunwell, P. (1980). Developmental language disorders at the phonological level. In F. M. Jones (Ed.), *Language disability in children*. Lancaster, PA: MTP Press.

Hall, B. J. C. (1990). Attitudes of fourth and sixth graders towards peers with mild articulation disorders. *Language, Speech, and Hearing Services in Schools, 22*, 344–340.

Handzic-Cuk, J., Cuk, V., Gluhinic, M., Risavi, R., & Stajner-Katusic, S. (2001). Tympanometric findings in cleft palate patients: Influence of age and cleft type. *Journal of Laryngology & Otology, 115*, 91–96.

Kent, R. D., Miolo, G., & Bloedel, S. (1994). The intelligibility of children's speech: A review of evaluation procedures. *American Journal of Speech-Language Pathology, 3*, 81–95.

Khan, L., & Lewis, N. (1986). *Khan-Lewis Phonological Analysis*. Circle Pines, MN: American Guidance Service.

Leonard, R. J., & Gillis, R. (1982). Effects of a prosthetic tongue on vowel intelligibility and food management in a patient with total glossectomy. *Journal of Speech & Hearing Disorders, 47*(1), 25–30.

Leonard, R. J., & Gillis, R. (1983). Effects of a prosthetic tongue on vowel formants and isovowel lines in a patient with total glossectomy (an addendum to Leonard & Gillis, 1982). *Journal of Speech & Hearing Disorders, 48*(4), 423–426.

Lewis, B. A. (1990). Familial phonological disorders: Four pedigrees. *Journal of Speech and Hearing Disorders, 55*, 160–170.

Lynch, J. I. (1990). Tongue reduction surgery: Efficacy and relevance to the profession. *ASHA, 32*, 59–61.

McReynolds, L. V. (1982). Functional articulation problems. In G. H. Shames & E. H. Wiig (Eds.), *Human communication disorders: An introduction*. Columbus, OH: Charles E. Merrill.

Messner, A. H., & Lalakea, M. L. (2002). The effect of ankyloglossia on speech in children. *Otolaryngology—Head and Neck Surgery: Official Journal of American Academy of Otolaryngology-Head and Neck Surgery, 127*(6), 539–545.

Moore, C. A., Yorkston, K. M., & Beukelman, D. R. (Eds.). (1991). *Dysarthria and apraxia of speech*. Baltimore: Paul H. Brookes.

Odding. E., Roebroeck, M. E., & Stam, H. J. (2006). The epidemiology of cerebral palsy: incidence, impairments and risk factors. *Disability and Rehabilitation, 28*(4), 183–191.

Peterson-Falzone, S. J., Hardin-Jones, M. A., & Karnell, M. P. (2001). *Cleft palate speech* (3rd ed.). St. Louis, MO: Mosby Year Book.

Prather, E., & Whaley, P. (1984). Articulation training based on coarticulation. In H. Winitz (Ed.), *Treating articulation disorders: For clinicians by clinicians*. Baltimore: University Park Press.

Ramig, L. O., Countyman, S., Thompson, L., & Horii, L. (1995). A comparison of two intensive speech treatments for Parkinson disease. *Journal of Speech and Hearing Research, 39*, 1232–1251.

Ricke, L. A., Baker, N. J., Madlon-Kay, D. J., & DeFor, T. A. (2005). Newborn tongue-tie: Prevalence and effect on breast-feeding. *Journal of the American Board of Family Practice, 18*(1), 1–7.

Ruscello, D. M. (2008). Treating articulation and phonological disorders in children. St. Louis, MO: Elsevier.

Ruscello, D. M., St. Louis, K. O., & Mason, N. (1991). School-age children with phonologic disorders: Coexistence with other speech/language disorders. *Journal of Speech and Hearing Disorders, 34*, 236–242.

Shelton, R. L., Furr, M. L., Johnson, A., & Arndt, W. B. (1975). Cephalometric and intraoral variables as they relate to articulation improvement with training. *American Journal of Orthodontics, 67*, 423–431.

Shprintzen, R. J., Siegal-Sadewitz, V. L., Amato, J., & Goldberg, R. B. (1985). Retrospective diagnosis of previously missed syndromic disorders among 1000 patients with cleft lip, cleft palate, or both. *Birth Defects, 21*, 85–92.

Shriberg, L., Austin, D., Lewis, B. A., McSweeny, J. L., & Wilson, D. L. (1997). The percentage of consonants correct (PCC) metric: Extensions and reliability data. *Journal of Speech Language and Hearing Research, 40*, 708–722.

Shriberg, L. D., & Kwiatkowski, J. (1988). A follow-up study of children with phonologic disorders of unknown origin. *Journal of Speech and Hearing Disorders, 53*, 144–155.

Shriberg, L. D., & Kwiatkowski, J. (1990). Self-monitoring and generalization in preschool speech-delayed children. *Language, Speech, and Hearing Services in Schools, 21*, 157–170.

Shriberg, L. D., Kwiatkowski, J., Best, S., Hengst, J., & Terselic-Weber, B. (1986). Characteristics of children with phonological disorders of unknown origin. *Journal of Speech and Hearing Disorders, 51*, 140–161.

Shriberg, L. D., Tomblin, J. B., & McSweeny, J. L. (1999). Prevalence of speech delay in 6-year-old children and comorbidity with language impairment. *Journal of Speech, Language, and Hearing Research, 42*, 1461–1481.

Square-Storer, P. (Ed.). (1989). *Acquired apraxia of speech in aphasic adults.* Salisbury, UK: Lawrence Erlbaum Associates.

Suter, V. G., & Bornstein, M. M. (2009). Ankyloglossia: Facts and myths in diagnosis and treatment. *Journal of Periodontology, 80*(8), 1204–19.

Wertz, R. T., LaPointe, L. L., & Rosenbek, J. C. (1984). *Apraxia of speech in adults: The disorder and its management.* Orlando, FL: Grune & Stratton.

Yorkston, K. M., Beukelman, D. R., & Bell, K. R. (1988). *Clinical management of dysarthric speakers.* Boston: College-Hill Press.

READINGS FROM THE POPULAR LITERATURE

Albom, M. (1998). *Tuesdays with Morrie.* New York: Doubleday. (amyotrophic lateral sclerosis [ALS], or Lou Gehrig's disease)

Fox, M. J. (2002). Lucky man: A memoir. New York: Hyperion. (Parkinson disease)

Gordon, S., & Tempel, L. (1992). *Parkinson's: A personal story of acceptance.* Boston: Branden. (Parkinson disease)

Graboys, T. & Zheutlin, P. (2008). Life in the balance: A physician's memoir of life, love, and loss with Parkinson's disease and dementia. Nottingham, UK: Union Square Press. (renowned cardiologist's experience with Parkinson disease and dementia)

Grady-Fitchett, J. (1998). *Flying lessons: On the wings of Parkinson's disease.* New York: Forge. (Parkinson disease)

Grealy, L. (1994). *Autobiography of a face.* New York: Harper Perennial. (facial cancer)

Handler, L. (1998). *Twitch and shout: A Touretter's tale.* New York: Dutton. (Tourette syndrome)

Hasse, J. (1996). *Break out: Finding freedom when you don't quite fit the mold.* Berea, OH: Quixote Publications. (cerebral palsy)

Kondracke, M. (2000). *Saving Milly: Love, politics and Parkinson's disease.* New York: Ballantine Books. (Parkinson disease)

McDermott, J. (2000). *Babyface: A story of heart and bones.* Bethesda, MD: Woodbine House. (Apert syndrome)

Montague, A. (1999). *Elephant man* (3rd ed.). New York: E. P. Dutton. (facial disfigurement)

Rabin, R. (1985). *Six parts love: One family's battle with Lou Gehrig's disease.* New York: Scribner. (ALS)

Reeve, C. (1997). *Still me.* New York: Random House. (spinal cord injury, ventilator dependency)

Robillard, A. B. (1999). *Meaning of a disability: The lived experience of paralysis.* Philadelphia: Temple University Press. (motor neuron disease)

Rummel-Hudson, R. (2008). *Schuyler's monster: A father's journey with his wordless daughter*. New York: St. Martin's Press. (rare brain malformation, alternative and augmentative communication device)

Sacks, O. (1973). *Awakenings*. New York: E. P. Dutton. (cases of diminished movement and communication related to Parkinsonism)

Segalman, B. (2009). *Against the current — My life with cerebral palsy*. Verona, WI: Full Court Press. (autobiography by Dr. Bob, who has two doctoral degrees, and his life with cerebral palsy. Available at www.drbobsautobiography.org)

Sienkiewicz-Mercer, R., & Kaplan, S. (1989). *I raise my eyes to say yes*. West Hartford, CT: Whole Health Books. (cerebral palsy)

Sinton, W. (2002). *I choose to live: A journey through life with ALS*. Gurnee, IL: Banbury Publishing. (ALS)

Stehli, A. (1995). *Dancing in the rain*. Westport, CT: Georgiana Organization. (stories by parents of children with special needs)

Webster, B. D. (1989). *All of a piece*. Baltimore: Johns Hopkins University Press. (multiple sclerosis)

Wexler, A. (1995). *Mapping fate*. New York: Times Books: Random House. (Huntington disease)

CHAPTER 5

Disorders of Fluency

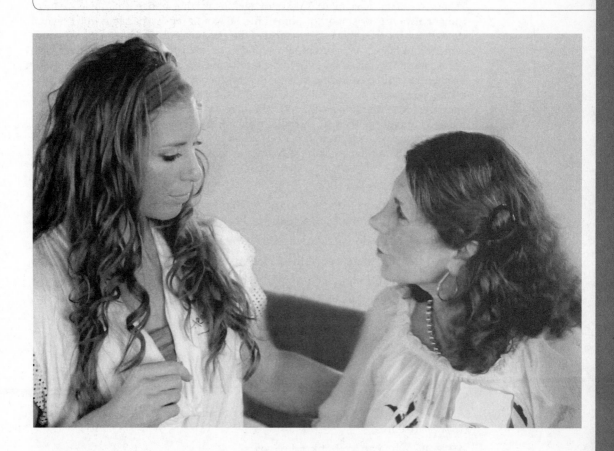

PREVIEW   The area of fluency and fluency disorders has been one of the most dynamic areas within the profession of speech-language pathology. Principal among disorders of fluency is the phenomenon of stuttering. The various definitions of stuttering reflect a wide range of perspectives that experts have brought to bear on trying to understand this disorder of communication. Developmental, familial, psychological, neurological, and motoric factors all appear to interact in cases of stuttering. Although stuttering is the most common fluency disorder, there are other disorders characterized by changes in fluency. We will briefly consider a fluency disruption called cluttering as well as cases of acquired stuttering in adults.

When Abraham[1] was about 3 years of age, his mother noticed that his sentences did not always flow smoothly. Sometimes he would repeat the same word several times before he was able to get the rest of the sentence out. There were pauses mid-sentence. In fact, at times Abraham sounded quite disfluent. This concerned both of his parents because they each had a family history of **stuttering**. The mother's brother had stuttered during most of his childhood, although he was described as completely fluent as an adult. The father's sister began stuttering as a child and continued to stutter into adulthood. Abraham's parents did not want him to struggle to communicate the way their siblings had, and they were naturally concerned when Abraham went through periods when he seemed particularly disfluent. At age 3 years, 3 months, we had the following conversation with him:

AUTHOR: What's Wishbone?

ABRAHAM: Um, he's one of the shows that I watch. He's a dog. The story of Wishbone is really . . . um, really a show.

AUTHOR: He's a dog. And he has his own show?

ABRAHAM: No, there's a . . . there's a boy in it.

AUTHOR: What do they get to do?

ABRAHAM: They do everything. But only in the show, they get to do . . . I don't know. (Abraham notices the barnyard toys and goes to them.)

AUTHOR: Let me see what's in this barn. There's a lot of animals in here.

ABRAHAM: Yeah, I . . . (Silence)

AUTHOR: All right. Well, there's a cow. And there's a baby cow. That's a . . . that's a brown cow.

ABRAHAM: No, that's a white cow. That's called . . . that's called . . . These two are cows.

AUTHOR: Oh yeah? What kind of cows?

---

[1]We follow the speech and language development of Abraham in Chapters 3 and 7.

ABRAHAM: Black ones and white ones.

AUTHOR: Black ones and white ones. And this is a dog.

ABRAHAM: This is . . . This is a dog.

AUTHOR: Do you think he's a sheep dog?

ABRAHAM: Nooo.

AUTHOR: Do you think he's a cow dog? Does he have to watch out over the cows?

ABRAHAM: (Nods in agreement)

AUTHOR: Well, I've got some hay. (Picks up a cow) Do you think he's a hay eater?

ABRAHAM: Yes he is. I'll put hay on his . . . in his . . . in his . . . in there so he can't eat anything. (Abraham puts animals in the hay loft.)

AUTHOR: Now, we have two cows in the hay.

ABRAHAM: Is this one the . . . the . . . the . . . the baby one?

AUTHOR: I don't know. It's kind of small. Maybe he is a baby one.

During this brief conversation, we were able to observe a number of interruptions in the flow of communication. These included whole word repetitions ("the . . . the . . . the . . . the baby one"), phrase repetitions ("This is . . . this is a dog"), and interjections ("um"). However, Abraham seemed completely unfazed by his disfluencies. His focus was on the toys and our play, and he was probably unaware of his own speech patterns. Notice, too, that Abraham was not the only one to show speech repetition. The author repeated part of a sentence ("That's a . . . that's a brown cow") during the conversation as well. In fact, everyone experiences a minor interruption in the flow of speech at some time or another. Differentiating between "normal" disfluencies and stuttering is an ongoing challenge to those working in the area of fluency disorders.

It is not always easy to distinguish an episode of disfluency that characterizes stuttering from an episode that is a momentary lapse of fluency. This is particularly true in the case of young children. As children are learning to put together sentences, it is very common to hear them make false starts (I . . . he did it!), revise midsentence ("He's in . . . he's on TV"), hesitate over the next word to come ("I want . . . juice") We often get the sense that these interruptions in fluency have more to do with the child's partial grasp of the language than any struggle to get the words out. Likewise, we have all heard a child so excited that word or phrase repetitions came pouring forth ("Mommy! Mommy! Mommy! Mommy! Mommy! Can I, can I, can I have one?!"). For most children, these episodes reflect normal development, rather than the onset of stuttering. In fact, for Abraham, this proved to be the case. As he continued to develop speech and language skills, the episodes of disfluency decreased. By 4½ years, no one, including his parents, had any concerns about his speech fluency.

All speakers have some disruptions of speech fluency, which include word and phrase repetitions, hesitations, and interjections.

Stuttering refers to abnormal disruptions in speech fluency that include sound repetitions, prolongations, or blocks, and may include some associated nonspeech behaviors, such as blinking or grimacing.

Normal Disfluencies versus Stuttering

Conture (1990) noted that deciding who is and who is not stuttering is a relative rather than an absolute decision, in that there is no behavior that children who stutter display that normal children never exhibit. Although normally developing children (and adults on occasion) sometimes experience breakdowns in these speech parameters, the child who stutters exhibits those behaviors to a greater degree. For example, normal children such as Abraham may repeat words or phrases at the age of 3. However, by the age of 4½, children usually repeat utterances only when they wish to emphasize something (Curlee, 1980).

Early Signs of Stuttering

Although no method is foolproof for identifying the young child who will persist in stuttering, a number of behavioral signs are considered to be "red flags" (see Table 5.1). In true developmental stuttering, speech is characterized by changes in duration, rate, and rhythm, with frequent interruptions of fluency from sound to sound and from word to word. One distinction that has been suggested involves the unit of speech in which the disfluency occurs (Andrews et al., 1983; Wall, 1988). Normal disfluencies typically occur on whole words, phrases, or sentences; stuttering is more likely to affect single sounds and syllables. A child showing normal disfluency may say, "I want . . . I want it," whereas a child who stutters may say, "I wwwwwwant it." The frequency of disfluent episodes is also different for children with normal disfluencies than for those who stutter. Wingate (1962) found that nonstuttering children

TABLE 5.1   Signs Often Associated with Normal and Stuttered Speech

Normal Disfluencies	
Word repetitions	I like that . . . that book.
Phrase repetitions	I want a . . . want a big one!
Sentence repetitions	Watch me! Watch me! Watch me!
Hesitations	He took . . . my juice.
Interjections	We, um, got to go too.
Stuttering	
Syllable repetitions	We saw a vi-vi-vi-video.
Sound repetition	I g-g-g-got it from school.
Sound prolongations	Wwwwwwait for mmmme.
Sound blocks	[starts word but no sound comes out]
Nonspeech behaviors	[e.g., blinks, facial tension, limb movement]

seldom make repetitions for more than 3 percent of their total speech utterances; children who stutter were found to have a frequency of syllable disfluencies ranging from 7 to 14 percent.

The signs of stuttering are not restricted to interruptions of speech. Conture and Kelly (1991) reported that young children who stutter could be differentiated from nonstuttering children by the types of facial behaviors they exhibit. For example, children who stutter were likely to look away, blink their eyes, raise their upper lip, or press their lips together during periods of disfluency, whereas their fluent peers showed these behaviors less frequently. Stuttering children may show signs of struggle or tension while attempting to speak, whereas children with normal disfluencies typically seem unaffected by the disfluent episode.

Several investigators (Schwartz, Zebrowski, & Conture, 1990; Yairi & Ambrose, 1992) have examined the earliest signs of stuttering by studying the behaviors of young children whose parents reported stuttering of a recent onset (within the previous twelve months). Yairi and Ambrose (1992) interviewed parents concerning the age of their children and the characteristics of their disfluent speech when stuttering began. Parents reported that their children were sometimes quite young, between the ages of 20 months to 5 years of age, when stuttering was first observed. Just under half of the parents reported that their children began to stutter suddenly, whereas other parents remembered the onset as evolving gradually over the course of several weeks. Schwartz and colleagues (1990) recorded the speech of such children on videotape to assess the behaviors associated with the earliest stages of stuttering. The investigators reported that the disfluencies of these children included many sound prolongations (33 to 60 percent of all disfluent episodes). The children also exhibited frequent nonspeech behaviors, such as eye movements or eye closings during disfluent episodes. Somewhat surprisingly, the stuttering behaviors of children who were at the younger end of the age range did not differ remarkably from those at the older end. Although prolongations were somewhat more frequent for children who had been stuttering longer, the authors emphasized that there were more similarities than differences among the behaviors of children at different ages.

The signs that suggest the onset of stuttering, as opposed to developmental disfluencies, can vary between children and even within a single child. However, we have seen that there are some early indications that a child is struggling with more than just the normal disruptions of fluency that all children experience. These signs can be seen in the case of a young boy who was brought to the clinic for a fluency evaluation.

Jackson was 6 years old when he was first seen in the clinic. His mother brought him in because "he stutters." She reported that he had started stuttering two years before, but she had always assumed that he would grow out of it. Now that Jackson was in school, she was concerned that other children were teasing him. She had already noticed that Jackson seemed aware that his speech was different from other children. She reported that he sometimes got frustrated when trying to talk. As far as she knew, no one in her family had ever stuttered, and she couldn't recall anyone having had any kind of developmental problems.

When we talked with Jackson, it was apparent that his speech showed more than the typical amount of disfluency. In fact, sometimes it seemed as if he could hardly get his thoughts out. His speech was frequently disrupted by sound prolongations and blocks, when no sound came out at all. During these episodes, his mouth seemed to lock into a tense position from which he was unable to break free. His brows knit together, and sometimes he would blink or contort his face until the disfluent period passed and speech resumed its normal flow. When asked why his mother brought him to the clinic, he replied, "I-i-i-t's . . . because I t-t-t-t-t . . . alk . . . I can't talk."

In contrast to his disfluency, a formal assessment of Jackson's language showed average to above average skills. When he was not stuttering, he did not show problems with speech articulation. An examination of his oral mechanism (see Chapter 4) revealed normal structure, muscle tone, and nonspeech movements. Likewise, he could repeat nonsense words and say entire sentences in a fluent, sing-song cadence, which indicated he possessed the physical mechanisms to support normal speech.

Persistent Stuttering

A majority of children who show early disfluencies will eventually develop fluent speech. However, some children will not. Yairi and colleagues reported that children destined to recover from early stuttering-like behaviors may initially show more disfluencies than children who continue to be disfluent. However, the children who recover typically show reductions in the number of disfluencies within the first year after their stuttering-like disfluencies began. In contrast, children who failed to recover were relatively stable in their rate of disfluency (Yairi, Ambrose, Paden, & Throneburg, 1996). Although there is a chance that some of these children will recover still later in childhood, they are at risk for struggling with fluency throughout their lives. Let us look at the case of one such man:

> *Mr. Andrews*, age 32, has stuttered since childhood. Although he had received therapy several times, he continued to show a variety of stuttering signs. His stuttering consisted primarily of silent blocks, during which his mouth and face contorted as he struggled to speak. Occasionally, he also experienced part-word repetitions, in which the first sound of a word was repeated over and over. He had recently contacted the clinic because he thought that his stuttering was preventing him from advancing in his career. He expressed, "T———eam work is very important in my c-c-c-c-ompany, and I knnnnnnnnow that the others would rather not have me on the team b———cause of my stuttering. When I present m——y ideas, they d———on't take them as ssssseriously." He reported that he was able to speak fluently "most of the time" after his last experience with therapy in high school. However, to maintain fluency, Mr. Andrews felt he had to concentrate harder on how he was speaking than on what he was actually trying to say. Over time, his disfluency had slipped back to pretherapy levels. He was willing to try again to reduce his stuttering severity.

Adults who stutter may show some of the same characteristics seen in childhood stuttering. They may continue to produce sound repetitions and prolongations, along with silent interruptions, called blocks, in the flow of speech. "Secondary" characteristics of stuttering, which may have been present during childhood, may be more pronounced. These characteristics include facial tension, facial contortions, and extraneous movements during the stuttering episode. In addition, these adults typically have had years of frustration about being unable to communicate ideas with the ease that comes naturally to others. This frustration can become as problematic as the actual episodes of fluency breakdown.

It is not uncommon for nonstuttering individuals to stereotype those who stutter as having a variety of negative traits, including being anxious, tense, insecure, or nervous (Kalinowshi, Lerman, & Watt, 1987). Indeed, several studies have examined physiological correlates of stress and found evidence of increased levels of stress and anxiety among those who stutter (Blood, Blood, Bennet, Simpson, & Susman, 1994; Weber & Smith, 1990). An alternate explanation is that stuttering stress and anxiety are a consequence of repeated negative experiences with communication. Several studies suggest that this is the case. For example, Miller and Watson (1992) reported that their subjects who stuttered were no more anxious overall than nonstuttering subjects. However, the two groups differed in terms of their attitudes toward communication, with attitudes worsening with increased stuttering severity. Craig (1990) showed that, prior to treatment for stuttering, adults who stutter were significantly more anxious during a communication task than control subjects. After their level of disfluency was decreased through treatment of stuttering behaviors, their anxiety was reduced to a level characteristic of nonstuttering adults. Such findings have led to a shift in clinician perceptions concerning the role of personality traits such as anxiety or other negative affective states (Cooper & Cooper, 1996).

One of the more puzzling features of persistent stuttering is that speech can be completely fluent under certain speaking circumstances. Let us consider the following case:

> *Mr. Tirai*, age 27, was a graduate student who had come to this country to study engineering three years earlier. Although he spoke two other languages with native proficiency, he had only rudimentary English at that time. He spent his first academic year in the United States studying primarily for his English language proficiency exam. He needed to pass this exam to continue his program in engineering. An outgoing man, he also spent his time going to campus and community cultural events, through which he developed a number of American friends. Through his determined study, his circle of English-speaking friends, and a measure of talent for learning languages, he steadily gained proficiency in English. Other than his accent, his English seemed largely unremarkable. He had long since acquired the common grammatical forms of English. His vocabulary had grown to a point where he rarely needed to search for words in conversation. However, in his final years of study, he was beginning to show occasional episodes of stuttering-like disfluencies. Although "stuttering" was not a word he had acquired in English, he managed to convey that he had escaped from stuttering by speaking English, but that it appeared to have caught up with him just as he was feeling comfortable with his new language.

Mr. Tirai was fluent for an extended period of time while he was learning English. Others have discovered they can induce short-term fluency by adopting foreign accents or imitating voices. Fluency may be achieved under conditions of **delayed auditory feedback**. This involves use of instrumentation that presents the speaker's own voice, through headphones, at a slight time delay. So, as the speaker is talking, what he or she hears lags behind what is currently being said. Choral reading or speaking, during which people speak in concert, also tends to promote fluency. Likewise, intentional changes in the rhythm of speech, such as in chanting or singing, will produce fluency. All of these speaking conditions, from learning a foreign language to chanting, involve a change from the normal pattern of speech production. It appears that such changes may "override" whatever mechanisms may lead to disfluent episodes in regular speech. Unfortunately, as Mr. Tirai found, when speakers grow proficient with these "unusual" speaking conditions, stuttering may reappear.

> Singing is one of several conditions that tends to reduce or eliminate stuttering.

Stuttering in the Population

The **prevalence** of a disorder is the number of people in the population who have a particular problem at any given time. There have been several prevalence studies of stuttering over the years. The National Institute of Deafness and Other Communication Disorders (NIDCD; 2010) of the National Institutes of Health (NIH) estimated that approximately 3 million Americans stutter. This corresponds to a prevalence of approximately 1 percent of the United States population, but the percentage of people who stutter varies across the lifespan. Morley (1972) followed approximately 1,000 children in Newcastle-Upon-Tyne for fifteen years to examine various aspects of development. In this particular study, the **incidence** of stuttering, or the number of new cases identified during a period of time, was about 4 percent, or 1 in 25 children. NIDCD estimates that 1 in 30 children will go through a period of disfluency that lasts a minimum of six months.

> The incidence and prevalence statistics for stuttering confirm that many individuals recover from stuttering.

Stuttering is typically first identified before the age of 5 and many times resolves to normal fluency before puberty (Morley, 1972; Wingate, 1976). Wingate (1976) summarized fourteen studies and concluded that approximately 80 percent of children recover from stuttering. Although there has been some dispute about the exact number, it appears that for the majority of children who stutter at an early age, stuttering will disappear before they graduate from high school. Curlee (1980) came to the following conclusion: "if the incidence of stuttering among the general population does approximate 4 percent, a recovery rate of 80 percent would account for a 0.7 percent prevalence of stuttering" (p. 281).

In some respects, stuttering is an "equal opportunity" disorder. It affects people of all racial and socioeconomic backgrounds. However, it does appear that some individuals are at higher risk than others for developing the disorder. Stuttering affects more boys than girls (Hull et al., 1976; Morley, 1972; Yairi & Ambrose, 1992). NIDCD (2011) estimated that boys are three times more likely to stutter than girls. The male-to-female ratio tends to increase at older ages, which has led some to suggest that girls may show higher rates of recovery with age than boys (Yairi, Ambrose, & Cox, 1996).

In addition to the higher rate of stuttering for males than females, a family history of stuttering increases an individual's risk for the disorder. Although the population prevalence for stuttering is thought to hover around 1 percent, the prevalence among the relatives of an individual who stutters is much higher (Andrews & Harris, 1964; Howie, 1981; Kidd, 1980; Yairi & Ambrose, 1992; Yairi, Ambrose, & Cox, 1996). Yairi and Ambrose (1992) reported that almost half (46.6 percent) of their sample of young children who stutter had parents or siblings who also stuttered at one time. If blood relatives in the extended family were considered, two-thirds (66.3 percent) of the children had a positive family history for stuttering. The pattern of family aggregation for stuttering may signal the presence of a single major gene that contributes to expression of the disorder (Yairi et al., 1996). Additional support for the genetic basis of stuttering comes from recent research that demonstrated a specific genetic mutation associated with stuttering (Kang et al., 2010). However, the actual components that contribute to the development of stuttering may be more complex. Some have suggested that genetic factors may confer a risk for stuttering, but that certain environmental factors are needed to trigger the disorder (Andrews et al., 1983; Howie, 1981).

> It is not uncommon for stuttering to run in families, which is consistent with a genetic basis for stuttering.

Family history for stuttering may account for some of the variability seen among individuals who stutter. Janssen, Kraaimaat, and Brutten (1990) examined a variety of traits in subjects who stuttered with reference to family history for stuttering. One group had a positive family history for stuttering; the other did not. Those with relatives who stuttered had more sound prolongations and silent blocks in their speech. They also showed differences on measures of duration and variability in the acoustic stream from those without a positive family history. In contrast, the two stuttering groups did not differ on measures of reading, autonomic nervous system response, or responsiveness to therapy. Janssen and colleagues (1990) suggested that these results indicate that familial or genetic contributions to stuttering may have a greater impact on the motoric aspects of stuttering than on other associated features of the disorder.

Definitions of Stuttering

Definitions of stuttering are many and varied. Let us consider a few of the definitions that have appeared in the literature over the years.

1955, Johnson: "Stuttering is an anticipatory, apprehensive, hypertonic avoidance reaction" (p. 23). According to Johnson, stuttering is what speakers do when they expect stuttering to occur: dread it, tense in anticipation of it, and attempt to avoid doing it.

1977, World Health Organization: Stuttering includes "disorders in the rhythm of speech, in which the individual knows precisely what he wishes to say, but at the time is unable to say it because of an involuntary, repetitive prolongation or cessation of sound" (p. 227).

1978, Wingate: "Stuttering is characterized by audible or silent elemental repetitions and prolongations. These features reflect a temporary inability to move forward to the following sound" (p. 249).

1980, Perkins: "Stuttering is the abnormal timing of speech sound initiation."

1987, Speech Foundation of America: Stuttering is defined as "a communication disorder characterized by excessive involuntary disruptions or blockings in the flow of speech, particularly when such disruptions consist of repetitions or prolongations of a sound or syllable, and when they are accompanied by avoidance struggle behavior" (p. 183).

1991, Perkins, Kent, and Curlee: "Stuttering is a disruption of speech experienced by the speaker as a loss of control" (p. 734). They differentiate stuttering from nonstuttered forms of disfluencies by identifying the latter as "abnormal as well as normal sounding disfluency not experienced as loss of control" (p. 734).

1995, Cooper and Cooper: "Stuttering . . . is a clinical syndrome characterized by abnormal and persistent disfluencies in speech accompanied by characteristic affective, behavioral, and cognitive patterns" (p. 126).

2010, National Institute on Deafness and Other Communication Disorders: Stuttering is a speech disorder in which sounds, syllables, or words are repeated or prolonged, disrupting the normal flow of speech.

There is no one definition of stuttering that is uniformly accepted by experts in the field. The differences among these and other definitions available in the literature reflect the fact that stuttering is a complex disorder that is not simply characterized. These definitions highlight the differences in perspective among stuttering experts. Several of the definitions are limited to the description of stuttering behaviors (e.g., prolongations, repetitions) from a listener-based perspective. Three include the perspective of the individual who stutters by including his or her perception of it (i.e., loss of control) or reaction to it (e.g., apprehension, avoidance). The interpretation that disfluent episodes are involuntary in nature further reflects the perception of the person who stutters. A few definitions make inferences concerning the underlying cause of the disorder (e.g., psychological reaction to disfluency, timing disruptions). In all, the definitions reflect the changing trends within the field that have emphasized aspects of the disorder at different times.

Consider how the components of these various definitions might apply to a particular case.

Laura's parents report that she has stuttered since she was 3 years old. At the time of her speech evaluation at age 7, she was found to repeat the first sounds and syllables of many words at the beginning of a phrase or sentence. At times, she seemed to posture her mouth and blink, and no sound could be heard. She made

> no attempt to avoid talking and had moments of normal fluency; suddenly the fluency would end, seemingly without warning. During her stuttering, she would often purse her lips, close her eyes, and appear as if she were trying to push out the word she was attempting to say. Laura's parents reported that she has expressed frustration at times over her inability to speak fluently.

In this brief case description, we recognize some of the common components of many definitions of stuttering:

- Repetition and prolongation of sounds and syllables
- Sudden or involuntary fluency interruptions
- Often accompanied by physical signs of struggle
- Often perceived negatively by the speaker

Therefore, despite the differences in definitions of stuttering, it is possible to observe the various components that these definitions present within a single case.

Theories of Stuttering

There is probably no clinical area in speech-language pathology that has generated more controversy than our understanding of the cause and nature of stuttering. The number of causative theories is astonishing and reflects an evolution in thought over the last century. At any given time, one theoretical position becomes more popular as research advances and changing social mores shift the clinical perspective on this disorder. As Van Riper indicated in 1971, the pendulum of popular and clinical opinion tends to swing between physical and psychological causes. Despite these shifts in theoretical perspective over the years, we will clearly see the impact of these various theories reflected in approaches to intervention later in this chapter. Let us consider a few of the more prominent theoretical positions that have appeared over time.

Wendell Johnson is considered one of the founding fathers of the field of speech-language pathology. He spent his professional life studying the onset of stuttering. He concluded that the normal disfluencies experienced by many children were often labeled by their parents and other listeners as stuttering (Johnson, 1959). His **diagnosogenic theory of stuttering** was built on the belief that stuttering begins when normal disfluencies are labeled as stuttering. This theory recognized that normal children often pass through a period of nonfluent speech as they are in the process of language acquisition. Parents may hear their young children's normal episodes of disfluent speech and react negatively to them. They may call attention to their children's speech by telling them to "slow down" or to "take a deep breath and start over." Johnson suggested that these children are sensitive to their parents' reactions and become nervous or self-conscious about their speech. This leads them to become more disfluent in response, until stuttering becomes a learned behavior. Although there has never been any direct evidence in support of Johnson's theory, we continue to see its influence today. For example, some approaches to stuttering therapy involves indirect treatment methods that avoid calling attention to the stuttering behaviors themselves.

Johnson was also concerned with the psychological effects of disfluent speech. He believed the fear of stuttering could eventually become as great a problem as the actual stuttering episodes. As we saw earlier in this chapter, those who stutter can show physical signs of stress and anxiety (Blood et al., 1994; Weber & Smith, 1990) and may report higher levels of anxiety about possible speaking situations (Blood, Blood, Tellis, & Gabel, 2001). Signs of anxiety associated with speaking led to the idea that stuttering might be a manifestation of an underlying emotional conflict (Blanton, 1965; Glauber, 1958; Travis, 1971). In the mid-twentieth century, some recommended psychotherapy with the goal of uncovering hidden or repressed feelings that were thought to be at the root of stuttering. Today most speech-language pathologists reject the idea that stuttering is caused by a psychological disturbance. However, in some cases, sustained stuttering may cause significant psychological stress. Therapy approaches that include a component designed to address anxiety associated with stuttering episodes can produce long-term reductions in negative psychological consequences of stuttering (Blomgren, Roy, Callister, & Merrill, 2005). Likewise, many individuals derive benefit from participation in social support groups for persons who stutter (Yaruss et al., 2002).

In contrast to psychological explanations, some theories have proposed that stuttering has its roots in a form of neurological dysfunction. One early neurological theory was made popular by Orton in the 1920s. He proposed that a disturbance in the normal pattern of hemispheric specialization might account for disorders including stuttering (and also dyslexia). Early studies designed to examine cerebral functioning failed to identify any gross neurological deficit or robust differences between those who stutter and those who do not (see Andrews et al., 1983). However, advances in the techniques available to study brain structure and function have led to evidence of altered patterns of brain activation in adults who stutter. This includes overactivation in regions of the right hemisphere, typically the nondominant hemisphere for speech (e.g., De Nil, Kroll, Lafaille, & Houle, 2003; Fox, Ingham, Ingham, et al., 1996: Neumann et al., 2003). Furthermore, these anomalous patterns of activation may shift after successful participation in stuttering treatment (De Nil et al., 2003; Neumann et al., 2003), suggesting that altered speech is accompanied by altered patterns of brain activation in those who stutter. A neurological basis for stuttering was also supported by another line of research that demonstrated abnormal white matter connections in the left frontal lobe of individuals who stutter (Chang et al., 2011).

To date, the neurological findings for stuttering do not explain why the speech of those who stutter is sometimes fluent and sometimes disfluent, even within the same conversation. Perkins and colleagues (1991) attempted to address this enigma by proposing that stuttering occurs as the consequence of dysynchrony among any of the neural systems that support communication, including phonology and language, in addition to the control of speech movements. There is support for the idea that the linguistic aspects of speech do indeed affect the occurrence of stuttering. Stuttering is often first reported at an age when children are starting to formulate complete sentences. When young children first begin to stutter, they rarely do so on single-word utterances and often do at the beginning of sentences, clauses, and phrases (Bloodstein, 2006). In addition, young children are more likely to stutter on utterances that are relatively long compared to what they typically produce (Zackheim & Conture, 2003). These patterns suggest that individuals who stutter may have difficulty coordinating speech movements when language formulation is also demanding. This idea is supported by the finding that the conversational language of young children who stuttered was more advanced than expected during pretreatment language testing. Their posttreatment speech was both more fluent and closer to the language level expected for their age (Bonelli et al., 2000). However, not all studies show this same pattern. Several have indicated that language skills of children are unchanged by success in treatment (see Lattermann, Shenker, & Thordardottir, 2005, for a review).

Aspects of language are known to influence stuttering in adults. Adults are more likely to stutter on content words (i.e., nouns and verbs) and long words than on words that serve grammatical function (e.g., articles). This may reflect subtle problems in the ability to rapidly access specific word forms while the overall message is being formulated. Support for this idea comes from Prins, Main, and Wampler (1997), who showed an effect for one's speed at naming pictures that reflected the frequency with which words appear in the language. When words are relatively infrequent, and therefore less familiar, it took longer to retrieve the name. This effect was magnified for individuals who stutter. Furthermore, disfluencies are more likely to occur on low-frequency words than on high-frequency words (Dayalu, Kalinowski, Stuart, Holbert, & Rastatter, 2002), further reinforcing the idea that subtle difficulty with word retrieval may provoke stuttering episodes. Similarly, adults have shown a reduction in speech articulation rate following treatment to enhance fluency (Andrews et al., 1983), suggesting that initial faster articulation rates were taxing the speech production system sufficiently to result in stuttering.

> The linguistic demands on a speaker who stutters can affect whether a stuttering episode occurs.

Whether these interactions between language and stuttering reflect a dysynchrony between the neural systems that support speech and language is unknown. An alternate explanation is that speakers who are operating at the edge of their capacity for fluent speech may become disfluent when the demands for the speaking task exceed their capacity for producing the motor patterns for speech (Venkatagiri, 2005). Under this explanation, stuttering interacts with language, not because of mistakes in the coordination of the neural systems, but because use of more difficult language forms (e.g., complex sentences, less common vocabulary) is sufficiently demanding that language formulation interferes with automatic speech production. In contrast, speaking more slowly than usual, speaking in concert with other speakers, or singing forces the speaker to use a more deliberate rather than automatic means of programming speech, thus enhancing fluency. Therapy approaches that seek to reduce the demands on the speaker, so that his or her capacity for fluent speech is not exceeded, are consistent with this idea (e.g., Adams, 1990; Franken, Kielstra-Van der Schalk, & Bolens, 2005).

Evaluation of Developmental Stuttering

The broad goals of a fluency evaluation are to determine whether clinically significant disfluencies are present, to understand (to the extent possible) the nature and potential cause of these disfluencies, and to understand the impact of these disfluencies within the context of the client's life. As we have discussed throughout the chapter, everyone experiences disfluent speech from time to time, and many young children typically pass through a period of normal disfluency as they acquire language skills. One of the first jobs of the clinician is to assess the likelihood that the child's disfluencies fall outside the range of normal. Typically, the clinician will consider the types of disfluencies observed, their frequency and duration, associated nonspeech behaviors (e.g., struggle, avoidance), and the child's (or parents') attitudes toward the disfluent episodes. The clinician may need to assess fluency in more than one context, because stuttering severity can change remarkably depending on the situation. School-based clinicians, for example, may observe a child in the classroom or out on the playground or even request a recorded speech sample from home. Different task demands, such as making a phone call or providing an explanation, often alter the frequency of disfluent speech as well.

As we will see later in this chapter, there are other forms of disfluent speech besides stuttering. Disorders such as cluttering can produce disruptions in fluency that are qualitatively different from stuttering. The clinician must also differentiate between stuttering and the breakdowns in fluency that result from an expressive language disorder. A sudden disruption of fluency, particularly in later childhood or adulthood, may be the first sign of a neurological disorder, which would prompt referral to a neurologist. Formal and informal measures of speech and language, as well as a detailed case history, are invaluable in distinguishing among disorders that affect fluency. Failure to do so can lead to inappropriate treatment choices.

> There are many well-known individuals in politics, entertainment, and sports who have a history of stuttering, some of whom show little evidence of speaking difficulty today.

Finally, the perceptions and attitudes of individuals who stutter can have an enormous impact on the degree to which their lives are altered by stuttering and their readiness or motivation for change. Gaining this information is an ongoing process that starts with an initial interview and continues over the course of intervention. Clients and families may have very specific intervention goals ("I need to be able to conduct interviews for my job") or completely unrealistic ones ("I want my child to stop repeating himself all the time when he's excited"). A client's internal anxiety or lack of confidence about speaking may interfere with his or her ability to benefit from speech modifications. Unless we know what these attitudes and perceptions are, subsequent intervention may be fruitless or even offensive to the client.

Stuttering Therapy

Stuttering can be successfully treated. There are numerous reports in the literature that show that people who stutter can develop and maintain fluency over time (e.g., Blood, Blood, Tellis, & Gabel, 2001; Hasbrouck, 1992; Hewat, Onslow, Packman, & O'Brian, 2006; Onslow, Costa, Andrews, Harrison, & Packman, 1996; Packman, Onslow, & van Doorn, 1994). The primary questions regarding intervention are who should receive treatment, when it should begin, and what form it should take. For adults, the decision to seek treatment is a personal one. For children, a number of factors may influence parents' decisions to initiate treatment. Because many children who show early signs of stuttering will overcome this difficulty, some professionals have advocated vigilant waiting, with parent counseling and regular monitoring of the child's speech (Zebrowski, 1995). In contrast, Starkweather (1990) noted a growing emphasis on early intervention for stuttering. He also noted that a wait-and-see attitude is more risky than the cost of treatment for a child who would have recovered later on his or her own. In addition, he reported that recovery rates with treatment routinely exceed the rate of spontaneous recovery. Finally, there is some evidence to suggest that waiting to initiate treatment for the child who stutters is associated with more time in treatment. All these factors support the trend toward early intervention for children who show early signs of stuttering.

Parental Involvement

There are a number of components of fluency therapy. For children, one critical component may be parent and family attitudes. Family involvement in the therapy process may be key to its success (e.g., Healy, Scott, & Ellis, 1995; Rustin & Cook, 1995). Kelly (1995) noted that mothers and fathers often differ in terms of how they interact with their children and may require different advice and guidance in order to best improve their child's fluency. We can see the need to understand the parents' perspectives in the following case:

> *Gerry* and *Anna* had very different reactions to their 4-year-old son's periods of disfluency. Anna told of her anxiety whenever Gerry Jr. would stutter: "It hurts me to see him struggle. I don't want other kids teasing him, either." She went out of her way to "not call his attention to it." As a result, she would allow her son to interrupt her conversations with others, and she often intervened when she thought his brothers and sisters might upset him and cause him to stutter. Gerry Sr. interpreted his wife's actions as "spoiling the boy." He didn't see his son's disfluencies as a problem. If anything, he thought that stuttering was one way that Gerry Jr. could get more attention in a household that included four other children. Needless to

say, these differences in how each parent reacted to Gerry Jr.'s disfluencies were a source of friction between them. It was apparent that intervention would have to include the parents' reactions to their child's disfluencies. This began with discussions to help the parents differentiate between the actual disfluent episodes and their reactions to it. The parents were provided with weekly "homework assignments" designed to help them develop workable and appropriate means of responding to specific situations that were problematic from either a fluency or a social-interaction perspective (e.g., should Gerry Jr. be allowed to interrupt at will?). For these parents, this approach allowed them to develop new perspectives on their son's disfluencies.

Parents may have many roles in the intervention process. They are often the first ones to seek help on behalf of their children and should be involved in setting long- and short-term goals for their child. As we saw in Gerry's case, parents may hold a range of attitudes and beliefs about stuttering. They may need information about what changes they can reasonably expect from therapy (Healey et al., 1995). They can also become invaluable assets in the intervention process. A number of therapy methods involve training parents to promote fluency in the child as the primary means of intervention (e.g., Jones, Onslow, Harrison, & Packman, 2000; Stephenson-Opsal & Bernstein Ratner, 1988; Yarus, Coleman, & Hammer, 2006). Parents may also be asked to reinforce treatment goals outside of therapy. Some intervention programs have used parents as the primary service provider with success (e.g., Craig et al., 1996; Franken et al., 2005).

Treatment Approaches

Therapy approaches can be conceptualized as one of two types: indirect or direct. Indirect therapy methods are those that attempt to bring about fluent speech without direct instruction on how the person should modify his or her own speech. Indirect therapy may be selected because of the belief that calling attention to stuttering episodes only serves to raise the anxiety of the individual who stutters and may worsen stuttering as a consequence. This idea has its roots in Johnson's diagnosogenic theory, discussed earlier. Indirect therapy approaches may also be preferred with young children, who may not have the skills to think about how they are speaking as a separate phenomenon from what they are speaking about. Therefore, it may be difficult for young children to monitor or modify their own speech. Direct therapy approaches train specific techniques to modify or eliminate stuttering. These techniques require individuals to focus on how they are speaking as well as what they are speaking about.

Indirect Methods

Indirect treatment methods have taken several forms over time. In some cases, a clinician may work to reduce the person's anxiety about stuttering without addressing the stuttering directly. For children, the clinician may advise the parents concerning changes they can make to increase fluency in their child.

For example, parents can enhance fluency by slowing their own speaking rate in conversation with their child (Stephenson-Opsal & Bernstein-Ratner, 1988). Other indirect methods may call attention to the stuttering without offering explicit guidance in how to correct stuttering behaviors. One such example uses a time-out after a disfluent episode (e.g., Hewat et al., 2006; James, 1981; Martin, Kuhl, & Haroldson, 1972; Onslow, Packman, Stocker, van Doorn, & Siegel, 1997; Prins & Hubbard, 1988). For example, when the individual stutters, he or she may immediately hear a tone (James, 1981) or some other signal (e.g., Martin et al., 1972) that requires the client to stop speaking. The time-out may even be self-administered by the client (Hewat et al., 2006; James, 1983). Why these time-out episodes are effective in reducing stuttering is unknown. However, they appear to reduce stuttering frequency in both children and adults.

One of the best-studied forms of indirect therapy is the Lidcombe Program (e.g., Bonelli, Dixon, Bernstein Ratner, & Onslow, 2000; Franken et al., 2005; Harris, Onslow, Packman, Harrison, & Menzies, 2002; Harrison, Onslow, & Menzies, 2004; Lattermann et al., 2005). This is a parent-delivered therapy program for children who stutter. Parents are trained to explicitly acknowledge or even praise the fluent speech of their child. In addition, parents call attention to disfluent speech by acknowledging its occurrence and asking the child to repeat his or her message fluently. Other than verbally differentiating between fluent and disfluent speech, no explicit instruction is used to teach the child how to produce stutter-free speech. Despite the fact that this program requires parents to explicitly draw attention to their child's stuttering, children seem to tolerate the program without ill psychological effects (Woods, Shearsby, Onslow, & Burnham, 2002). The treatment reduces stuttering in children during the treatment period (Harris et al., 2002), and the improved fluency persists after treatment has ended (Lincoln & Onslow, 1997).

A final class of indirect methods includes devices that are known to produce fluency. These devices involve earpieces that cause the person who stutters to hear his or her own speech in some altered fashion (Armson, Kiefte, Mason, & Croos, 2006; Howell, El-Yaniv, & Powell, 1987; Kalinowski, Armson, Roland-Mieszkowski, Stuart, & Gracco, 1993). Commercially available devices resemble a hearing aid that is worn in the ear canal or behind the ear. One class of devices presents the speaker's voice with a short time delay. The effect of this is that the speaker hears his or her own words just after they are produced. This effect, called **delayed auditory feedback**, is known to produce fluent speech, at least temporarily, in people who stutter. Other devices present speech that is altered in terms of its frequency or tone or that masks the speaker's voice with noise. These devices may be used as the sole method of intervention or in conjunction with instruction to the client on how to modify speech (a combination of indirect and direct therapy methods). The devices may enhance fluency for some individuals, but not all clients derive the same degree of benefit (Armson et al., 2006). There are various reasons why these devices may provide at least temporary relief from stuttering. It is well known that those who stutter can become temporarily fluent when singing, talking in unison with others (choral speech), talking to the

Both direct and indirect treatment methods have been shown to improve fluency in individuals who stutter.

beat of a metronome, talking with a sing-song cadence, and the like. It may be that altered auditory feedback causes speakers to adopt slower speech or speech that is otherwise altered from their normal pattern. In addition, speaking in the presence of altered auditory stimuli may cause the speaker to use more deliberate speaking methods that enhance fluency (see Venkatagirir, 2005). One concern is whether the effect of these devices on fluency will be maintained as those who use them become accustomed to their influence.

Direct Methods

Direct therapy methods involve direct instruction to the client concerning speech production. Direct therapy methods can be divided into two basic approaches: those that modify stuttering to help the client stutter more fluently and those that modify speech to eliminate stuttering completely.

Modifying Stuttering.   Charles Van Riper, an early contributor to study and treatment of stuttering, concluded, "the stutterer already knows how to be fluent. What he doesn't know is how to stutter. He can be taught to stutter so easily and briefly that he can have very adequate communication skills. Moreover, when he discovers he can stutter without struggle or avoidance, most of his frustration and negative emotions will subside" (1990, p. 318). This statement implies that the primary goal of treatment is better communication skills; reduction of stuttering episodes is a secondary consideration. The philosophy behind stuttering modification approaches is that "the root of stuttering is in the struggle to be fluent" (Perkins, 1980).

Consequently, therapy to modify stuttering often involves two components. The first involves improving the client's attitude toward speaking, so that the client is not apprehensive about the possibility of stuttering, and the actual stuttering episodes are no longer associated with anxiety. The second involves learning to stutter with less effort and fewer secondary stuttering behaviors, such as tension or avoidance behaviors. Techniques used by clients may involve intentionally extending the number of part-word repetitions produced on a stuttered word so that the client gains control over his behavior. Clients may be taught to cease a word attempt when their speech is blocked (known as "cancellation") or to ease out of blocked sounds by using intentional prolongations on stuttered words. Because the aim of this form of therapy is not to eliminate stuttering, it is not surprising that it is not necessarily effective in reducing the number of episodes of stuttering, even though patients may feel better about their overall ability to communicate (Blomgren et al., 2005). This type of stuttering modification may be the therapy approach of choice for clients who have stuttered for many years and consider true fluency to be an unrealistic goal.

Modifying Speech.   In the treatment of stuttering during the mid-1970s, there was a shift away from modification of stuttering toward the shaping of fluent speech. The fluency-shaping approach came directly out of learning theory, in which behavior was modified by degrees until it reached the target of natural sounding, fluent speech. Clients may use any of a variety of methods, such as slowing their speech, changing the prosody of speech, using light contacts of the tongue and lips when forming sounds, or prolonging the vowel sounds in words. For children, these techniques may be described in easy-to-understand terminology to assist their comprehension of the desired behaviors. For example, Druce, Debner, and Byrt (1997) taught young children a technique they referred to as "sleepy talk" to represent the slow, easy nature of the speech they wanted children to produce. The client, whether a child or adult, may apply the fluency-shaping techniques at first to very short utterances, on which they are highly likely to produce fluent speech, and then systematically increase the length of utterances (e.g., Druce et al., 1997; Riley & Ingham, 2000).

One problem with the techniques used to modify speech is that they can result in somewhat unnatural-sounding speech. For example, if clients are asked to slow or prolong their speech in order to attain fluency, the slow speech may be as disruptive to communication as the original stuttering was. Individuals who stutter may be reluctant to speak in an unnatural manner and may revert to stuttering (Martin, Haroldson, & Triden, 1984). Therapy may include a component that further shapes the clients' speech to be more natural sounding (Ingham, Sato, Finn, & Bekknap, 2001; Onslow, Costa, Andrews, Harrison, & Packman, 1996). Attention to speech naturalness, in addition to fluency, appears to improve overall outcomes for those who stutter.

A common component of programs designed to modify speech is transfer of the trained behaviors to settings outside the clinic or therapy setting. The clinician may use activities, such as telephone calls or field trips, during which the client is asked to use the fluent speech he or she has developed through treatment. This phase may be completed in the company of a clinician or through homework assignments. In either case, the client must eventually take responsibility for maintaining fluency outside of the therapeutic setting in order for fluency to be long lasting.

Other Disorders of Fluency

Cluttering

Another clinical disorder associated with altered fluency is **cluttering**. Like those who stutter, children who are described as clutterers have abnormally high frequencies of word and phrase repetitions. In contrast to stuttering, however, cluttering involves fewer sound- or syllable-level disfluencies (e.g., prolongations, sound repetitions). In addition, cluttering usually occurs without the signs of struggle, tension, or avoidance that are common in stuttering (St. Louis, Hinzman, & Hull, 1985). However, there are reports of both cluttering and stuttering occurring in the same individual, indicating that signs of both disorders may coexist (Craig, 1996; Williams & Wener, 1997). Although the prevalence of cluttering is unknown, speech-language pathologists in the United States tend to report few cases of cluttering in their practices.

Wood (1971) defined cluttering as "rapid, nervous speech marked by omissions of sounds and syllables" (p. 10). This definition gives equal prominence to the symptoms of rapid rate and articulatory errors and is similar to that of Wingate (1978), who defined cluttering as "a fluency disorder of unknown origin characterized by sporadically excessive rate and incomplete and distorted articulation" (p. 268). In an early monograph written on the topic, Arnold (1966) reviewed literature from Europe that described cluttering as involving rapid rate, faulty articulation, and related reading and writing problems. Wall (1988) said that cluttering is characterized by rapid speed and disordered articulation but added this important part to the definition: "a lack of awareness of the problem on the part of the speaker" (p. 637). It would appear that most clutterers, unlike stutterers, are not upset by their continuing disfluency.

Clutterers speak much faster than stutterers; in fact, the word *tachyphemia*, which is sometimes used as a synonym for cluttering (although it is not), literally means "rapid speech." Clutterers may be differentiated from stutterers by the former's slurred and omitted phonemes, periods of unusually rapid rate of speech, lack of awareness of their poor speech, and the fact that they neither avoid nor feel tense about the act of speaking. In addition, clutterers are often observed to exhibit disorganized thought processes, some problems in language formulation and comprehension, and problems in reading and writing (St. Louis et al., 1985; Teigland, 1996). Such problems may require services for language and learning disabilities during the school years (St. Louis & Hinzman, 1986). By combining the views of several writers, let us define cluttering:

> *Cluttering* is speech characterized by rapid rate, disfluencies, and articulation errors, often accompanied by spoken and written language difficulties. These signs usually occur without the speaker's awareness or concern.

Treatment of Cluttering.   Although both stuttering and cluttering involve disfluencies, the differences between the two disorders dictate very different treatment approaches. St. Louis and Meyers (1995) offered a series of working principles to guide treatment of cluttering. St. Louis and Meyers begin with a recognition that stuttering and cluttering are, in fact, independent disorders. For the child who clutters, disfluencies are a direct combination of fast speaking rate combined with a weak ability to handle the phonologic, syntactic, or semantic aspects of spoken language.

Children who clutter can increase their fluency by slowing their rate. However, as anyone who has tried to change his or her speaking rate knows, sustaining a slower speaking rate while thinking about what to say is difficult. We can use direct methods to address speaking rate. The speaker might pace his or her speaking rate with a metronome to raise awareness about rate of speech. Later, a clinician might provide visual feedback, such as an arrow to signal whether speech is too fast, too slow, or just fine. The following case illustrates an indirect method of addressing rate, having the speaker alter loudness (which later can be reduced to normal levels when rate has been reduced). This 17-year-old was asked to listen to a recording of himself followed by one of a normal male speaker near the client's age:

CLINICIAN: I bet you talk twice as fast as that other kid. Did you hear him?

CLIENT: He donna wanna go fatter than me.

CLINICIAN: Maybe if we just had you talk a little louder, like this: "I'm going to speak loudly for a bit." That sure makes me sound better, doesn't it?

CLIENT: Talin' loud is easy for me. I tal' loud at home and they all hear me.

CLINICIAN: Well, let's make a recording of you talking louder, and we'll see how that sounds.

Rather than working on the components of rate and articulation, both of which were far from normal in this case, the clinician elected to work holistically on making the patient aware that he could "speak better" by changing his speaking habits. Given a tangible method of changing his speech, that patient could monitor his loudness, which served to slow the rate of speech and improve his articulation.

Sometimes, indirect methods can be used to decrease rate by concentrating on another element of speech or language. For example, if a child's poor articulation contributes to cluttering, exercises designed to remediate articulation may have the side effect of reducing speaking rate. Likewise, if fluency breakdowns are occurring because of linguistic deficits such as word-finding problems or difficulty with syntactic constructions, then it makes sense to remediate these linguistic problems directly. In many cases, improved fluency is a side effect of a linguistic approach.

St. Louis and Meyers (1995) pointed out that a synergistic approach that focuses on improved communication may be best. Language formulation problems may be aided when rate is slowed, because the individual has more time to organize his ideas and give them linguistic structure. Improved self-monitoring may help the individual concentrate on correct articulation, which in turn will tend to slow speaking rate. Word-finding strategies may help prevent semantic breakdowns that reduce fluency. This dynamic approach may also include services coordinated with others (e.g., family members, teacher, psychologists) who can help to manage social and educational aspects associated with cluttering.

Acquired Neurogenic Disfluency

Most adults who stutter have a history of childhood stuttering. There are, however, cases of previously fluent adults who have an abrupt onset of stuttering (Market, Montague, Buffalo, & Drummond, 1990). In most instances, acquired stuttering is associated with neurological disease or exposure to toxins (Helm-Estabrooks, 1998; Ringo & Dietrich, 1995). Less frequently, acquired stuttering may have a psychological origin related to anxiety, depression, or other psychological disturbance (Baumgartner & Duffy, 1997). Although the symptoms of neurogenic and psychogenic stuttering may be difficult to distinguish from one another, a review of the patient's history is usually helpful in determining the cause of the disfluencies. We were asked recently to help interpret the disfluencies of a 69-year-old man.

Mr. Nelson was referred by his neurologist after a series of transient ischemic attacks or possibly small strokes. The most recent episode was followed by what appeared to be stuttering. The disruption of speech was a concern to Mr. Nelson, who was a highly educated, articulate man and a frequent public speaker as president of a volunteer organization. Despite his neurological history, the referral letter from the neurologist described Mr. Nelson's disfluency as "a functional acquired stuttering, possibly secondary to some sort of depression or anxiety."

Prior to his visit, Mr. Nelson was asked to write a narrative of his recent medical history and to describe any changes in his speech or language. His description clarified that he had experienced two episodes two years apart involving neurological signs. The first episode included persistent numbness and tingling on the left side of his body that lasted for about a week. The second included a more dramatic onset of right-sided weakness and some problems speaking. Mr. Nelson was hospitalized following the second episode and put on blood-thinning medication because of his risk for a stroke. He wrote that he was recovering fully from the second episode, but within a month he began to have increasing difficulty talking. He had some trouble coming up with the names of things, but his most vexing problem was stuttering, which he described as having "a lot of hesitation" in his speech.

An evaluation of Mr. Nelson's speech revealed many disfluencies. For example, as he read a 100-word passage aloud, he was disfluent on ten words: five were tense pauses, three were sound prolongations, and two were sound repetitions. His conversational speech was similarly disrupted by pauses—although his articulators were postured correctly to produce a word, he seemed unable to proceed. No secondary stuttering characteristics such as facial grimacing, hand clenching, or head movements were observed. In fact, Mr. Nelson appeared to be annoyed by his disfluencies but not overly upset by them.

> The fact that some individuals acquire stuttering after brain damage lends support for a neurological basis of developmental stuttering.

Mr. Nelson's disfluencies and his medical history suggested that he had acquired neurogenic stuttering. Although an MRI brain scan revealed some small areas of white matter changes, and it was not clear that Mr. Nelson had suffered a stroke, his medical history clearly indicated some compromise of his neurological functions. Neurogenic stuttering is not limited to damage to a particular region of the brain but has been related to left- and right-hemisphere and cortical and subcortical damage, as well as damage to the cerebellum and brainstem. About one-third of individuals with neurogenic stuttering also exhibit an aquired language impairment (Baumgartner & Duffy, 1997). In Mr. Nelson's case, he evidenced some mild word-finding problems (**anomia**), but his overall performance was excellent for spoken and written language.

Neurogenic versus Developmental Stuttering. Neurogenic stuttering refers to an acquired disruption of fluency that can be linked with an identifiable neurological event, such as a stroke or head injury. This is in contrast to developmental stuttering, which may also have an underlying neurological component, as described earlier. The disruptions in normal speech production that are observed in neurogenic disfluency are similar in some ways to developmental stuttering, but there are some differences. Whereas instances of disfluency in developmental stuttering occur more often on words that start with consonants than with vowels, neurogenic stuttering occurs equally often on words beginning with either consonants or vowels (Ringo & Dietrich, 1995). Likewise, neurogenic stuttering occurs equally often on substantive and function words, whereas content words are more likely to be disfluent for adults who have stuttered since childhood. As was true with Mr. Nelson, most individuals with neurogenic stuttering are notably free of anxiety about their speech and lack characteristics such as accessory behaviors and facial tension that are common in stuttering having a developmental origin.

Neurogenic versus Psychogenic Stuttering.   Mr. Nelson's disfluencies differed from psychogenic stuttering in several ways. Although psychogenic stuttering can be similar to neurogenic stuttering, Baumgartner and Duffy (1997) found several distinguishing features. Unlike neurogenic stuttering, psychogenic stuttering may be intermittent and associated with specific speaking situations. In addition, struggle behaviors and other signs of anxiety are not uncommon in psychogenic stuttering, and unusual or bizarre speech patterns that are not observed in other speech or language disorders are often present (e.g., using "me" for the pronoun "I"). Moreover, psychogenic stuttering usually responds quickly to behavioral treatment.

Intervention.   After we determined that Mr. Nelson's disfluencies were consistent with those of a neurogenic origin, we needed to decide whether treatment was warranted. Cases reviewed in the literature indicated that neurogenic stuttering often resolves on its own without treatment within a month or two of onset. Therefore, we assured Mr. Nelson that his stuttering appeared to be related to the neurological episodes he had experienced and told him that we suspected his fluency would improve on its own. He was scheduled for a follow-up visit six weeks later, at which time he showed considerable improvement in fluency. Some brief pauses were still observed as he spoke, but they were relatively subtle, and he reported that they were not as bothersome to him. In fact, he said that he was most annoyed by his occasional word-finding difficulty at that time, a problem he had minimized during his initial visit.

Had Mr. Nelson's stuttering persisted and had he wanted treatment, we might have treated it behaviorally in much the same way as developmental stuttering. Approaches that enhance fluency, such as slowed speaking rate and easy onset of voicing, have been used with success in neurogenic stuttering (Market et al., 1990). Fluency can also be facilitated by pacing speech production so that it is not disrupted by hesitations, prolongations, or repetitions (Helm-Estabrooks, 1998). In some cases, medications have been shown to improve neurogenic stuttering, although other cases of acquired disfluency appear to have been caused by medication (reviewed in Helm-Estabrooks, 1998). Thus, a careful review of a patient's history and medications are essential in instances of adult-onset disfluency.

Clinical Problem Solving

Annette first came to the attention of the school speech-language pathologist through a phone call from the district director of special education. Annette's parents had been phoning the director's office and home requesting that their daughter be treated for her stuttering. Annette's father was an adult stutterer, and both parents wanted Annette's speech to be "corrected before her stuttering became permanent." They also reported that Annette began speaking somewhat late, but they had no concerns about her speech or language other than the stuttering. Annette was enrolling in kindergarten that fall. After school began, the clinician was able to observe Annette on several occasions in the classroom, during which her speech was consistently fluent. The clinician reported her observations to the parents, advising them to allow Annette time to settle into the school routine. The parents were adamant that Annette stuttered frequently at home and were insistent that she be treated through the school. At the parents' urging, the clinician set up a classroom monitoring program to permit the classroom teacher to systematically document Annette's speech. From September to December, only two disfluent episodes were noted. After receiving this news, the parents sent the clinician a recorded sample of Annette's speech at home. The recording revealed frequent episodes of disfluent speech, including part-word repetitions, sound prolongations, and silent episodes, which may well have reflected blocks.

1. Do you think that Annette does stutter? What makes you think so/not?
2. What risk factors for stuttering appear in Annette's history?
3. Select two theories and discuss how this case profile might relate to each theory.
4. Speculate on the reasons why Annette may stutter at home but not in her new kindergarten.
5. Do you think that Annette should receive therapy for stuttering? If so, what factors would you consider in developing a plan of intervention for Annette?

REFERENCES

Adams, M. R. (1990). The demands and capacities model I: Theoretical elaborations. *Journal of Fluency Disorders, 15*, 135–141.

Andrews, C., Craig, A., Feyer, A., Haddinott, S., Neilson, M., & Howle, P. (1983). Stuttering: A review of research findings and theories circa 1982. *Journal of Speech and Hearing Disorders, 48*, 226–245.

Andrews, C., & Harris, M. (1964). *The syndrome of stuttering.* London: Heinemann Dynamic Medical Books.

Armson, J., Kiefte, M., & Mason, J. (2006). The effect of SpeechEasy on stuttering frequency in laboratory conditions. *Journal of Fluency Disorders, 31*, 137–152.

Arnold, C. (1966). *Studies in tachyphemia: An investigation of cluttering and general language disability.* New York: Speech Rehabilitation Institute.

Baumgartner, J., & Duffy, J. R. (1997). Psychogenic stuttering in adults with and without neurologic disease. *Journal of Medical Speech Language Pathology, 5,* 75–95.

Blanton, S. (1965). Stuttering. In D. Barbara (Ed.), *New directions in stuttering.* Springfield, IL: Charles C. Thomas.

Blomgren, M., Roy, N., Callister, T., & Merrill, R. M. (2005). Intensive stuttering modification therapy: A multidimensional assessment of treatment outcomes. *Journal of Speech, Language, and Hearing Research, 48,* 509–523.

Blood, G. W., Blood, I. M., Bennett, S., Simpson, K. C., & Susman, E. J. (1994). Subjective anxiety measurements and cortisol responses in adults who stutter. *Journal of Speech and Hearing Research, 37,* 760–768.

Blood, G. W., Blood, I. M., Tellis, G., & Gabel, R. (2001). Communication apprehension and self-perceived communication competence in adolescents who stutter. *Journal of Fluency Disorders, 26,* 161–178.

Bloodstein, O. (2006). Some empirical observations about early stuttering: A possible link to language development. *Journal of Communication Disorders, 39,* 185–191.

Bonelli, P., Dixon, M., Bernstein Ratner, N., & Onslow, M. (2000). Child and parent speech and language and the Lidcombe Program of early stuttering intervention. *Clinical Linguistics and Phonetics, 14,* 427–446.

Chang, S.-E., Horwitz, B. , Ostuni, J., Reynolds, R., Ludlow, C. L. (2011). Evidence of left inferior frontal-premotor structural and functional connectivity deficits in adults who stutter. *Cerebral Cortex, 11,* 2507–2518.

Conture, E. G. (1990). Childhood stuttering: What is it and who does it? *ASHA Report Series, 18,* 2–14.

Conture, E. G., & Kelly, E. M. (1991). Young stutterers' nonspeech behaviors during stuttering. *Journal of Speech and Hearing Research, 34,* 1041–1056.

Cooper, E. B., & Cooper, C. S. (1995). Treating fluency disordered adolescents. *Journal of Communication Disorders, 28,* 125–142.

Cooper, E. B., & Cooper, C. S. (1996). Clinicians' attitudes toward stuttering: Two decades of change. *Journal of Fluency Disorders, 21,* 119–135.

Craig, A. (1990). An investigation between anxiety and stuttering. *Journal of Speech and Hearing Disorders, 55,* 290–294.

Craig, A. (1996). Long-term effects of intensive treatment for a client with both a cluttering and stuttering disorder. *Journal of Fluency Disorders, 21,* 329–335.

Craig, A., Hancock, K., Chang, E., Mccreay, C., Shepley, A., Mccaul, A., Costello, D., Harding, S., Kehren, R., Masel, C., & Reilly, K. (1996). A controlled clinical trial for stuttering in persons age 9–14 years. *Journal of Speech and Hearing Research, 39,* 808–826.

Curlee, R. F. (1980). A case selection strategy for young disfluent children. *Seminars in Speech, Language, Hearing, 1,* 277–287.

Dayalu, V., Kalinowski, J., Stuart, A., Holbert, D., & Rastatter, M. P. (2002). Stuttering frequency on content and function words in adults who stutter: A concept revisited. *Journal of Speech, Language, and Hearing Research, 45,* 858–870.

De Nil, L. F., Kroll, R. M., Lafaille, S. J., Houle, S. (2003). A positron emission tomography study of short- and long-term treatment effects on functional brain activation in adults who stutter. *Journal of Fluency Disorders, 28,* 357–380.

Druce, T., Debner, S., & Byrt, T. (1997). Evaluation of an intensive treatment program for stuttering in young children. *Journal of Fluency Disorders, 22,* 169–186.

Fox, P. T., Ingham, R. J., Ingham, J. C., Hirsch, T., Downs, J. H., Martin, C., Jerabek, P., Glass, T., & Lancaster, J. L. (1996). A PET study of the neural systems of stuttering. *Nature, 382,* 158–162.

Franken, M-C. J., Kielstra-Van der Schalk, C. J., & Boelens, H. (2005). Experimental treatment of early stuttering: A preliminary study. *Journal of Fluency Disorders, 30,* 189–199.

Glauber, I. P. (1958). The psychoanalysis of stuttering. In J. Eisenson (Ed.), *Stuttering. A symposium.* New York: Harper and Row.

Harris, V., Onslow, M., Packman, A., Harrison, E., & Menzies, R. (2002). An experimental investigation of the impact of the Lidcombe Program on early stuttering. *Journal of Fluency Disorders, 27,* 203–213.

Harrison, E., Onslow, M., & Menzies, R. (2004). Dismantling the Lidcombe Program of early stuttering intervention: Verbal contingencies for stuttering and clinical measurement. *International Journal of Language and Communication Disorders, 39,* 257–267.

Hasbrouck, J. M. (1992). FAMC intensive stuttering treatment program: Ten years of implementation. *Military Medicine, 157,* 244–247.

Healey, E. C., Scott, L. A., & Ellis, G. (1995). Decision making in the treatment of school-age children who stutter. *Journal of Communication Disorders, 28,* 107–124.

Helm-Estabrooks, N. (1998). Stuttering associated with acquired neurological disorders. In R. F. Curlee (Ed.), *Stuttering and related disorders of fluency* (pp. 255–268). New York: Thieme Medical.

Hewat, S., Onslow, M., Packman, A., & O'Brian, S. (2006). A Phase II clinical trial of self-imposed time-out treatment for stuttering in adults and adolescents. *Disability and Rehabilitation, 28,* 33–42.

Howell, P., El-Yaniv, N., & Powell, D. J. (1987). Factors affecting fluency in stutterers. In H. F. M. Peters & W. Hulstijn (Eds.), *Speech motor dynamics in stuttering* (pp. 361–369). New York: Springer.

Howie, P. M. (1981). Concordance for stuttering in monozygotic and dizygotic twin pairs. *Journal of Speech and Hearing Research, 24,* 317–321.

Hull, F. M., Mielke, P. W., Willeford, J. A., & Timmons, R. J. (1976). *National speech and hearing survey.* Final Report, Project 50978. Washington, DC: Office of Education, Bureau of Education for the Handicapped, Department of Health, Education, and Welfare.

Ingham, R. J., Sato, W., Finn, P., & Belknap, H. (2001). The modification of speech naturalness during rhythmic stimulation treatment of stuttering. *Journal of Speech, Language, and Hearing Research, 44,* 841–952.

James, J. (1981). Behavioral self-control of stuttering using time-out from speaking. *Journal of Applied Behavioral Analysis, 14,* 25–37.

James, J. (1983). Parameters of the influence of self-initiated time-out from speaking on stuttering. *Journal of Communication Disorders, 16,* 123–132.

Janssen, P., Kraaimaat, F., & Brutten, G. (1990). Relationship between stutterers' genetic history and speech-associated variables. *Journal of Fluency Disorders, 15,* 39–48.

Johnson, W. (1955). A study of the onset and development of stuttering. In W. Johnson & R. R. Leutenegger (Eds.), *Stuttering in children and adults.* Minneapolis: University of Minnesota Press.

Johnson, W. (1959). *The onset of stuttering.* Minneapolis: University of Minnesota Press.

Jones, M., Onslow, M., Harrison, E., & Packman, A. (2000). Treating stuttering in young children: Predicting treatment time in the Lidcombe Program. *Journal of Speech, Language, and Hearing Research, 43,* 1440–1450.

Kalinowski, J., Armson, J., Roland-Mieszkowski, M., Stuart, A., & Gracco, V. L. (1993). Effects of alterations in auditory feedback and speech rate on stuttering frequency. *Language and Speech, 36,* 1–16.

Kalinowski, J., Lerman, J., & Watt, J. (1987). A preliminary examination of the perceptions of self and others in stutterers and nonstutterers. *Journal of Fluency Disorders, 12,* 317–331.

Kang, C., Riazuddin, S., Mundorff, J., Krasnewich, D., Friedman, P., James C. Mullikin, J. C., & Drayna, D. (2010). Mutations in the lysosomal enzyme–targeting pathway and persistent stuttering. *New England Journal of Medicine, 362,* 677–685.

Kelly, E. M. (1995). Parents as partners: Including mothers and fathers in the treatment of children who stutter. *Journal of Communication Disorders, 28,* 93–106.

Kidd, K. K. (1980). Genetic models of stuttering. *Journal of Fluency Disorders, 5,* 187–202.

Lattermann, C., Shenker, R. C., & Thordardottir, E. (2005). Progression of language complexity during treatment with the Lidcombe Program for early stuttering intervention. *American Journal of Speech-Language Pathology, 14,* 242–253.

Lincoln, M. A., & Onslow, M. (1997). Long-term outcome of early intervention for stuttering. *American Journal of Speech-Language Pathology, 6,* 51–58.

Market, K. W., Montague, J. C., Buffalo, M. D., & Drummond, S. S. (1990). Acquired stuttering: Descriptive data and treatment outcome. *Journal of Fluency Disorders, 15,* 221–233.

Martin, R. R., Haroldson, S. K., & Triden, K. A. (1984). Stuttering and speech naturalness. *Journal of Speech and Hearing Disorders, 49,* 53–58.

Martin, R., Kuhl, P., & Haroldson, S. (1972). An experimental treatment with two preschool stuttering children. *Journal of Speech and Hearing Research, 15,* 743–52.

Miller, S., & Watson, B. C. (1992). The relationship between communication attitude, anxiety and depression in stutterers and nonstutterers. *Journal of Speech and Hearing Research, 34,* 789–798.

Morley, M. F. (1972). *The development and disorders of speech in childhood.* Edinburgh: Churchill Livingstone.

National Institutes of Deafness and Other Communication Disorders (NIDCD). (2010). *NIDCD Fact Sheet: Stuttering.* Bethesda, MD: Author. Retrieved from www.nidcd.nih.gov/staticresources/health/voice/StutteringFactSheet.pdfNeumann, K., Euler, H. A., von Gudenberg, A. W., Giraud, A-L., Lanfermann, H., Gaul, V., & Preibisch, C. (2003). The nature and treatment of stuttering as revealed by fMRI: A within- and between-group comparison. *Journal of Fluency Disorders, 28,* 381–410.

Neumann, K., Euler, H. A., von Gudenberg, A. W., Giraud, A-L., Lanfermann, H., Gaul, V., & Preibisch, C. (2003). The nature and treatment of stuttering as revealed by fMRI: A within- and between-group comparison. *Journal of Fluency Disorders, 28,* 381–410.

Onslow, M., Costa, L., Andrews, C., Harrison, E., & Packman, A. (1996). Speech outcomes of a prolonged-speech treatment of stuttering. *Journal of Speech and Hearing Research, 39,* 734–749.

Onslow, M., Packman, A., Stocker, S., van Doorn, J., & Siegel, G. (1997). Control of children's stuttering with response-contingent time-out: Behavioral, perceptual, and acoustic data. *Journal of Speech, Language, and Hearing Research, 40,* 121–133.

Packman, A., Onslow, M., & van Doorn, J. (1994). Prolonged speech and modification of stuttering: Perceptual, acoustic, and electroglottographic data. *Journal of Speech and Hearing Research, 39,* 724–737.

Perkins, W. H. (1980). Disorders of speech. In T. Hixon, L. Shriberg, & J. Saxman (Eds.), *Introduction to communication disorders.* Englewood Cliffs, NJ: Prentice Hall.

Perkins, W. H., Kent, R. D., & Curlee, R. F. (1991). A theory of neuropsycholinguistic function in stuttering. *Journal of Speech and Hearing Research, 34,* 734–752.

Prins, D., & Hubbard, C. (1988). Response contingent stimuli and stuttering: Issues and implications. *Journal of Speech and Hearing Research, 31,* 696–709.

Prins, D., Main, V., & Wampler, S. (1997). Lexicalization in adults who stutter. *Journal of Speech Language and Hearing Research, 40,* 373–384.

Riley, G. D., & Ingham, J. C. (2000). Acoustic duration changes associated with two types of treatment for children who stutter. *Journal of Speech Language and Hearing Research, 40,* 965–978.

Ringo, C. C., & Dietrich, S. (1995). Neurogenic stuttering: An analysis and critique. *Journal of Medical Speech-Language Pathology, 3*(2), 111–122.

Rustin, L., & Cook, F. (1995). Parental involvement in treatment of stuttering. *Language, Speech, and Hearing Services in Schools, 26,* 127–137.

Schwartz, H. D., Zebrowski, P. M., & Conture, E. G. (1990). Behaviors at the onset of stuttering. *Journal of Fluency Disorders, 15,* 77–86.

Speech Foundation of America. (1987). *Self-therapy for the stutterer* (6th ed.). Publication 12. Memphis, TN: Author.

St. Louis, K. O., & Hinzman, A. R. (1986). Studies of cluttering: Perceptions of cluttering by speech-language pathologists and educators. *Journal of Fluency Disorders, 11,* 131–149.

St. Louis, K. O., Hinzman, A. R., & Hull, F. M. (1985). Studies of cluttering: Disfluency and language measures in young possible clutterers and stutterers. *Journal of Fluency Disorders, 10,* 151–172.

St. Louis, K. O., & Meyers, F. L. (1995). Clinical management of cluttering. *Language, Speech, and Hearing Services in Schools, 26,* 187–195.

Starkweather, C. W. (1990). Current trends in therapy for stuttering children and suggestions for future research. *ASHA Report Series, 18,* 82–90.

Stephenson-Opsal, D., & Bernstein Ratner, N. (1988). Maternal speech rate modification and childhood stuttering. *Journal of Fluency Disorders, 13,* 49–56.

Teigland, A. (1996). A study of pragmatic skills of clutterers and normal speakers. *Journal of Fluency Disorders, 21,* 201–214.

Travis, L. E. (1971). The unspeakable feelings of people with special reference to stuttering. In L. D. Travis (Ed.), *Handbook of speech pathology and audiology* (2nd ed.). Englewood Cliffs, NJ: Prentice Hall.

Van Riper, C. (1971). *The nature of stuttering.* Englewood Cliffs, NJ: Prentice Hall.

Van Riper, C. (1990). Final thoughts about stuttering. *Journal of Fluency Disorders, 15,* 317–318.

Venkatagiri, H. S. (2005). Recent advances in the treatment of stuttering: A theoretical perspective. *Journal of Communication Disorders, 38,* 375–393.

Wall, M. J. (1988). Disfluency in the child. In N. J. Lass, L. V. McReynolds, J. L. Northern, & D. E. Yoder (Eds.), *Handbook of speech-language pathology and audiology.* Philadelphia: B. C. Decker.

Weber, C. M., & Smith, A. (1990). Autonomic correlates of stuttering and speech assessed in a range of experimental tasks. *Journal of Speech and Hearing Research, 33,* 690–706.

Williams, D. F., & Wener, D. L. (1997). Cluttering and stuttering exhibited in a young professional. *Journal of Fluency Disorders, 21,* 261–269.

Wingate, M. E. (1962). Personality needs of stutterers. *Logos, 5,* 35–37.

Wingate, M. E. (1976). *Stuttering theory and treatment.* New York: Irvington.

Wingate, M. E. (1978). Disorders of fluency. In P. Skinner & R. Shelton (Eds.), *Speech, language, hearing: Normal processes and disorders.* Reading, MA: Addison-Wesley.

Wood, K. S. (1971). Definitions and terms. In L. D. Travis (Ed.), *Handbook of speech pathology and audiology* (2nd ed.). Englewood Cliffs, NJ: Prentice Hall.

Woods, S., Shearsby, J., Onslow, M., & Burnham, D. (2002). The psychological impact of the Lidcombe Program of early stuttering intervention: Eight case studies. *International Journal of Language and Communication Disorders, 37,* 31–40.

World Health Organization (WHO). (1977). *Manual of the international statistical classification of diseases, injuries, and causes of death* (Vol. I). Geneva: Author.

Yairi, E., & Ambrose, N. (1992). Onset of stuttering in preschool children: Selected factors. *Journal of Speech and Hearing Research, 35,* 782–788.

Yairi, E., Ambrose, N. G., & Cox, N. (1996). Genetics of stuttering: A critical review. *Journal of Speech and Hearing Research, 39,* 771–784.

Yairi, E., Ambrose, N. G., Paden, E. P., & Throneburg, R. N. (1996). Predictive factors of persistence and recovery: Pathways of childhood stuttering. *Journal of Communication Disorders, 29,* 51–77.

Yaruss, J. S., Coleman, C., & Hammer, D. (2006). Treating preschool children who stutter: Description and preliminary evaluation of a family-focused treatment approach. *Language, Speech, & Hearing Services in Schools, 37,* 118–136.

Yaruss, J. S., Quesal, R. W., Reeves, L., Molt, L. F., Kluetz, B., Caruso, A. J., Mclure, J. A., & Lewis, F. (2002). Speech treatment and support group experiences of people who participate in the National Stuttering Association. *Journal of Fluency Disorders 27,* 115–134.

Zackheim, C. T., & Conture, E. G. (2003). Childhood stuttering and speech disfluencies in relation to children's mean length of utterance: A preliminary study. *Journal of Fluency Disorders, 28,* 115–142.

Zebrowski, P. M. (1995). The topology of a beginning stutterer. *Journal of Communication Disorders, 28,* 75–92.

READINGS FROM THE POPULAR LITERATURE

Bobrick, B. (1996). *Knotted tongues.* New York: Kodansha International.

Jezer, M. (1997). *Stuttering: A life bound up in words.* New York: Nasic.

Logue, M., & Conradi, P. (2010). *The King's speech.* London, UK: Quercus.

Shields, D. (1998). *Dead languages.* New York: Random House. (novel)

St. Louis, K. O. (2001). *Living with stuttering.* Morgantown, WV: Populore.

6 CHAPTER

Disorders of Voice and Swallowing

Julie Barkmeier-Kraemer

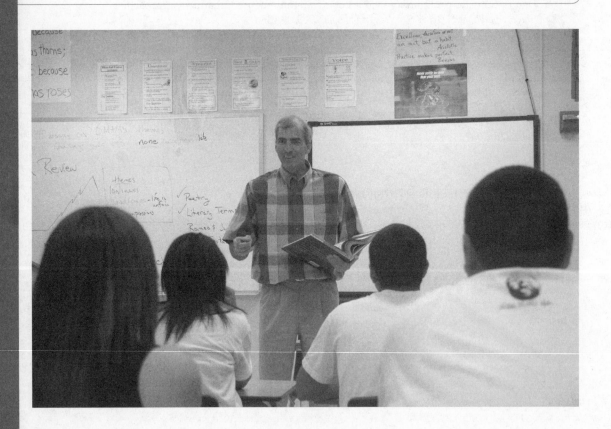

The larynx is the source of our voice for speaking, but it also serves to protect the airway during eating. Damage to the larynx or structures of the vocal tract may result in voice or swallowing problems. Most people experience problems with their voice due to improper voicing habits. Such voice disorders can usually be treated or improved by therapy that identifies and changes damaging vocal behaviors and facilitates healthy ways of voicing. Voice disorders related to physical damage to the laryngeal structure(s) may also be treated effectively with voice therapy; however, in some cases, medical intervention is needed. Swallowing problems can occur as a result of normal aging effects, neurological conditions, cancer, psychological problems, or structural abnormalities associated with birth defects or subsequent to surgery of the head and neck. Swallowing problems may be corrected by changing the consistency of food or making postural adjustments. Exercises are sometimes used to strengthen oral and pharyngeal structures for safe and effective eating. More recently, sensory stimulation and electrical stimulation have been studied for facilitating improved swallowing. Medical management in the form of pharmaceutical or surgical treatment may also be necessary to help individuals with swallowing problems. In most clinical practice settings, voice and swallowing disorders are evaluated and managed using a multi-disciplinary approach.

Voice Disorders

As described in Chapter 2, vocal fold vibrations produce sound that is further modified by the vocal tract. Individual differences in the vocal mechanism and its resonance characteristics contribute to the unique characteristics of each person's voice. Many temporary conditions, such as a stuffy nose or the effects of prolonged yelling, can change the voice. These types of problems tend to resolve on their own and typically do not require professional attention. However, permanent changes to the voice may occur with damage or disease. These conditions often require professional intervention.

The exact number of individuals who experience voice disorders in the population is not known. The National Institute on Deafness and Other Communication disorders estimates that 7.5 million Americans have trouble using their voices (around 2–3 percent of the U.S. population; NIDCD, 2011), but several studies place the estimates closer to 6–7 percent of the population. A large cross-sectional study in the United Kingdom found that about 6 percent of children have a problem with their voice (Carding, Roulstone, Northstone, & ALSPAC Study Team, 2006). When considered over time, as many as 23 percent of children have had a voice disorder at some point (Silverman & Zimmer, 1975). Similarly, the prevalence of voice disorders in adults is about 7 percent, and about 30 percent of adults report having had a voice disorder during their lifetime (Roy, Merrill, Gray, & Smith, 2005). The cause and persistence of voice disorders varies, and is related to patterns of voice use and demands, as well as conditions such as colds, sinus problems, and gastric problems that cause esophageal reflux (Roy et al., 2005). Voice problems are even more common in older adults (over age 65), where the prevalence is close to 30 percent, with more than half of the people in this age group reporting chronic voice problems lasting at least four weeks in duration (Roy, Stemple, Merrill, & Thomas, 2007).

As might be expected, some occupations carry a high risk for developing voice problems due to the intense communication demands. Classroom teachers have the highest incidence (and prevalence) of voice disorders, with about half of all teachers reporting a voice disorder at some point (Fritzell, 1995; Roy, Merrill, Thibeault, Gray, & Smith, 2004; Roy, Merrill, Thibeault, Parsa, Gray, & Smith, 2004; Smith, Gray, Dove, Kirchner, & Heras, 1997; Thibeault, Merrill, Roy, Gray, & Smith, 2004). A study conducted at the University of Wisconsin indicated that teachers represented 20 percent of the voice disorders caseload, followed by singers (11 percent), salespeople (10 percent), clerks (9 percent), administrators and managers (7 percent), and factory workers (6 percent) (Titze, Lemke, & Montequin, 1997). A majority of voice patients report that their problem had a negative impact on their career options, social interactions, and other aspects of their daily lives (Smith et al., 1996; Roy et al., 2004).

> The most common cause of voice disorders is overuse or improper use of the voice.

Voice disorders can be described as problems related to pitch, loudness, voice quality, and resonance. These problems may stem from vocal misuse, disease, congenital defects, laryngeal trauma, aging effects, and neurological disorders. Emotional and psychological factors may also contribute to acquired voice disorders (Dietrich, Verdolini-Abbott, Gartner-Schmidt, & Rosen, 2008; Roy, Bless, & Heisey, 2000). Treatment usually requires the combined specialties of the ear-nose-throat doctor (otolaryngologist) and a speech-language pathologist with experience in assessing and treating voice disorders.

Voice Disorders Related to Vocal Fold Tissue Changes

Most voice disorders arise from overuse or frequent improper use of the voice, which can result in tissue changes that disrupt normal fold vibration.

> *Susan*, age 17, was a cheerleader for her high school varsity football team for three years. During her first two years as a cheerleader, she experienced temporary bouts of hoarseness following each game. These usually subsided in a couple of days. During her third year as a cheerleader, however, she began to experience longer periods of hoarseness that did not fully resolve before the next game. By the end of the football season, her voice almost always sounded hoarse, and she had difficulty being heard in the football stands. Eventually, she was no longer able to cheer.

> An otolaryngologist found bilateral nodules on her vocal folds (see Figure 6.1). Vocal nodules are calluses that typically result from chronic vocal misuse. The size of Susan's nodules prevented her vocal folds from coming together unless she

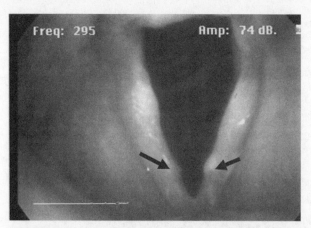

FIGURE 6.1 The vocal folds viewed from above showing bilateral vocal nodules, indicated by arrows. Note that the larynx is oriented with the front of the structure at the bottom of the figure (i.e., the bottom is anterior and the top is posterior).

increased her loudness. She was discouraged from participating in cheerleading until the vocal nodules diminished. She was also referred to a speech-language pathologist for voice therapy. The speech-language pathologist helped Susan identify other habits that were contributing to physical damage of the vocal folds, such as coughing, clearing her throat frequently, and yelling at her younger brother when he teased her. Susan reduced the frequency of these behaviors and learned better ways to produce her voice. After one month, the size of the vocal nodules had reduced dramatically, and Susan's voice was significantly improved.

Traumatic Laryngitis

In the early stages of her voice disorder, Susan experienced repeated episodes of **traumatic laryngitis**. This condition is characterized by swollen and red vocal folds resulting from excessive yelling, screaming, or other behaviors that involve forceful use of the voice (see Figure 6.2). Traumatic laryngitis is common and usually resolves within days of its onset. It often results from continuous vocal misuse such as yelling or cheering throughout an exciting athletic event. In such situations, yelling at high intensity over loud environmental noise causes the vocal folds to slam together at high velocities. This results in trauma to the vocal fold tissue at the site of impact. As a result, the vocal folds become swollen and irritated (Brodnitz, 1971). Tissue swelling along the length of the vocal folds changes their mass and disrupts the normal pattern of vibration so that it is no longer nicely symmetrical. These changes in the structure and function of the vocal folds affect the voice quality so that it typically sounds hoarse. In severe cases, there may be a complete loss of voice (**aphonia**). The best treatment for traumatic laryngitis is to rest the voice, allowing the vocal folds to heal. After two to five days, depending on the extent of damage, vocal fold swelling and

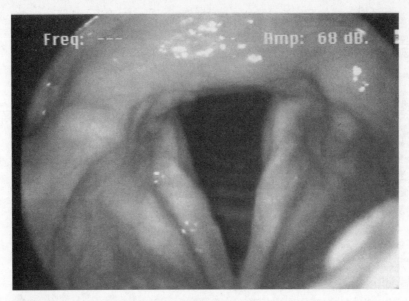

FIGURE 6.2 An example of the appearance of traumatic laryngitis, obtained using videoendoscopy. Notice the swollen and irregular borders of the vocal folds.

irritation typically resolve, and the normal voice returns. In Susan's case, she experienced this cycle of trauma and recovery during her first two years of cheerleading.

If the vocal misuse continues, however, vocal fold irritation can become chronic. The tissue that covers the vibrating portion of the vocal folds may thicken. Chronic irritation may result from attempts to talk over environmental noise (e.g., machinery noise in a factory or the cheering and other crowd noise that occurs at an athletic event) or talking for long periods of time. Changes in daily voice use are needed to prevent further permanent damage and to allow healing. Voice therapy may be necessary to identify poor vocal habits and teach improved techniques for using the voice.

> Onset of laryngitis after a night of yelling and screaming at a sports event or a concert is usually caused by swollen vocal folds.

Vocal Nodules

Vocal nodules are small bumps that develop on the medial border of the vocal folds (see Figure 6.1). These bumps consist of fibrous tissue (Gray, Hammond, & Hanson, 1995), much like calluses that develop on the hands or feet. Nodules occur along the anterior one-third of the vocal folds as a result of persistent improper voicing patterns, such as excessive yelling or sustained overuse of the voice. Although vocal nodules certainly are not life-threatening, they can result in significant voice problems. The symptoms of vocal nodules arise gradually and manifest as increasing hoarseness and difficulty projecting the voice. Vocal nodules can occur on one vocal fold, but most frequently they develop on both vocal folds at the site of impact. In early stages, nodules may appear as small swollen areas on the vocal folds. In later stages, the nodules become hard and impair normal vocal fold vibration. If the nodules become large enough, they can prevent the vocal folds from coming together completely, as occurred with Susan. She also demonstrated signs of traumatic laryngitis that preceded the development of nodules. She could have prevented the development of vocal nodules with modification of her voice use. Instead, Susan's vocal fold tissue adjusted to the continual irritation and traumatic impact by developing vocal nodules. This condition can be treated effectively with voice therapy that identifies voice misuse and teaches improved voicing habits (McCrory, 2001; McFarlane & Watterson, 1990; Yamaguchi et al., 1986) including better methods for producing and projecting the voice.

> Vocal nodules are like calluses that develop after chronic misuse of the vocal folds.

Vocal Polyps

Vocal polyps are small, fluid-filled sacs that develop on the vocal folds as a result of yelling and other excessive uses of the voice (Johns, 2003; Kleinsasser, 1979, 1990). Compared to nodules, which are fibrous and usually bilateral, polyps are soft and compliant and typically occur on one side only. They may appear anywhere in the larynx, including on the vocal folds or ventricular folds or between the arytenoids. In contrast to the prolonged vocal misuse that leads to nodules, it is believed that a single event of vocal misuse, such as screaming or even intense coughing, can lead to development of a polyp (McFarlane & Von Berg, 1998).

> *Mrs. Delvechio*, age 56, began to experience a gradual onset of hoarseness after an upper respiratory infection with severe coughing episodes. She was seen by an otolaryngologist who identified a polyp located near the posterior segment of the vibrating portion of the left vocal fold. The physician suspected the polyp had resulted from traumatic vocal fold impact during repeated episodes of coughing. The physician referred Mrs. Delvechio to a speech-language patholo-gist for counseling concerning excessive coughing and throat clearing. During counseling, Mrs. Delvechio also mentioned that her husband was hard of hearing and she often tried to talk to him over the television or from another room in the house. She was encouraged to speak at comfortable loudness and not to speak over noise. In addition, she was instructed to talk to her husband only when they were in the same room. After six weeks, her polyp was reduced in size, and her voice was almost completely normal.

A vocal polyp may result in significant voice problems, including breathi-ness or hoarseness. The polyp may also cause each vocal fold to vibrate at a dif-ferent rate, causing a double voice, or **diplophonia**. Treatment for a vocal polyp frequently entails identification of the behaviors that led to the problem (e.g., yelling, throat clearing, coughing). In Mrs. Delvechio's case, once she became aware of the behaviors that were contributing to the voice problem, she could eliminate those habits. Subsequently, the polyp reduced in size as the laryngeal tissue healed. In some cases, the individuals may need specific therapeutic instruction by a speech-language pathologist to improve use of the voice. In still other cases, surgical removal of a polyp by an otolaryngologist is necessary (Johns, 2003; Kleinsasser, 1979, 1990).

Laryngeal Papilloma

Papillomas are wart-like growths found along the vocal tract and respiratory system. If they develop on or near the vocal folds, they can disrupt normal vocal fold vibration, so that the voice typically sounds breathy or hoarse. The growths are caused by a variant of the human papilloma virus (HPV) and are more commonly found in children than adults (Derkay & Darros, 2006). Although not common (occurring in about 3–4/100,000 children and 1–4/100,000 in adults), the papilloma warts are of particular concern if they grow large enough to impede or obstruct the airway. In such cases, a whistling sound (called stridor) may be heard, and there may be breathing difficulties. Papilloma may be treated with laser surgery, but it grows back quickly, and multiple surgeries may be necessary. Unfortunately, frequent laser surgeries may result in vocal fold scarring that cannot be repaired. In extreme cases, the vocal folds may become so scarred that the voice cannot be produced due to the stiffness of the vocal fold tissue. Voice therapy can sometimes help these individuals make the best of their voices after surgery. Other forms of treatment include chemotherapy and antibiotic treatments.

Laryngeal Cancer

Cancer, or **carcinoma**, of the larynx can be a life-threatening disease if not identified during its early stages. Persistent hoarseness is the most common symptom associated with laryngeal cancer. Other warning signs include swallowing problems, swelling in the throat and neck regions, and persistent throat pain.

> *Mr. Mahr*, age 45, smoked a pack of cigarettes per day for twenty-five years. He also enjoyed a cigarette along with several drinks during cocktail hour every night before dinner. Over a period of six months, his voice became increasingly hoarse. He did not report any illness during this time, although he noticed that he experienced more fatigue than usual and sometimes felt as though he could not breathe in enough air. Mr. Mahr loved his work as an attorney and usually had a lot of energy. He finally went to see an otolaryngologist, who discovered that his vocal folds were covered with a whitish mass that impaired their normal movement. The physician scheduled surgery to remove a piece of the mass and determine its pathology. The biopsy revealed that it was cancer. Mr. Mahr was told that the cancer had invaded much of the laryngeal region and that the entire larynx would need to be removed. After surgery, Mr. Mahr also needed to undergo a series of radiation treatments to reduce the risk that the cancer would recur. Fortunately, Mr. Mahr's laryngeal cancer was caught early enough that survival was likely. However, the treatment cost him his voice. Mr. Mahr was referred to a speech-language pathologist to explore alternatives for generating a new voice after the laryngectomy.

As in Mr. Mahr's case, those who develop laryngeal cancer usually smoke and drink alcohol (McKenna, Fornataro-Clerici, McMenamin, & Leonard, 1991; Rafferty, Fenton, & Jones, 2001). When caught in its early stages, laryngeal cancer frequently can be treated using conservative medical approaches. These include radiation, chemotherapy, and surgery to remove the cancer, leaving the larynx as intact as possible (Mendenhall, Parsons, Stringer, Cassisi, & Million, 1988). In its later stages, laryngeal cancer is typically treated by surgical removal of the entire larynx.

When the larynx is removed, the trachea is attached to a permanent opening in the neck called a **tracheostoma** (or stoma, for short). After his laryngectomy, Mr. Mahr will be able to breathe normally except that the air will enter and exit the body through an opening in his neck rather than the nose and mouth (see Figure 6.3). Food and drink are still taken by mouth, although the sense of taste is diminished because airborne odors are no longer breathed through the nose.

After laryngectomy surgery, a speech-language pathologist will work with the individual to develop alternative ways of generating a sound source for speech. One method is esophageal speech. To use this method, an individual

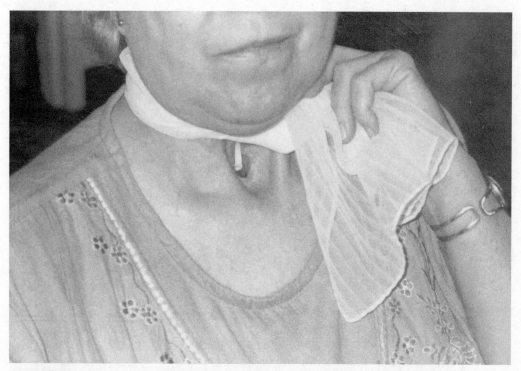

FIGURE 6.3　This woman is showing the location of the airway opening in her neck, called a tracheostoma. Since undergoing a laryngectomy, she now breathes through the tracheostoma. The white tab attached to the skin outside the tracheostoma secures a one-way valve. This valve shunts airs into the esophagus to create voice by vibrating esophageal tissue in a similar, but less predictable, way than the vocal folds.

If the larynx is removed, the normal sound source for voicing is no longer available. You may be surprised to learn that the esophagus provides an alternative voice, which is like talking on a burp.

must learn to trap air in the mouth and push it into the esophagus (McKenna et al., 1991). Once the air is trapped in the esophagus, it is belched back up, creating a sound source by vibration of the esophageal tissues. This sound is transformed into words by the articulatory movements of the teeth, tongue, and lips, as with normal speech.

A second method of speech production involves an electronic device called an **electrolarynx**, or artificial larynx (Casper & Colton, 1993). The electrolarynx is a handheld device that makes a buzzing sound that substitutes for vocal fold vibration. The device is placed against the neck so that the sound travels through the skin into the vocal tract, providing a "voice" that is then modified into speech by mouthing words (see Figure 6.4). The speech-language pathologist provides therapy to help improve speech intelligibility using the electrolarynx.

A popular method to provide voice is a tracheo-esophageal puncture. This surgical procedure creates a hole for the placement of a small tube into the tissue that divides the trachea from the esophagus. The tube has a one-way valve that shunts air from the trachea into the esophagus when the tracheostoma is covered

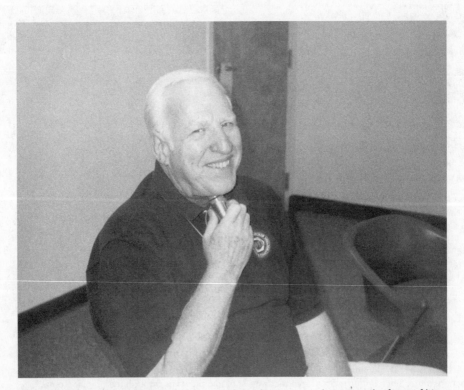

FIGURE 6.4 This gentleman is holding an electrolarynx securely against the front of his neck to provide his "voice" for speech.

by the individual's thumb or finger (see Figure 6.3). The shunted air vibrates the esophageal tissue in the same way the belching does in esophageal speech, resulting in voice.

Whichever method Mr. Mahr uses to communicate, he will need training and practice to maximize speech intelligibility. Many individuals like Mr. Mahr are grateful that they have another chance at life and resume their activities with great enthusiasm. Others may fall into depression and need professional counseling to help them deal with the psychological and social issues that arise.

Neurological Voice Disorders

Mrs. Finley, age 45, developed a voice problem after undergoing surgery to remove her thyroid gland. After the surgery, her voice was breathy, and she choked whenever she drank liquids too quickly. She was evaluated by an otolaryngologist, who diagnosed paralysis of the right vocal fold. The doctor suggested that the nerve serving the vocal fold had probably been injured during thyroid surgery. Because this nerve may recover from such damage, the physician decided to wait six months before considering surgical intervention. In the meantime, Mrs. Finley was referred to a speech-language pathologist to learn techniques for stimulating the left vocal fold to vibrate against the paralyzed right vocal fold. In addition, the speech-language pathologist provided Mrs. Finley with strategies for swallowing that would reduce her choking episodes.

Through voice exercises, Mrs. Finley learned to produce a soft voice instead of a breathy one. She was able to avoid choking by taking small sips of liquid while tilting her chin toward her chest. At five months post surgery, her voice had become stronger and closer to normal, indicating that innervation to the nerve was returning. By six months, her voice was clear and strong. The otolaryngologist re-examined her larynx at that time and determined that her right vocal fold had regained near-normal function.

Vocal Fold Paralysis

The recurrent laryngeal nerve is a branch of cranial nerve X (the vagus nerve). It provides neural input to muscles that move the vocal folds during voicing and swallowing (see Chapter 2). Vocal fold paralysis may result from damage to one or both recurrent laryngeal nerves on either side of the larynx. Unilateral vocal fold paralysis is most common. As in Mrs. Finley's case, damage to the nerve can occur when it is cut or compressed during surgery. Nerve damage can also result from a tumor or viral infection. In some cases, there is no known cause for nerve damage. Once the nerve to the laryngeal muscles is damaged, the vocal fold on the same side as the nerve is immobilized. Because the vocal folds cannot close completely, the

> The vocal folds are controlled by the right and left cranial nerve X (the vagus nerve), so nerve damage can affect the ability to move the vocal folds for breathing or speech.

voice is breathy, and patients often choke on liquids. In many cases, the impaired nerve recovers or regenerates within six months, resulting in recovery of the voice (Hockauf & Sailer, 1982; Mu & Yang, 1991).

To compensate for the paralyzed vocal fold, patients are taught to use greater effort to increase the movement of the unaffected vocal fold. With increased exertion, the healthy vocal fold may be able to vibrate against the paralyzed vocal fold to produce voicing. If the impaired nerve does not recover within six months, several surgical procedures are available to improve voice production. The surgical procedures move the immobile vocal fold to a more medial position so that the working vocal fold can vibrate against it. This was not necessary in Mrs. Finley's case because her vocal fold function recovered over time.

Paralysis of both vocal folds is a more serious problem than one-sided vocal fold paralysis. This disorder is typically caused by a problem within the central nervous system, such as a tumor or stroke that interferes with the generation of the neural signals that control movement of the vocal folds. Bilateral paralysis may result in difficulty breathing if the vocal folds are paralyzed in the closed (or nearly closed) position. Surgical intervention is usually necessary to create an open airway adequate for breathing.

Spasmodic Dysphonia

Spasmodic **dysphonia** is a rare voice disorder often characterized by a strained-strangled voice quality. The cause of this disorder was once believed to be related to psychological dysfunction (Arnold, 1959). It is currently thought to result from a dysfunction of the neural signals that control the vocal folds during speaking (Ludlow, 1995b). There are two types of spasmodic dysphonia: *adductor* and *abductor*. The adductor type occurs when the vocal folds close together too tightly during voiced speech sounds, resulting in a strained-strangled voice quality. The abductor type occurs when the vocal folds spasm apart during production of speech, resulting in excessive breathiness. Thus, the difference between the two types of spasmodic dysphonia can be remembered by these two rules:

1. The "AD" part of *adductor* means that the vocal folds spasm together.
2. The "AB" part of *abductor* means that the vocal folds spasm apart.

Adductor spasmodic dysphonia is characterized by intermittent onset of the strained-strangled voice quality, or voice stoppage. Additional muscular force is needed to move the folds from the midline, resulting in effortful voice production. The abductor type of spasmodic dysphonia occurs less frequently than the adductor type and is characterized by intermittent bursts of breathy voice quality. The breathiness results from spasms that keep the vocal folds apart during speech. Thus, these individuals may complain that they cannot make their voice loud enough to be heard.

Mr. Sparks, age 42, began to experience a catch in his voice while giving business reports to his employer. When this first began, he thought it was related to being nervous. However, he noticed the catches in his throat occurred more frequently over time. They also occurred at times when he was not nervous, such as after a church service or at home. Over the course of a year, the condition worsened. He put such effort into forcing his voice to function that he often became exhausted after a short period of talking. As the voice problem increased, his employer became displeased with Mr. Sparks's productivity and inability to provide regular business presentations. In desperation and frustration, Mr. Sparks went to see his doctor.

Mr. Sparks's primary care physician thought the problem was related to stress but agreed to refer him to a speech-language pathologist specializing in voice disorders. The speech-language pathologist recognized Mr. Sparks's problem as spasmodic dysphonia. Voice therapy was initiated to modify some of the problematic voice patterns he had developed as compensation for his uncooperative larynx. The speech-language pathologist also recommended consultation with an otolaryngologist for further evaluation. The otolaryngologist diagnosed Mr. Sparks with adductor spasmodic dysphonia and recommended medical treatment that consisted of injections of a toxin (Botox®) into the muscles of the vocal folds to reduce spasms during talking.

The injection of toxin into the vocal folds is the current treatment of choice for adductor-type spasmodic dysphonia. The toxin is botulinum type A, most often referred to as Botox. Botox impairs the ability of nerve endings to cause contraction of the vocal fold muscles. This results in weakened vocal folds that can no longer spasm closed during talking. However, the vocal folds may be so weak that they cannot come together to create a strong voice or protect the airway during swallowing. After a few weeks the Botox is absorbed by the body, and new nerve endings grow. At this point, the vocal folds begin to move normally, resulting in an improved voice quality. After three to six months, the Botox wears off, and the symptoms of spasmodic dysphonia typically return, requiring reinjection of Botox to maintain an improved voice.

> You have probably heard of the use of Botox® to reduce facial wrinkles, but you may not realize that it is also used to reduce unwanted muscle contractions in the larynx.

In some individuals, Botox does not effectively weaken the vocal fold muscles. In those cases, an alternative is surgery to cut one of the laryngeal nerves, creating unilateral vocal fold paralysis (Dedo & Behlau, 1991; Dedo & Izdebski, 1983; Weed et al., 1996). Although the resulting voice is slightly breathy, it allows the individual to function more normally in daily communication. In approximately 20 percent of individuals who undergo surgical cutting of the laryngeal nerve, the nerve regrows, and symptoms of adductor spasmodic dysphonia return within one to three years after the surgery (Dedo & Behlau, 1991). Although cutting the nerve is a treatment of last resort, newer methods show promise for more successful long-term benefits for those who do not respond well to Botox treatment (Weed et al., 1996).

Despite its successes in the treatment of adductor-type spasmodic dysphonia, Botox injections are not as effective with abductor spasmodic dysphonia. Botox treatment is typically attempted with abductor spasmodic dysphonia to see if it will effectively weaken the laryngeal muscles that pull the vocal folds apart during a spasm. However, the improvement is usually minimal and lasts only two to four weeks. In addition, these individuals often experience an extremely breathy voice for several weeks after treatment before their voice improves (Ludlow, 1995a). Presently, there is no consistently effective way to treat abductor spasmodic dysphonia.

Voice Assessment

The goal of a voice evaluation is to determine the nature of the problem, its probable cause, and the options available to treat the disorder. Some people go to their primary care physician first, who then refers them to an otolaryngologist or speech-language pathologist. Others seek help on their own and go directly to the otolaryngologist. Otolaryngologists with specialized interest in voice disorders often work with a speech-language pathologist with similar interests. Thus, medical evaluation and treatment may be augmented by voice therapy from a speech-language pathologist. Depending on the setting and equipment available for assessing the voice problem, various methods of evaluation may be used.

Voice evaluations begin with gathering information about the history of the problem and the symptoms present at the time of the examination. This information influences the evaluation procedures as well as the treatment.

Ms. Norwood worked as a real estate agent for the past six years and was one of the top salespeople in her company. The company relocated to a new building two years ago. Since the relocation, numerous renovation projects were necessary, such as putting in new carpeting and painting. She noticed that whenever she worked in her new office, her voice became increasingly hoarse over the course of the day. When her productivity dropped significantly and she felt increasingly anxious about her work, she sought medical help from an otolaryngologist.

The otolaryngologist looked at Ms. Norwood's larynx and noted that both vocal folds were swollen and red and did not vibrate normally during voicing. Thinking that she probably developed improper voicing patterns that led to changes in the vocal folds, the otolaryngologist referred her to a speech-language pathologist for voice therapy. The speech-language pathologist documented events leading to Ms. Norwood's voice disorder and discovered her problems began after her office was relocated to the new building. More specifically, her voice problems coincided with the new carpet and paint in her office. The speech-language pathologist suspected that Ms. Norwood was sensitive to chemicals in the air from the renovations. She also had begun to cough frequently and clear her throat because it felt like something was in her throat. Furthermore, she reported drinking a lot of coffee and only small amounts of water each day. The caffeine from the coffee and the low amount of other fluids may have caused dehydration that exacerbated her voice disorder. The speech-language pathologist helped Ms. Norwood monitor and eliminate the daily habits that were irritating her voice and taught her techniques to improve the sound of her voice. In addition, she was instructed to avoid the office for two weeks to determine whether the chemicals from the new carpet and paint were irritating her vocal folds.

Ms. Norwood's voice improved dramatically over the two weeks she was away from her office. Upon her return, the voice problem returned despite her efforts to use the techniques she learned from the speech-language pathologist. Thus, it appeared that Ms. Norwood's voice problem was caused by her sensitivity to the chemicals in her office. She decided to work from home to avoid exposure to the chemical fumes until the renovation was completed.

In the example above, the true source of Ms. Norwood's voice problem was uncovered after all the information related to the onset of her voice disorder was obtained. The physical appearance of her larynx was similar to that associated with chronic improper and effortful use of the voice. However, use of the following case history guidelines helped to determine the probable causes of the voice problem and, consequently, influenced the course of treatment:

1. Obtain the client's description of the voice problem.
2. Determine whether the onset of the voice problem was associated with an illness, accident, or other significant circumstance.
3. Note the duration and consistency of the symptoms of the voice problem.
4. Note patterns or variability in the reported symptoms or severity of the voice problem on a daily, weekly, monthly, and seasonal basis.
5. Obtain a description of the client's daily voice use.
6. Obtain a description of the client's work, home, and social activities.
7. Note whether the client's voice changes across different environments, speaking situations, or times of the day.

The case history provides information concerning development and impact of the voice disorder on the individual's life. It also provides an opportunity for the speech-language pathologist to get to know the client as an individual, which is important for designing successful behavioral therapy. In Ms. Norwood's case, an examination of the circumstances leading to the voice problem helped reveal the true cause of the voice problem, resulting in an effective voice treatment plan.

> A careful case history may reveal the likely cause of a voice disorder.

In addition to the case history, a voice evaluation also includes examination of the vocal mechanism. In Ms. Norwood's case, the otolaryngologist examined the larynx to determine whether vocal pathology was present. To observe the pharynx and larynx, the physician may use a tongue depressor, a light to illuminate the structures, and a laryngeal mirror to reflect their image. Other ways of viewing the soft palate and throat utilize fiberoptic equipment to obtain a video recording of the soft palate or throat. This procedure is called videoendoscopy. Videoendoscopy can be performed using a scope placed through the mouth or nose. The scope inserted through the nose (i.e., **nasoendoscope**) is a small tube with fiberoptic cables that illuminate and allow viewing of the nasal passages, soft palate, pharynx, and larynx. The type of scope inserted through the mouth is a rigid scope that looks like a steel rod with a lens on the end. It acts like a periscope in that it is placed over the tongue and provides a view of the larynx from just beyond the back of the

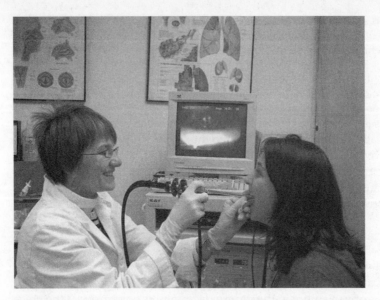

FIGURE 6.5   The vocal folds are viewed from above using a rigid scope placed at the back of the mouth. Note the image of the healthy vocal folds on the video monitor.

tongue (see Figure 6.5). The image obtained by either scope is displayed on a monitor and can be recorded on videotape. The rigid scope obtains a closer view of the vocal folds than the flexible scope, but the client cannot talk with the rigid scope in his or her mouth. The flexible scope is a good way to obtain a recording of the structures in the throat during speech. The lighting used for both scopes can be changed into a strobe light while the client sustains a vowel sound such as "ee." The strobe light illuminates only a fraction of the vocal fold vibrations so that they appear to occur in slow motion and are easier to evaluate.

The voice evaluation should include assessment of the facial muscles, lips, teeth, soft and hard palate, tonsils, and pharynx, because these structures may contribute to a voice disorder. Other components of a voice evaluation include respiration testing, acoustic measurements of the voice (e.g., frequency and intensity), and descriptions of the voice quality (e.g., breathy, hoarse) as perceived during different speaking tasks. The combined information from observation and measurements helps the speech-language pathologist determine the best approach for treating the client's voice problem. They can also be compared to findings after therapy.

Ms. Alvarez worked as a kindergarten teacher. During the first six months of her job, she began experiencing increased hoarseness that worsened from morning to night. By the end of each week, she could barely make herself heard in the classroom. Ms. Alvarez became frightened that she might have laryngeal cancer, so she went to see an otolaryngologist. The otolaryngologist looked at Ms. Alvarez's larynx and noted the presence of two vocal nodules. In addition, her vocal folds were red and swollen. Ms. Alvarez was referred to a speech-language pathologist for further evaluation of her voice and voice therapy.

To assess vocal fold vibration, the speech-language pathologist performed videoendoscopy on Ms. Alvarez using the rigid scope and a strobe light. The speech-language pathologist also tape-recorded Ms. Alvarez's voice during sustained phonation of "ah" and "ee" and while reading. The speech-language pathologist asked Ms. Alvarez about her work, family, and social life to obtain a better idea of how she uses her voice in different environments. From this information, the speech-language pathologist determined that Ms. Alvarez's problems were primarily related to how she used her voice at work. She often needed to shout above noise to get the children's attention. The speech-language pathologist suggested using a microphone system so that Ms. Alvarez could project her voice above the noise without much effort. In addition, they discussed instructional strategies such as using a whistle to get attention and using more visual aids to help preserve her voice. Finally, the speech-language pathologist taught Ms. Alvarez how to project her voice without straining. After one month, Ms. Alvarez's voice had improved noticeably. On reexamination, the vocal nodules appeared smaller than they had been initially.

In Ms. Alvarez's case, the strain on her voice at work led to the development of vocal nodules. The speech-language pathologist knew that vocal nodules usually occurred with chronic misuse of the voice. The therapy implemented with Ms. Alvarez included the following:

1. Elimination of harmful daily vocal habits.
2. Learning new techniques to effectively use the voice without strain.

As discussed earlier, these are the two primary approaches used to treat voice disorders resulting from harmful vocal habits. In severe cases, surgical removal of the vocal nodules may be necessary; however, more frequently, voice therapy is successful in treating clients such as Ms. Alvarez and Ms. Norwood.

Dysphagia

Eating is vital to maintaining life and providing the energy for basic bodily functions. The process of ingestion begins with chewing and swallowing food, a complex process that we do not often think about. However, when swallowing is impaired, we become more aware of how large a role eating plays in our lives. In addition to providing nutrition, eating serves as the focus of many social functions. Impaired eating, called **dysphagia** (pronounced dis-fay-jah), may create such difficulties that eating becomes an unpleasant activity and social occasions are avoided.

Although individuals diagnosed with dysphagia can be of any age, most are over 55 years old. In that age group, the prevalence is estimated at between

> We rarely think about what processes are involved in swallowing, but if the ability to eat and drink are impaired, it quickly becomes a major concern.

16 to 22 percent (Bloem et al., 1990; Kjellen & Tibbling, 1981). This includes a wide range of problems with eating that are related to stroke, neuromuscular problems, traumatic brain injury, progressive neurological diseases, surgery to structures involved with ingestion of food, gastroesophageal reflux, head and neck cancer, and cognitive problems such as dementia. In young people, dysphagia primarily relates to illness, trauma, surgeries of the head and neck, severe reflux, or congenital malformations.

In order to understand dysphagia, one must appreciate the components of normal eating. There are four phases involved, any of which may be impaired in someone with dysphagia. Figure 6.6 illustrates the sequence of the phases of swallowing.

The Normal Swallow

Phase One.   The first phase of eating is referred to as the *oral preparatory phase* (see Figure 6.6A). This phase is important for preparing food in the mouth for transport to the stomach. During this phase, the lips, tongue, and soft palate play a major role in holding the food within the oral cavity. The tongue moves the food around so that it can be chewed and then gathered into a central groove formed by the tongue prior to swallowing. The collection of food held together by the tongue is referred to as a food **bolus**. Saliva produced by glands in the mouth begins the digestion process. Saliva coats the food so that it is moist, and the digestive chemicals soften the food prior to swallowing. Problems with the oral preparatory phase may arise because of congenital malformations of the oral structures or changes related to age, surgery, trauma, or neurological problems.

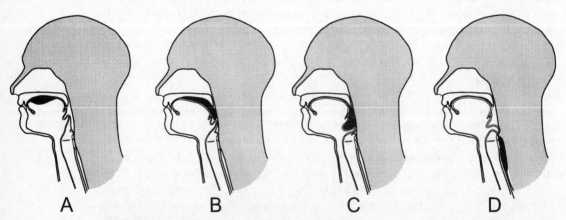

FIGURE 6.6   The four phases of eating are shown: (A) the oral preparatory phase, (B) the oral transport phase, (C) the pharyngeal phase, (D) and the esophageal phase. The black shape represents the food bolus as it travels from the oral cavity to the esophagus.

Mrs. Baker, age 71, had lost all of her teeth and had not replaced them with dentures. As a consequence, she was unable to eat any food that required chewing, such as meat, popcorn, salad, or fruit. Her self-imposed diet was restricted to soups, applesauce, oatmeal, and fluids. Over time, Mrs. Baker lost considerable weight and became malnourished. She sought help from her doctor, who recognized that her health issues were related to her diet and chewing problems. Mrs. Baker was admitted to the hospital, where she received intravenous fluids to rehydrate and rebalance her body chemistry. She was seen by a dietician, who recommended supplemental drinks to increase Mrs. Baker's daily intake of calories and fluid. Mrs. Baker was also seen by a dentist to consider purchasing dentures to allow her to eat a normal diet. Once Mrs. Baker began to gain more weight and was more normally nourished, she was released from the hospital and instructed to check back with her doctor and dietician periodically for monitoring of her health and diet.

> Go get a snack, maybe a cookie or cracker. As you eat it, take note of what you are doing as you chew and prepare the food to swallow. Place your hand lightly on your throat as you swallow. What do you feel happening?

In this example, Mrs. Baker's lack of teeth resulted in difficulty chewing, which limited her food options. She did not make wise food choices to ensure adequate nutritional and caloric intake. As a consequence, she lost weight and jeopardized her health due to poor nourishment. Mrs. Baker's situation was easily remedied by high-calorie drink supplements and by obtaining dentures. However, if dentures were not an option for her, Mrs. Baker would need to consider using long-term nutritional supplemental drinks to balance her diet and ensure adequate caloric intake.

Phase Two.   Once food is chewed and ready to be swallowed, the tongue gathers it into a cohesive bolus held between the tongue and hard and soft palate. The tongue propels the bolus into the pharynx by pressing up against the hard palate and pushing the bolus backward. This phase of transporting the bolus from the oral cavity into the pharynx is called the *oral transport phase* of the swallow (see Figure 6.6B).

Mr. Roswell, age 85, suffered a stroke that impaired his ability to control tongue and lip movements. As a consequence, it was difficult to control the food in his mouth while chewing. Food and fluids often spilled out of his mouth because his lips were too weak to keep them in his oral cavity. Mr. Roswell also had difficulty collecting the food in his mouth into a cohesive bolus for swallowing. After swallowing, some food remained in his mouth.

The speech-language pathologist assessed Mr. Roswell while he ate and determined that his primary difficulty was controlling food in the mouth. A procedure called *flexible endoscopic examination of swallowing* (FEES) was performed to visualize the pharynx while he swallowed measured amounts of milk and then applesauce. FEES involves the placement of a fiberoptic tube in the nose to allow viewing of the pharynx from above. This exam showed that after a teaspoon of milk was placed in Mr. Roswell's mouth the milk ran back into the pharynx before he initiated a swallow. Milk also spilled through his lips. Mr. Roswell was able to control the applesauce so that it did not spill into the pharynx or out through his lips. He was able to swallow all of the applesauce so that none remained in his mouth.

The speech-language pathologist recommended that Mr. Roswell's wife try thickening liquids and soups using cornstarch or a food-thickening product. This allowed Mr. Roswell to place a spoonful of food with a consistency similar to applesauce on his tongue and immediately swallow without having to chew first. Adding thickener to liquids also allowed Mr. Roswell improved oral control so that liquids did not spill out of his mouth or into his throat before initiating a swallow. Treatment included exercises to strengthen his tongue, lips, and jaw and to increase the range of their motion in order to control food in his mouth. The combination of strengthening exercises and the use of foods with preferred consistencies helped Mr. Roswell recover most of his oral control so that he could enjoy a wider variety of foods.

As seen in the example of Mr. Roswell, difficulty with the oral transport phase can prevent an individual from moving food out of the oral cavity to be swallowed. However, simple measures can be taken to help compensate for this problem by restricting foods to those the individual can manage best. In addition, weakness of the oral musculature may be improved by strengthening and range-of-motion exercises for the tongue, lips, and jaw (Logemann, 1983).

Phase Three.   The *pharyngeal phase* of swallowing is characterized by movement of the food bolus through the pharynx and into the esophagus (see Figure 6.6C). The bolus is propelled into the pharynx, and, as it passes over the back of the tongue, muscles of the pharynx contract to continue the propulsive action initiated by the tongue. As the superior portion of the pharynx contracts, the airway closes and the larynx elevates. This raised position during the swallow maximizes protection from *aspiration* of food into the airway. After the bolus enters the esophagus, the pharyngeal structures return to their resting positions. This phase is less than one second in duration.

Mrs. Lasser, age 65, began having difficulty swallowing. She felt as though there was something caught in her throat, and she needed to drink extra fluid to clear the food that was stuck. In addition, she experienced choking on the fluids she drank as she tried to clear her throat. Her swallowing difficulties required so much time and effort that she stopped enjoying meals and was embarrassed to eat in front her friends. As a result, she reduced the amount of food eaten and declined invitations to join friends for meals. After losing weight and becoming malnourished, Mrs. Lasser went to see her doctor.

Mrs. Lasser's doctor referred her for a swallowing examination, which was performed jointly by a radiologist and speech-language pathologist. During the test, Mrs. Lasser experienced all of the swallowing difficulties described earlier. The examination revealed that Mrs. Lasser's pharyngeal muscles appeared weak and her larynx was not elevating as it should during swallowing. The food she swallowed was not cleared completely from her throat. The speech-language pathologist showed Mrs. Lasser a way to swallow while tilting her chin downward. Mrs. Lasser used this posture while eating and found swallowing less difficult. However, she still needed to follow each bite of food with water or juice to clear her throat completely.

As shown in this case, impairment of the pharyngeal phase of the swallow can often be compensated for by simple posture changes. If food does not clear the throat during this phase of the swallow, the individual risks aspiration of food into the airway. This can lead to inflammation of the lungs, which is a potentially serious illness called aspiration pneumonia.

> Speech-language pathologists trained in the area of dysphagia play a central role in the diagnosis and management of swallowing disorders.

A team assessment by the radiologist and speech-language pathologist is the best way to assess the pharyngeal phase of swallowing. Using a procedure called a modified barium swallow, the patient is given food or liquid mixed with a radio-contrast material, barium, which is detected using an X-ray procedure called **videofluoroscopy**. Videofluoroscopy allows visualization of the pharyngeal structures and their movement during swallowing. It also allows identification and estimation of the amount of food aspirated into the airway before, during, and after the swallow. In addition, videofluoroscopy permits determination of whether changes in posture or food consistency improve the clearance of food from the mouth and throat.

Phase Four.   The final, *esophageal phase* of swallowing involves transportation of the bolus to the stomach by the esophagus (see Figure 6.6D). The esophagus pushes the bolus toward the stomach using muscle contractions, called **peristaltic contractions** that squeeze each portion of the esophagus from the top to the bottom. This muscle action is similar to that used by a worm as it moves along the ground. That is, each muscle segment surrounding the esophagus contracts in sequence from the upper esophagus to the stomach so that the bolus is moved into the stomach.

> *Rocco*, age 6 months, began spitting up copious amounts after drinking a bottle of formula. When he spits up, he tends to exhibit gagging behaviors and difficulty breathing. More recently he has developed a wet cough and appears to have stopped gaining weight. His crying voice and cooing voice appeared hoarse. Rocco's mother also reports frequent occurrence of hiccups and frequent burping. However, there was no sign of a fever or loss of hunger or thirst. Rocco's mother sought help from a pediatrician. The pediatrician suspected that Rocco exhibited a severe form of gastrointestinal **reflux**. The severity of Rocco's reflux warranted referral to a pediatric gastroenterology specialist. The gastroenterologist confirmed the diagnosis of reflux using a barium swallow examination to assess Rocco's esophagus and digestive tract. This radiologic test entailed swallowing a liquid barium contrast while videofluoroscopy was used to monitor the path of the barium. The test revealed that any food swallowed by Rocco was propelled back into the esophagus from the stomach within minutes of being swallowed. The gastroenterologist prescribed a medication to increase the rate at which the stomach empties. He also recommended a different formula that did not contain lactose, in case Rocco had a food sensitivity. Strategies for positioning Rocco during eating were offered by the occupational therapist and speech-language pathologist. The occupational therapist also recommended using a special bottle that reduced the amount of air swallowed during feeding sessions. The combined strategies were successful in reducing the degree and frequency of Rocco's reflux. In fact, within one month, he was happily feeding, with minimal regurgitation, and had gained three pounds.

As all of these cases demonstrate, dysphagia occurs when there is a problem with any or all of the four phases of swallowing. Common signs of dysphagia include the following:

- Difficulty initiating a swallow
- Difficulty chewing food due to poor dentition (as in Mrs. Baker's case)
- Difficulty controlling food in the oral cavity, such that it spills out of the mouth or into the airway before the larynx closes to protect the airway (as in Mr. Roswell's case)
- Choking when swallowing food, and food sticking in the throat (as Mr. Lasser experienced)
- Reflux of food from the esophagus or stomach back up to the throat or mouth (as in Rocco's case)

Various methods exist for assessing the swallow, as described in the above examples. Imaging techniques such as the FEES method (Langmore, Schatz, & Olsen, 1988) and the modified barium swallow (Logemann, 1993) are most frequently used to visualize the oral, pharyngeal, and esophageal structures. Although the speech-language pathologist can perform the FEES method if properly trained, an otolaryngologist may obtain FEES images while the speech-language pathologist administers the test food substances. During a modified barium swallow, the radiologist or radiology technician performs the videofluorographic imaging while the speech-language pathologist administers the barium contrast substances and determines which postures or consistencies appear to be successfully swallowed during testing. The gastroenterologist and radiologist are best trained to assess esophageal and other digestive organs during the barium swallow.

Assessing and providing care to someone with dysphagia may involve many professionals, including a speech-language pathologist, radiologist, gastroenterologist, otolaryngologist, neurologist, dentist, nurse, social worker, dietician, occupational therapist, and psychologist. The speech-language pathologist plays a major role in the assessment procedures, making recommendations to compensate for the dysphagia and referring the individual for further assessment by other dysphagia team members. Treatment of dysphagia most frequently entails simple measures such as changing the posture of the head and body during eating and swallowing, altering the consistency of the foods eaten, changing the temperature of foods to improve initiation of the swallow, and performing exercises to increase strength and range of motion of oral structures. Other treatment methods provided by medical specialists include the use of drugs to improve smooth muscle contraction, non-oral feeding using a nasogastric or gastric tube, and surgical intervention.

Clinical Problem Solving

Mrs. Hepple, age 65, underwent surgery to remove a portion of her esophagus that was cancerous. After surgery, her voice was breathy, and she choked every time she drank water. In addition, the food she swallowed came back up.

She was sent to an otolaryngologist, who examined her vocal folds and noted that the left vocal fold was not moving during voicing. She was referred to a speech-language pathologist, who used rigid videoendoscopy with a strobe light to further evaluate her voice. Mrs. Hepple's vocal folds did not come together completely when vibrating. The speech-language pathologist was concerned about Mrs. Hepple's difficulties with swallowing and suggested a modified barium swallow study. During this test, the speech-language pathologist noted that liquids entered Mrs. Hepple's trachea during the pharyngeal phase of the swallow. Subsequently, she choked and coughed to clear the liquid from her airway.

1. Why does Mrs. Hepple have a breathy voice quality?
2. What do you think caused her left vocal fold to stop moving?
3. How might the speech-language pathologist try to help improve her voice quality?
4. Might the voice problem go away with voice therapy?
5. What phase of the swallow is impaired?

REFERENCES

Arnold, G. E. (1959). Spastic dysphonia: I. Changing interpretations of a persistent affliction. *Logos, 2*, 3–14.

Bloem, B. R., Lagaay, A. M., van Beek, W., Haan, J., Roos, R. A. C., & Wintzen, A. R. (1990). Prevalence of subjective dysphagia in community residents aged over 87. *British Medical Journal, 300*, 721–722.

Brodnitz, F. S. (1971). *Vocal rehabilitation*. Rochester, MN: Whiting Press.

Carding, P. N., Roulstone, S., Northstone, K., & the ALSPAC Study Team (2006). The prevalence of childhood dysphonia: A cross-sectional study. *Journal of Voice, 20(4)*, 623–630.

Casper, J. K., & Colton, R. H. (1993). *Clinical manual for laryngectomy and head and neck cancer rehabilitation*. San Diego: Singular Publishing Group.

Dedo, H. H., & Behlau, M. S. (1991). Recurrent laryngeal nerve section for spastic dysphonia: 5- to 14-year preliminary results in the first 300 patients. *Annals of Otology, Rhinology, and Laryngology, 100(4)*, 274–279.

Dedo, H. H., & Izdebski, K. (1983). Intermediate results of 306 recurrent laryngeal nerve sections for spastic dysphonia. *Laryngoscope, 93*, 9–16.

Derkay, C. S., & Darrow, D. H. (2006). Recurrent respiratory papillomatosis. *Annals of Otology, Rhinology, & Laryngology, 115(1)*, 1–11.

Dietrich, M., Verdolini Abbott, K., Gartner-Schmidt, J., & Rosen, C. A. (2008). The frequency of perceived stress, anxiety, and depression in patients with common pathologies affecting voice. *Journal of Voice, 22(4)*, 472–488.

Fritzell, B. (1995). *Occupation and voice problems*. Paper presented at the Proceedings from XXIII World Congress of IALP [abstract].

Gray, S. D., Hammond, E., & Hanson, D. F. (1995). Benign pathologic responses of the larynx. *Annals of Otology, Rhinology, and Laryngology, 104(1)*, 13–18.

Hockauf, H., & Sailer, R. (1982). Postoperative recurrent nerve palsy. *Head and Neck Surgery, 4*, 380–384.

Johns, M. M. (2003). Update on the etiology, diagnosis, and treatment of vocal fold nodules, polyps, and cysts. *Current Opinion in Otolaryngology Head and Neck Surgery, 11*(6), 456–461.

Kjellen, G., & Tibbling, L. (1981). Manometric oesophageal function, acid perfusion test and symptomatology in a 55-year-old general population. *Clinical Physiology, 1*, 405–415.

Kleinsasser, O. (1979). *Microlaryngoscopy and endolaryngeal microsurgery: Technique and typical findings.* Baltimore: University Park Press.

Kleinsasser, O. (1990). Restoration of voice in benign lesions of the vocal fold by endolaryngeal microsurgery. In R. T. Sataloff (Ed.), *Voice perspectives.* San Diego: Singular Publishing.

Langmore, S. E., Schatz, K., & Olsen, N. (1988). Fiberoptic endoscopic examination of swallowing safety: A new procedure. *Dysphagia, 2*, 216–219.

Logemann, J. A. (1983). *Evaluation and treatment of swallowing disorders.* Austin, TX: Pro-Ed.

Logemann, J. A. (1993). *Manual for the videofluorographic study of swallowing* (2nd ed.). Austin, TX: Pro-Ed.

Ludlow, C. (1995a). Treating the spasmodic dysphonias with botulinum toxin: A comparison of results with adductor and abductor spasmodic dysphonia and vocal tremor. In J. Tsui & D. Calne (Eds.), *The dystonias.* New York: Dekker.

Ludlow, C. L. (1995b). Management of the spasmodic dysphonias. In J. S. Rubin, R. T. Sataloff, & G. S. Korovin (Eds.), *Diagnosis and treatment of voice disorders* (pp. 436–434). New York: Igaku-Shoin.

McCrory, E. (2001). Voice therapy outcomes in vocal fold nodules: A retrospective audit. *International Journal of Language and Communication Disorders, 36*(Suppl.), 19–24.

McFarlane, S. C., & Von Berg, S. (1998). Facilitative techniques in intervention for dysphonia. *Current Opinion in Otolaryngology and Head and Neck Surgery, 6*, 161–165.

McFarlane, S. C., & Watterson, T. L. (1990). Vocal nodules: Endoscopic study of their variations and treatment. *Seminars in Speech and Language, 11*, 47–59.

McKenna, J. P., Fornataro-Clerici, L. M., McMenamin, P. G., & Leonard, R. J. (1991). Laryngeal cancer: Diagnosis, treatment and speech rehabilitation. *American Family Physician, 44*(1), 123–129.

Mendenhall, W. M., Parsons, J. T., Stringer, S. P., Cassisi, N. J., & Million, R. R. (1988). T1-T2 vocal cord carcinoma: A basis for comparing the results of radiotherapy and surgery. *Head and Neck Surgery, 12*, 204–209.

Mu, L., & Yang, S. (1991). An experimental study on the laryngeal electromyography and visual observations in varying types of surgical injuries to the unilateral recurrent laryngeal nerve in the neck. *Laryngoscope, 101*, 699–708.

National Institute on Deafness and Other Communication Disorders. (2011, September 15). Statistics on voice, speech, and language. Retrieved from www.nidcd.nih.gov/health/statistics/vsl.asp

Rafferty, M. A., Fenton, J. E., & Jones, A. S. (2001). The history, aetoiology and epidemiology of laryngeal carcinoma. *Clinical Otolaryngology, 26*(6), 442–446.

Roy, N., Bless, D.M., & Heisey, D. (2000). Personality and voice disorders: A multitrait-multidisorder analysis. *Journal of Voice, 14*, 521–548.

Roy, N., Merrill, R. M., Gray, S. D., & Smith, E. M. (2005). Voice disorders in the general population: Prevalence, risk factors, and occupational impact. *The Laryngoscope, 115*, 1988–1995.

Roy, N., Merrill, R. M., Thibeault, S., Gray, S. D., & Smith, E. M. (2004). Voice disorders in teachers and the general population: Effects on work performance, attendance, and future career choices. *Journal of Speech, Language, and Hearing Research, 47*, 542–551.

Roy, N., Merrill, R. M., Thibeault, S., Parsa, R. A., Gray, S. D., & Smith, E.M. (2004). Prevalence of voice disorders in teachers and the general population. *Journal of Speech, Language, and Hearing Research, 47*, 281–293.

Roy, N., Stemple, J., Merrill, R. M., & Thomas, L. (2007). Epidemiology of voice disorders in the elderly: Preliminary findings. *The Laryngoscope, 117*, 626–633.

Silverman, E., & Zimmer, C. (1975). Incidence of chronic hoarseness among school-age children. *Journal of Speech and Hearing Disorders, 40*, 211–215.

Smith, E., Gray, S., Dove, H., Kirchner, L., & Heras, H. (1997). Frequency and effects of voice problems in teachers. *Journal of Voice, 11*, 81–87.

Smith, E., Verdolini, K., Gray, S., Nichols, S., Lemke, J., Barkmeier, J., Dove, H., & Hoffman, H. (1996). Effect of voice disorders on quality of life. *Journal of Medical Speech-Language Pathology, 4*(4), 223–244.

Thibeault, S. L., Merrill, R. M., Roy, N., Gray, S.D., & Smith, E. M. (2004). Occupational risk factors associated with voice disorders among teachers. *Annals of Epidemiology, 14*, 786–792.

Titze, I. R., Lemke, J., & Montequin, D. (1997). Populations in the U.S. workforce who rely on voice as a primary tool of trade: A preliminary report. *Journal of Voice, 11*(3), 254–259.

Weed, D. T., Jewett, B. S., Rainey, C., Zealear, D. L., Stone, R. E., Ossoff, R. H., & Netterville, J. L. (1996). Long-term follow-up of recurrent laryngeal nerve avulsion for the treatment of spasmodic dysphonia. *Annals of Otology, Rhinology, Laryngology, 105*(8), 592–601.

Yamaguchi, H., Yotsukura, Y., Kondo, R., Horiguchi, S., Imaizumi, S., & Hirose, H. (1986). Nonsurgical therapy for vocal nodules. *Folia Phoniatrica, 38*, 372–373.

READINGS FROM THE POPULAR LITERATURE

Fox, M. J. (2002). *Lucky man*. New York: Hyperion. (Parkinson disease)

Rehm, D. (1999). *Finding my voice*. New York: Alfred A. Knopf. (spasmodic dysphonia)

Reid, R. J. (2004). *In a strange land*. Twickenham, UK: Athena Press. (laryngectomy)

Language

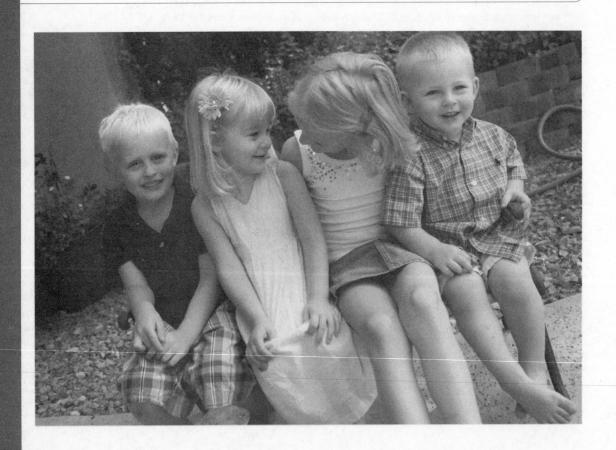

Human communication includes a wide range of activities. Much of it is nonverbal: A pointed stare or a strategic clearing of the throat is often sufficient to convey an emotion or prompt the recipient to respond. A speaker's body posture and hand gestures convey aspects of attitude, emphasis, and emotion. Often, these nonverbal forms of communication are unintentional and nonspecific. When a specific message must be conveyed, people typically employ language. Language, whether spoken, written, or signed, uses a system of symbols to convey meaning. Language involves the interaction of many skills that combine for effective communication. A speaker must know the rules for combining sounds into words and words into sentences. The speaker uses both sentence structure and word meanings to convey the content of the message. Finally, the speaker must appreciate the rules of social discourse to use language effectively for communication. These are skills that emerge from infancy onward, and continue to be refined throughout childhood. To illustrate normal acquisition, we will follow the progression of language skills in a typically developing preschool child.

PREVIEW

Human communication provides an opportunity for the exchange of feelings, knowledge, and wants between two or more people. In the first year of life, a baby communicates primarily through changes in the voice with accompanying facial expressions and gestures. These nonverbal vocalizations in the early part of life, primarily expressions of internal biological states, are affective in nature, and are interpreted by those around the baby as communicating emotion. The vocalizations soon begin to take on the melody of speech. When we left our discussion of infant vocalization in Chapter 3, Abraham, a child whose development we have been following, was just beginning to say his first words.

The Components of Language

As effortless as language appears to be for most people, effective use involves the interaction of many skills. To understand the nature of language better, it is sometimes useful to examine the skills that contribute to overall language functioning. Bloom (1988) suggested that language skills can be described in terms of form, content, and use. **Form** includes phonology, syntax, and morphology. **Content** includes the meaning, or **semantics**, of words and utterances. **Use** includes pragmatic skills such as the rules of social discourse and the speaker's purpose for communication.

Language performance can be characterized by its content, form, and use.

Form

Phonology.   **Phonology** is the study of the sounds of speech. Linguists have been studying the phonological development of children since the early 1900s (Ingram, 1981). Much of current phonological investigation focuses on uncovering the rules

Did you even realize that you use /z/ to pluralize *bed*, but you use /s/ to pluralize *bets*? Why do you think we follow that rule?

required for combining speech sounds (or phonemes) to form syllables and words. As we saw in Chapter 1, any given language contains only a subset of the possible sound combinations that can be produced. For example, the phonology of English permits the /st/ blend at either the beginning or end of words, but /str/ can only appear at word beginnings. Likewise, there are specific rules for voicing or unvoicing in pluralization. If we were to pluralize the words *hat* and *hit*, we would add the unvoiced consonant /s/. Pluralization of a noun ending in a voiced consonant requires the use of the voiced cognate of /s/, the phoneme /z/. So, if we were to pluralize the word *bed*, we would add the /z/ phoneme, writing the word in phonetics as [bɛdz]. Such rules for how sound is used are part of the phonology of the language.

Syntax. **Syntax** refers to the structure of sentences. The structure can be described in terms of hierarchically ordered components, as illustrated in Figure 7.1. A syntactic theory describes the rules by which words may be combined into grammatically acceptable sentences. For example, in English, the subject of a declarative sentence (a noun or noun phrase) must precede the predicate (a verb or verb phrase). Therefore, a sentence such as "He is swinging" is acceptable, whereas "Is swinging he" is not. Syntactic rules also describe the constraints in combining words and phrases of particular types. For example, for the predicate "is swinging," there are a limited number of phrases that might follow it in a sentence. We might say, "He is swinging wildly," or "He is swinging on the porch swing," or "He is swinging the baby." The predicate "is swinging" belongs to a class of verbs that can be followed by an adverbial phrase, prepositional phrase, or noun phrase. For most people, the rules for combining words into sentences are unconscious and automatic. Knowledge of these syntactic rules allows

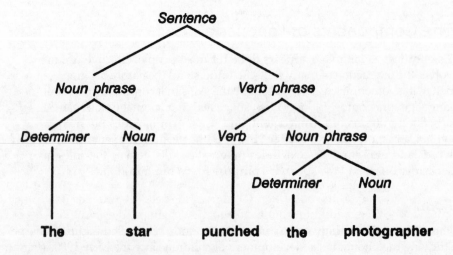

FIGURE 7.1 The syntactic structure of a sentence.

a speaker to produce grammatical utterances effortlessly. In any language, there is a limited number of acceptable syntactic structures. Therefore, knowledge of these structures allows listeners to anticipate the words they will hear and draw conclusions about how the words relate to one another to convey meaning. For example, in "Jamie asked Adelida . . ." there is a high probability that the sentence will continue with either a prepositional phrase (e.g., "about . . .") or a verb infinitive (for example, "to go . . ." or "to call . . ."). The listener, from the conversational context, may even be able to anticipate the precise phrase. Given the complete sentence "Jamie asked Adelida to go," the syntactic rules tell the listener that Jamie is doing the asking and that Adelida is being asked to go. In this way, the syntax has represented the general meaning of the utterance in a structured, rule-governed way. This phenomenon is referred to as mapping a deep structure (meaning) to a surface structure (syntax).

We will talk more about syntax in the next section of this chapter when we discuss language acquisition. Problems in syntactic comprehension and production in language-impaired children and adults will be presented in Chapters 8 and 9.

Morphology.   **Morphology** refers to how meaning is represented by the use of words, affixes, various grammar tenses (such as past tense), and plurality. A **morpheme** is the smallest unit of a language that has meaning. It can be a whole word, one of several parts of a word, the beginning of a word (i.e., a prefix, such as *un-*), or a word ending (i.e., a suffix, such as *-ing*). The following words contain one morpheme; they cannot be divided into any smaller units and still carry meaning:

> quick   (one morpheme)
>
> build   (one morpheme)
>
> structure   (one morpheme)

Words that can stand alone are called *free morphemes.* A second class of morphemes is called *bound morphemes* because they must be attached to other words. Bound morphemes include the suffixes *-ly*, *-er*, and *-ed* in:

> quickly   (two morphemes)
>
> builder   (two morphemes)
>
> structured   (two morphemes)

Each of these words contains two morphemes, one free and one bound. Notice that the bound morpheme changes the meaning of the word in each case. In some words the addition of a morpheme actually changes its syntactic classification. The addition of *-ly* changes *quick* from an adjective to an adverb. The addition of *-er* changes *build* from a verb to a noun. The addition of *-ed* to *structure* can change it from a noun to an adjective. In other cases, morphemes add meaning without changing the class of the word (e.g., *dog* versus *dogs*).

Children's acquisition of morphology seems to follow predictable stages. After analyzing the utterances of children over time, Brown (1973) developed five stages of sentence construction that seem to parallel (or mirror) overall language development. The five stages correspond to the average of number of morphemes a child says per utterance, known as the MLU, or mean length of utterance, in morphemes:

Stage I (1.75 morphemes). The child is using single words and is starting to put noun-verb sequences together, such as "Car go."

Stage II (2.25 morphemes). The child starts to use bound morphemes as part of his or her grammar, as in "Cars going."

Stage III (2.75 morphemes). The child begins to use questions and imperatives, for instance, "That a car?"

Stage IV (3.5 morphemes). The child begins to use complex sentences, for example, "Where's the car going?"

Stage V (4 morphemes). The child may use connectors and more functions, as in "Mom and Dad can come."

Although there is obvious overlap between successive stages, Brown and his colleagues conducted a number of studies over time that showed a progression from saying a single word to the two-word utterance to the telegraphic sentence, with the gradual refinement of grammar leading to complete sentences compatible with the adult model.

Content

Content includes the meanings of individual words and words in combination. The study of word meanings is sometimes referred to as **semantics**. Our basic use of language as a tool for communication is to transmit meaning to someone else. Hubbell (1985) noted, "Meaning is the bridge between the thoughts and experiences of individuals and the sequences of sounds they produce to symbolize those thoughts and experiences. Words symbolize concepts, and concepts represent experiences or reality" (p. 33).

As young children learn their native language, they attach meaning to a particular phonological sequence they have been hearing. The context in which they hear the word is critical to this process. As children hear words associated with particular actions and behaviors in social contexts, they begin to assign meaning to those words. Eventually, a word stands for those actions and feelings, without the need for the original context. As the child develops cognitively through various experiences, there is a greater coupling of words with meaning. The child begins to use "words to refer to or represent external objects and events" (Clark, 1979, p. 193).

Two kinds of meaning may develop for words, denotative and connotative. Denotative meaning is the literal meaning of the word. For example, for the word *milk*, we can use the dictionary definition of "a whitish fluid that is secreted by the mammary glands of female mammals for the nourishment of their young" as a literal, denotative meaning. Connotative meanings also reflect concepts associated with particular words, but they imply or suggest additional information that offers subtle overtones that distinguish words of very similar meanings. For example, if we associate *milk* with the concept of physical nourishment, we can make the connection to spiritual nourishment to understand an alternate meaning of milk in the metaphorical "milk of human kindness." Speakers learn the rules of the semantic system by hearing and using words in ways appropriate to both their connotative and denotative meanings. Although the differences in meaning are sometimes hard to explain, it is clear that we understand and associate feelings with certain words. A case in point: We would probably prefer to be called "unique" or even "unusual" rather than "atypical" or "abnormal." Connotative meanings often set an affective tone. For example, "Children may sometimes be unruly" has a more formal tone than "Kids can be squirrelly."

The sentence context influences the specific meanings that we attach to individual words. The meanings of nouns and verbs are modified by the use of adjectives and adverbs. The listener's expectations about the meaning of a sentence may change as later words cause it's meaning to shift. For example, the noun *shoe* typically produces in the mind of the listener a picture of a leather covering of the foot mounted on a thicker sole. We can see how the sentence context is used to produce many different meanings for this word:

If the shoe fits, wear it.	(a nonliteral, proverbial meaning)
It fits like an old shoe.	(from experience, old shoes feel good on the foot)
Make a ringer with a horseshoe.	(*horse* morpheme changes the meaning of *shoe*, and *ringer* requires specialized knowledge of horseshoe game)
You can't stop with worn shoes.	(a car's brake shoe is ineffective when worn)

In the preceding examples, we see that the noun *shoe* (which we may first think of as the object we wear on a foot) can have many other meanings. We understand the particular meaning in the context in which the utterance was made. Disagreements in interpreting what someone intended to say may sometimes relate to different interpretations of word meaning.

Use

How we use words, and in which situations, is the focus of language use, or pragmatics. Bates (1976) and Bruner (1975) pointed out that the human interaction a baby experiences in the first year of life establishes various pragmatic roles long before the baby is using language. The preverbal behaviors described in Chapter 3 are employed by babies to control and manipulate their environment. After the first

The social use of language is referred to as *pragmatics*. Our varied experiences with people foster growth of our pragmatic skills throughout life — maybe until we are too old to care what people think anymore.

six months of life, spontaneous vocalization begins to be replaced with intentional vocalization accompanied by expression and gesture (Oller, 1980). From about the age of 9 months, the baby enjoys interaction with the caregiver, using vocalization appropriately for such games as pat-a-cake and peek-a-boo. In these early games, the child is using vocalizations, to interact with others. Bates (1976) calls these "preverbal performatives," (p. 426). Even between 12 and 18 months, the baby uses single-word responses like "bye-bye" more as part of a physical interaction with the caregiver than as true words that represent specific concepts. These utterances are called "performative acts" by Bates. The performative act serves a communicative purpose for the child, such as declaring, promising, asking questions, and so forth (Bates, Benigni, Bretherton, Camaioni, & Volterra, 1977).

The speech acts theory, developed by Searle (1969), focuses on the speaker's intention rather than on the words used. Searle described three types of intents: *asserting, requesting,* and *ordering.* These categories focus on how the speaker is using language rather than on the specifics of what was said. Assertions are almost as varied as topics of communication, whereas requests are usually for some kind of action or information. Others have elaborated on this focus with additional functions that language serves. Lahey (1988) provided a description of many functions that children's language serves. Some examples follow:

1. Comment (I did it!)
2. Rejection (No anchovies!)
3. Pretend (Barbie goes in her dream house. . . .)
4. Obtain information (What's that?)
5. Routine (I pledge allegiance to the flag. . . .)

As young children grow, so does their verbal repertoire, enabling the use of language forms that meet the demands of particular situations. Children learn to communicate (verbally and nonverbally) one way to their peers, another way to their parents, and another way to the teacher or the doctor. The child learns that the situation or context of the communication has much to do with how things are phrased. The specific decision about what to say and how and when to say it is shaped by the success the child experiences in conversation. For example, the child soon learns that he can call his cousins by their first names but he'd better use "Aunt" or "Uncle" with their parents, even though the adults address each other by first name alone. Furthermore, the child soon understands that Grandmother likes to use baby talk and that Grandfather uses a very adult language form. Bilingual children learn which language to communicate with the different individuals in their lives. In Chapter 3, we saw the use of "child-directed speech" by Abraham's parents when addressing their infant son. However, it is unlikely that these parents speak to their bosses or coworkers in this style of speech. Instead, they adjust their speech to match the age and social status of their listener.

Early Language Development

Within the first four years of life, most children become quite proficient users of their native language. There is active and vigorous debate among those who study language acquisition concerning how this is accomplished. Some hold that the fact that these young children accomplish this feat without explicit instruction is evidence that humans come into the world with an innate capacity for language, or are even biologically preprogrammed with the basic parameters of language from birth (e.g., Chomsky, 1988; McNeill, 1970; Pinker, 1984; Poeppel & Wexler, 1993).

Others reject the idea that human infants are endowed with an inborn competence specifically for language. Instead, they hold that language acquisition reflects the application of broader cognitive processes that are supported by the human brain (Bates, 1999; Karmiloff-Smith, Plunket, Johnson, Elman, & Bates, 1998). From this perspective, language acquisition occurs because the infant brain is capable of such skills as associating events and perceiving patterns (Gómez & Gerken, 2000). Infants learn words because they can perceive the reoccurring

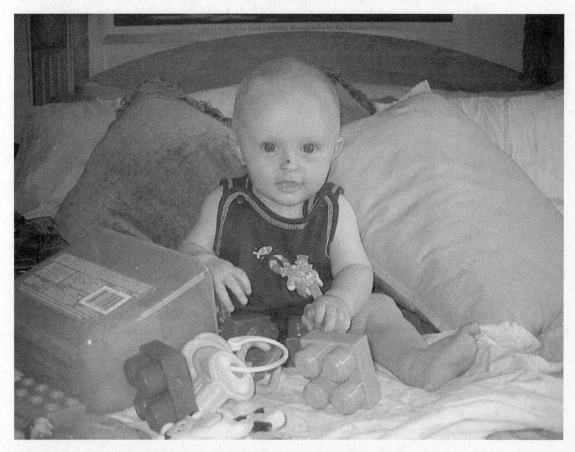

FIGURE 7.2 Infants have a remarkable ability to track features of language well before they produce their first words.

patterns of sounds that make up individual words and associate those specific sound sequences with particular objects, actions, and attributes. They likewise perceive other patterns involving syllables and words that provide syntactic structure and morpheme use.

Although the question of how language is acquired is a long way from being resolved, it has sparked interest in what very young children can show us about their capacity for language. New methods for studying language acquisition have demonstrated that infants not only know a considerable amount about their native language, but they have a remarkable capacity to learn simply by listening to the speech around them. Infants appear to be remarkably tuned to auditory input from the start and their auditory experiences provide the building blocks for language. Early on, infants are able to distinguish between the prosodic characteristics of their native language and those of an unfamiliar language (Mehler, Jusczyk, Lambertz, Halsted, Bertoncini, & Amiel-Tison, 1988; Nazzi, Jusczyk, & Johnson, 2000). Some have suggested that infants actively use prosodic information as a way to "chunk" a nearly continuous auditory speech stream into linguistically relevant units such as phrases or words. For example, in English, many words have a strong-weak stress pattern (e.g., "table," "peaches," "running," "open," "eager"). Although there are exceptions to this rule (e.g., "event," "describe"), a strong-weak pattern is prevalent enough that infants can use stress cues to make hypotheses concerning where words begin and end (e.g. "baby | is" is a more likely division of words than "ba | byis"). Infants can segment words with strong-weak stress from running speech at seven and a half months of age, and can segment weak-strong words by ten and a half months (Jusczyk, Houston, & Newsome, 1999).

Prosody is not the only information that infants use to learn spoken words. By eight months of age, infants are able to recognize that certain sound sequences co-occur in predictable sequences (Saffran, Aslin, & Newport, 1996; Pelucchi, Hay, & Saffran, 2009). Researchers refer to this as "statistical learning" because the infants appear to track which sequences of sounds have a high statistical probability of co-occurrence. For example, the sound /d/ is much more likely to be followed by /og/ than any other sounds in utterances like "good dog," "dogs bark," "The dog jumps," "My dog chews." The ability to track statistical information provides a means for infants to learn specific sound sequences that comprise individual words. These accomplishments occur months before infants begin to say their first words, between 10 and 12 months of age. Infants continue to use both this statistical information as well as prosodic information during their first year of life (Johnson & Seidl, 2008, Thiessen & Saffran, 2003).

As we saw in Chapter 3, when an infant begins to produce his or her first words, they do not always sound like the words an adult would use. Likewise, an infant may use a single sound sequence ("ma") to convey multiple meanings (e.g., "mommy," "milk," "mine"). These initial word forms are referred to as **protowords** (see Chapter 3) because they lack specificity in both phonological form and meaning relative to words adults use. Over time, the child will refine these early protowords so that they take on the standard pronunciation and meaning.

Young children show us that they understand something about the syntax and morphology of their language as they begin combining single words into two-word phrases. Rather than random word combinations (e.g., "talk you"), we see that these early combinations are simplified versions of adult-like grammar (e.g., "you talk"). However, this is not the beginning of morphosyntactic development. Infants are able to learn and recognize features of language form before they begin to produce it. In a series of experiments, researchers familiarized infants with a novel language and then tested the infants concerning what they had learned about the form of those languages. At twelve months of age, infants can learn the rules for simple two-word combinations (Gómez & Lakusta, 2004). This ability to recognize when words are correctly arranged emerges well before children are routinely producing three word phrases at 36 months (Miller, 1981a). By 15 months, infants can recognize syntactic patterns that underlie three-word phrases (Gómez & Maye, 2005). Sixteen-month-old infants can recognize certain forms of morphology and recognize when bound morphemes are correctly or incorrectly attached to words (Gerken, Wilson, & Lewis, 2005). This is also earlier than children typically use bound morphemes expressively (Miller, 1981b). In fact, it is the case that receptive skills are more advanced than expressive skills as language develops.

> Infants have extraordinary capabilities for learning about language, and are actively engaged in this process as they encounter spoken language in their environment.

As infants are actively engaged in the language-learning process, they receive help from the way adult speak to them. Adults commonly speak to infants and young children with exaggerated intonation referred to as *child-directed-speech* or, sometimes, *motherese* (see Chapter 3). This mode of speech may highlight the prosodic cues that infants use to learn new words. Adults also tend to use short and simple utterances with their children, so that the problem of discovering syntax has been simplified as well. Parents frequently direct their child's attention to an object before naming it, or they name objects the child are currently showing an interest in. This type of interaction creates the conditions under which a label and its referent co-occur so that new word meanings are acquired. We will see this in action as we examine the language development of Abraham, the young boy whose early speech development we considered in Chapter 3. We saw Abraham's communicative development progress from his first exposure to the sounds of language to the point where he was able to produce sound sequences recognizable as single words. This, in fact, was the onset of his expressive language. As you now know from this chapter, his language was also developing from birth, concurrently with the development of his speech. Here we pick up with Abraham at the onset of his first words.

Twelve to Eighteen Months

Abraham's parents note that he has been recognizing certain words for a couple of months now. When his mother looks at him and asks "Milk?," Abraham raises his arms to her in anticipation. She thinks that he has begun to use "Ma" to refer to her, but she isn't sure of this until he is a year old. This is his true first word.

Once the first word appeared, others soon followed. A child's first words reflect his or her environment. The family dog's name may be learned, and the word *dog* itself will follow. If there is no cat, however, that word will take longer to appear. Sometimes these first words are highly context specific. For example, Abraham could name animals from his Noah's ark book that he did not name at the zoo. Nonetheless, with each day and every new experience, there were opportunities to learn new words and refine his understanding of words recently acquired. For Abraham's parents, it seems like every day brings new words into his vocabulary. When children know about 50 words, they begin the process of combining them into simple phrases.

Twenty-one Months

Abraham visited us at the language clinic at 21 months of age. When he entered the large playroom, he was immediately attracted to the crayons and paper that we had set out on a child-size picnic table. He loved to color, which at this point consisted of light marks scribbled mostly on the page and occasionally on the table. At this age, Abraham's attention span for any one activity was fairly short. When he began to color, his mother had the following conversation with him:

MOTHER: You like to color, huh?

ABRAHAM: Gah!

MOTHER: Yeah, you like to color, huh?

ABRAHAM: Ah deh. Out.

MOTHER: Want to get out? (She lifts him out from between the table and bench.) You want to go look in that bag? Bring your bag. Bring the bag over here. (Abraham brings the bag.) All right! (Laughs) What's in there?

(Abraham and Mother look into the bag.)

ABRAHAM: Bribee [baby].

MOTHER: Yeah.

ABRAHAM: Beebee [baby].

MOTHER: That's your baby. (Takes it out)

ABRAHAM: Night night. Deh coo.

MOTHER: Blanket for the baby.

ABRAHAM: Deh yi gah.

MOTHER: Yeah, that's your grrrr bear. (Takes it out)

(Abraham wanders off . . .)

MOTHER: Where are you going, hun?

ABRAHAM: Ow meh.

MOTHER: You're coming here?

ABRAHAM: Eeehhh [yes].

MOTHER: What else is in the bag?

ABRAHAM: Ehhh off. (Abraham pulls at the vest he is wearing.)

MOTHER: Oh, we're gonna leave it on. Look how nice you look.

ABRAHAM: Ah hah.

MOTHER: Very handsome.

This short conversation illustrates many aspects of Abraham's current stage of language acquisition. The first thing we notice is that, although he is now using words, we don't always understand what he is saying. Even his parents do not always understand everything he says. However, when the context gives clues to the meaning of the words (e.g., pulling objects out of a bag), his mother can translate his attempts into actual words. In fact, parents provide indirect feedback about the form of their children's language by repeating and expanding on their children's utterances (Demetras, Post, & Snow, 1986).

At this age, Abraham's language consists mostly of single words. He is just beginning to use two-word combinations and an occasional three-word utterance. Abraham's production of single words, with few multi-word combinations, is reflected by an overall MLU (mean length of utterance in morphemes) of 1.49. These utterances consist almost exclusively of content-rich words (e.g., nouns, verbs). Completely absent are any of the grammatical morphemes (e.g., articles, plurals, verb tense markers). Like most children his age, Abraham can comprehend much longer utterances than he is able to produce. For example, his mother's direction to him ("Oh, we're gonna leave it on") is longer than what he produced.

Abraham has between fifty and hundred different words in his language repertoire. However, his understanding of the meanings of words may be different from those of an adult. This is the age when toddlers point to strange men in grocery stores and exclaim, "Daddy!" For them, the word *Daddy* may be broadly defined as including all adult males. The narrower meaning of, *Daddy* as "my male parent" will develop later. Conversely, other words may have too narrow a definition. *Doggie* may be used only with the household pet, and not for other dogs. Still other words are actually social routines (e.g., *Night night*) or parts of songs, which may not be used outside of that specific context. As children grow in both experience and cognitive maturity, their understanding of the meaning of words will become more refined and adultlike.

Despite the fact that most of his language consists of single words, Abraham gets a lot of "mileage" out of those single words. He is actually able to convey a range of meanings with similar utterances, depending on the situational context and his intonation. When we look at his utterances from the perspective of language content and use, we can see this flexibility of expression.

MOTHER: We got a bunch of different books here.

ABRAHAM: Elmo book! Elmo book! (Content: item name) (Use: requests an action [reading])

MOTHER: You want to read the Elmo book?

ABRAHAM: Elmo book. (Content: item name) (Use: confirmation)

(They read.)

MOTHER: Who's that?

ABRAHAM: Gower. (Content: character name) (Use: labeling; reply to mother)

MOTHER: Grover.

ABRAHAM: Gower coffee. (Content: possession) (Use: comment)

Twenty-eight Months

At 2 years of age, Abraham is quite the conversationalist. At this point, Abraham can be understood well by both family members and those who hear him speak less frequently. We can see an example when Abraham talks about his toddler gymnastics class.

MOTHER: What did you get to do at class?

ABRAHAM: Jump!

MOTHER: You get to jump. On what?

ABRAHAM: Trampoline.

AUTHOR: Did Mommy get to jump on the trampoline?

ABRAHAM: Yeah.

MOTHER: Did I jump on that trampoline?

ABRAHAM: No.

MOTHER: No.

AUTHOR: No? Why not?

ABRAHAM: She want to get off.

MOTHER: Who else got to jump on it?

ABRAHAM: Other boy turn.

MOTHER: Yeah. You guys shared, didn't you?

ABRAHAM: Yeah. (Abraham crouches and makes a funny face.) Went nnnnngggggggggg.

MOTHER: Is that what he said?

ABRAHAM: Yeah. I say that.

As this conversation illustrates, Abraham is talking in single words and short sentences. We hear the major content words (e.g., nouns, main verbs). We also hear the earliest-acquired grammatical morphemes (e.g., "com*ing* our house!" "Flower*s*."). However, most other grammatical units tend to be missing. In this early stage of language development, it is common to hear such "telegraphic speech" (Brown, 1976). Abraham's MLU on the day this conversation took place was 2.03, which is about average for children at this age.

We sometimes have difficulty understanding what Abraham says, not because the words themselves are mispronounced, but because he does not always provide enough information or background to convey the general context. For example, the word "jump" does not necessarily bring to mind bouncing on a trampoline when it is first said. In this case, Abraham's mother was filling in the background information and structure of the conversation by cueing him as to what information should be given next. In addition, children at this stage are likely to agree with what adults say, regardless of its actual truth, as we see here. Pragmatically, they understand that a positive response will continue the conversation, without appreciating that the listener's understanding has diverged from their own. Although Abraham's mother gets the conversation back on track, we can see that this tendency in young children can also lead to miscommunications.

Despite these limitations in form and content, Abraham is exhibiting a range of language use. During a play visit to the author at the clinic, we observed various pragmatic functions. The following is a small sample of these:

> By age 3, children are learning information about the world through language, not just what they observe in the here-and-now.

What that?	(request for information)
Mommy do it!	(request for action)
A doll.	(labeling)
Now him sad.	(commenting)
No! No!	(negating)

Thirty-nine Months.   Children's speech changes rapidly between the ages of 2 and 4. In twelve months, we can already see changes in the form of Abraham's language. We recorded this interaction between Abraham and his mother when Abraham was 39 months.

MOTHER: Oh, you know what? I should have brought your pictures of you and Christopher to show. They were so pretty. Remember?

ABRAHAM: You forgot?

MOTHER: I forgot to bring them. They were really neat.

ABRAHAM: The pictures that I made and colored?

MOTHER: Yep.

AUTHOR: You colored them by yourself?

ABRAHAM: Mmmhmm. I made 'em mixed with for the sky.

MOTHER: Yep, you mixed the color of the sky.

ABRAHAM: And I made the clouds inside.

MOTHER: You sure did.

ABRAHAM: But the 'nuther one was messed up.

MOTHER: Well, yeah. You did make one that you didn't like much.

> **ABRAHAM:** It was messed up.
>
> **MOTHER:** It was. But you really liked it because you put legs and feet and arms and hands.
>
> **ABRAHAM:** There wasn't enough room for the legs.

Although we still see a few form errors (e.g., "the 'nuther one" for "another one") we see noteworthy gains as well. Abraham increased the length of his utterances. His MLU on this day was 5.28. This is actually above average for his age. MLUs for children at this age typically range between 2.71 and 4.23 (Miller, 1981b). Abraham's MLU fluctuates from day to day as well. In a sample collected one month later, his MLU was 4.03. Other aspects of language form are entirely appropriate for Abraham's age. Most of his utterances now are complete sentences with nouns and verbs serving as subjects and predicates. Notice that Abraham now uses both content words and a number of grammatical morphemes (e.g., past tense -*ed*, plural *s*, articles *the* and *a*). Occasionally, we see complex sentences (e.g., "The pictures that I made and colored?").

Compared with the conversation we saw at age 28 months, Abraham's contributions carry much more content. Instead of just providing input when prompted, he is now contributing new information spontaneously. There are still instances in which his meaning is not entirely clear (e.g., "And I made the clouds inside"), but most of the time others can follow his conversations with little effort.

We can clearly see how form, content, and use have developed and interact by revisiting some of the pragmatic functions we saw at 28 months and looking at the form and content now being used to code those functions at 39 months.

What does mine do?	(request for information)
Buy some at the store.	(request for action)
It is a tool.	(labeling)
That looks like a robot.	(commenting)
Mickey doesn't have shoes.	(negating)

At this age, Abraham is using language not just for communication with others but for imaginative uses as well. He talks about what he is doing even when there is no one to hear or respond to him. The following excerpt was recorded while Abraham played alone with a large doll house and a family of dolls. What we hear is a verbal monologue of his ongoing thoughts as he plays. In this case, he is using language as a tool to organize and encode his thoughts and experiences in a pretend situation.

> Oh, wow, oh man, I need all these guys. There's a bunch of people. I don't want the bunch of people, just a little bit. A little bit means, this is a little bit. Yeah, this is a little bit. (Looks at one figure.) Gross. I don't want you. Well, get your mom and dad. I'll get the mom. I'll get the dad. (Talks for the boy figure.) Mom, could we go to the park? Dad, could we go to the park? This is the park already. Okay, I want to sit right . . . Let's go over . . . let's take . . . take a nap. Our bed. Oh wow. Your bed

> is . . . my bed is right down . . . your bed is right down there. That's right. These are not the big people's. No, these are ours. The baby's is right there where his is. Mommy and Daddy are busy down there. You guys, you can't wait to go to the nap like that. You need someone to help you get into bed. You guys already got back into bed and get the baby.

Forty-four Months

By age 4, children's language is adultlike in many respects. We rarely hear violations of language form, although we do hear false starts and revisions (even adults produce these periodically). At 44 months, Abraham's MLU is now 5.35, which indicates no increase in utterance length compared to five months before. In fact, Abraham has now passed the age where MLU is sensitive to gains in language acquisition. This is because his sentences are becoming more complex rather than simply becoming longer. We hear complex verb phrases ("He *wants to get* in there") and conjoined sentences ("But not the boy, *'cause* he's hiding in a hiding place up there").

The content of language continues to be dictated by experience. Children must hear new words to learn them (later, reading will contribute significantly to vocabulary growth). When children read a new book, play with others, go new places, or watch television programs, they are exposed to new words. Therefore, the words that children know depend, in large part, on their range of experience, which provides a context for new words to be learned. Once words are acquired, they are available to the child to help frame his or her future experiences and to support further learning. We can see the role of experience in building vocabulary when Abraham's preschool class made a trip to a local fire station. Although Abraham had never been there before, it was clear that he already had some very specific concepts about what a fire station is like and vocabulary to go along with the experience. In his case, a likely source of this vocabulary was a book that had been read to him many times. A home video of the field trip captured the following conversation:

(The children enter the fire station.)

ABRAHAM: What is . . . What's that? A fire truck. An old fire truck.

(The children go through the living areas.)

ABRAHAM: We don't have one right here? We don't have a pole here?

FIREFIGHTER: We don't have a pole. There's only one or two left in the country that still has a pole and we don't. . . .

ABRAHAM: Whoa! Look at this. This is where the firefighter sleeps.

(The children look at the ambulance.)

ABRAHAM: I have a question.

FIREFIGHTER: I have an answer. What can I do for you?

ABRAHAM: These are the people that drive the ambulance?

FIREFIGHTER: That's right. Do you know I can drive this ambulance? That's my job.

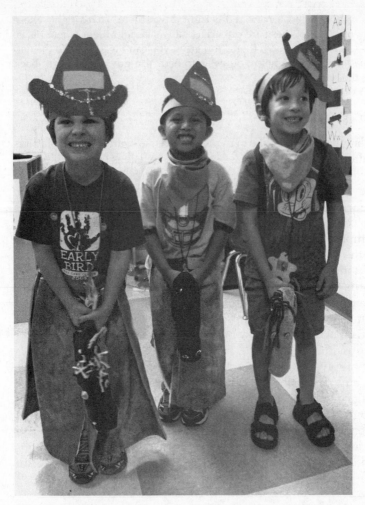

FIGURE 7.3 Children build vocabulary through their experiences. Here preschool children learn about concepts through thematic play activities.

In this conversation, we can see that Abraham is quite confident talking to others, although other children at this age may be shy. He is also beginning to show some of the subtleties of language use. For example, he uses the indirect "I have a question" before asking the actual question. We also see that his use of conversational conventions is still not perfect. Earlier, he asked a question and interrupted the adult before receiving the full answer. He will continue to refine skills within the domain of language use as he grows (see Figure 7.3).

In four short years, Abraham has gone from an infant, whose only means of expression was crying, to a preschooler, whose language contains many of the features one would see in an adult speaker. In this

Four-year-old children have typically mastered the basics of the language used in their environment.

chapter, we have seen the development of language *form* as he progressed from word attempts that were only approximations of the adult phonological form to fully intelligible speech. We saw single words progress to multiword phrases to sentences containing clauses and complex verbs. We saw increased use of morphology as phrases and sentences emerged. We saw language *content* grow from the restricted meanings of the first few words to the multitude of words whose meanings approximate adult versions. Finally, we saw improvement in the *use* of language for a variety of communication functions. By age 4, Abraham's language is already a remarkable tool for communication.

Later Language Development

By 4 years of age, typically developing children have little difficulty communicating, even with those who do not know them well. However, the job of language development will continue for many years. For example, although 4-year olds can discuss a wide range of topics, the sentences they use are relatively simple in terms of syntax. As these children continue to develop, they learn to combine thoughts in more sophisticated ways. Consider the following sentences about a trip to the zoo:

1. There was a tiger. There was a leopard. Leopards have spots. He was asleep the whole time.
2. There was a tiger and there was a leopard. The leopard was asleep the whole time.
3. There was both a tiger and a leopard. The leopard, which was the one with spots, slept the whole time.

All three groups of sentences convey the same information. However, the first set of sentences, which are typical of those produced by children at age 4, are fairly simple. As children continue to develop, they are capable of combining separate ideas into a single sentence. An early strategy for combining is to join whole sentences using conjunctions like "and" or "but" (see example 2, above). By late elementary school and middle school, typically developing children are also capable of combining ideas using more sophisticated syntax. In the third set of sentences, we see that the initially separate sentences about the tiger and leopard are combined without repeating "there was." The idea that leopards have spots is conveyed by a clause embedded in the middle the second sentence. By age 5, children are capable of producing sentences that contain these kinds of clauses (Diessel, 2004). The use of these complex sentence forms will continue to increase well into early adulthood (Nippold, Mansfield, & Billow, 2007).

Not only are children able to produce more complex sentences as they mature, they also are better at comprehending complex syntax. Although preschool children are sometimes confused by passive sentences (e.g., "The dog was chased by the cat"), older children and adolescents have no problem figuring out who did what to whom in these types of sentences. Children also begin to be able to think about the structure of a sentence independent of the communicative intent of the sentence. Preschool children cannot reliably make judgments about whether a sentence is grammatically correct (e.g., Is "The cats runs away" a good sentence?). As children mature, they become increasingly proficient in identifying these types of errors (Kail, 2004).

The ability to think about the form of language, apart from the message it communicates is a **metalinguistic** skill. Metalinguistic skills are particularly important for school. Being able to define a word requires children to think explicitly about word meanings independent of how they might use a word in conversation. We also see a strong role for metalinguistics in reading and writing. When children learn to read, they need to start thinking about the individual sounds that make up words, instead on just considering words as a whole unit. Writing, particularly revising written text, requires a number of metalinguistic skills. Writers must be able to spot ungrammatical sentences and recognize what makes the sentence ungrammatical in order to correct it (*metasyntax*). They need to consider if a word means precisely what they intend to communicate in the text (*metasemantics*). Finally, they need to consider the reader's perspective and whether the tone and organization will assist the reader in understanding what the text is attempting to convey (*metapragmatics*). All these skills are ones that emerge in rudimentary form early in childhood, but continue to develop with both experience and formal education.

> School-age children are able to think about language and language use in a way that younger children do not. These metalinguistic skills open the door to many years of verbal humor.

Later language development is not confined to language form. Language content and use also continue to develop. Vocabulary growth continues throughout life. A quick look at the glossary of this text will reveal words that are unknown to the average adult. However, these new words are incorporated into the corpus of words known to the reader as they master the content of the text. Likewise, new inventions and cultural phenomena introduce terms that were unknown a decade earlier (e.g., "blog," "skype," "ipad") or provide new meanings for old words (e.g., "twitter"). For this reason, it is not wise to challenge your grandparents to Scrabble, as they have had decades longer than you to expand their vocabularies.

It is not just the number of words in children's vocabularies that changes with age. Their ability to appreciate the connotative meanings of words also improves. With time, children develop an ability to appreciate and use nonliteral language. This includes comprehension of similes and metaphors, in which a conceptual comparison helps to communicate meaning (e.g., "her hair shone like sunlight"). During the grade school years, many children are taught explicitly how to recognize and create these language forms. Similarly, children become increasingly proficient in picking up the meaning of idioms from context as they progress from grade school to high school (Nippold & Taylor, 1995) and may receive explicit instruction on their nature as part of the school curriculum. Idioms, in which the literal meaning of words do not convey the meaning intended (e.g., "the short end of the stick," "blown away") require experience to develop. We become familiar with the idioms common to our own culture (e.g., "dog tired"), but can be baffled by those from other cultures (e.g., "I'm a potato." [I'm flexible]).

Nonliteral language also plays a strong role in humor. Small children often perceive the social value of jokes, even if they don't get what makes a joke funny. An example of joke telling at age 3 follows:

ABRAHAM: Knock knock.

PARENT: Who's there?

ABRAHAM: (Laughs).

It is only later that children grasp what makes a joke funny. Jokes and puns can rely on a play on the sounds of common words ("cashew," . . . "God bless you"). Other jokes rely on being able to appreciate multiple meanings of a key word (Why can't a leopard hide? Because he is always spotted.). Both of these skills are metalinguistic in nature, in that they reflect an appreciation of the phonological or semantic properties of language. Therefore, it is not surprising that these skills continue to develop with age.

Nonliteral language has important social functions. We use jokes to entertain or to make light of difficult situations. Teens of every generation generate slang that differentiates their communication from the adults in their lives. Email is rife with nonliteral language (Whalen, Pexman, & Gill, 2009). Children become more proficient in their social use of these forms with time. For example, many of us have had the experience of a misinterpreted email or text message that was meant to be ironic or sarcastic. We learn that these forms of nonliteral language do not translate well in print format because tone of voice is critical for determining when "Oh, I really like that" is meant in a literal or sarcastic way. These types of refinements in language use continue throughout life.

The Development of Literacy

In addition to spoken language skills, children develop skills for reading and writing their language. Like spoken language, the foundations for reading and writing may begin in early infancy and emerge over time. If the child is read to frequently, the development of early literacy skills may be as natural to the child as the development of spoken language. Let us look at Abraham's development of literacy skills.

Abraham was born to parents who value and enjoy reading. They purchased baby books and began reading to him shortly after his birth. This was part of their daily routine and provided an opportunity for baby and parents to interact. A typical book session involved his mother or father holding Abraham so that both could see the book. After reading a page, they would point out and name the things pictured on the pages before turning to the next page. By 12 months, Abraham was actively joining in this activity. We saw him waiting for his father to read the words before pointing to the picture and babbling. Then he helped to turn to the next page. When the book was closed, he babbled two syllables remarkably like "the end" would have sounded if he had said real words. By 2 years, Abraham wanted the same

In many homes, literacy experiences begin long before a child is formally taught to read and write, simply by the repeated experience with book-reading routines.

few books read over and over again. He would bring books to his mother during play times and was always read one of these stories before going to sleep. If his mother paused when reading the text, Abraham would fill in the final words. By 3, his mother started to point not only to pictures on the page but also to each word as she read. Some time after that, Abraham started to recognize words that occurred frequently in his favorite books. He was also given an alphabet book at this point and began to learn the names of the letters. Although his alphabet book associated letters with words ("A" with *apple, ants*), he showed no sign of recognizing that the letters made specific sounds that went with the items pictured on the page. However, he can recognize a handful of words in his favorite books. These tend to be those words that occur most frequently in the story, like *the,* a, or the name of the main character.

Abraham's experiences are typical of many children who are raised in households where reading is a common activity and where parents consider it their role to introduce their children to books (see Figure 7.4) (Weigel, Martin, & Bennett, 2006). Before such children even enter kindergarten, they have many preliteracy skills that will facilitate learning to read and write. It is evident that children who are read to develop social routines for books. They know how to hold them, know that the reader says some words, everyone looks at the picture, the page is turned, and the routine repeats until the end. Their experience with books teaches them that individual letters have names and that the groups of letters the reader points to correspond to the words said,

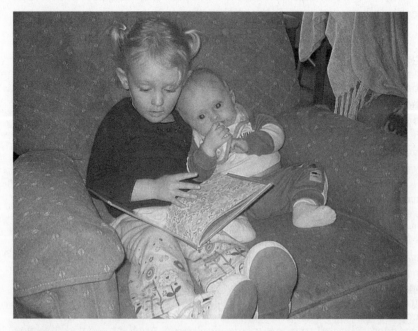

FIGURE 7.4   Literacy skills have their earliest roots in children's first experiences with books.

and the words correspond to the pictures on the page. Perhaps most importantly, these children see book reading as an enjoyable activity. These children have a strong advantage when they enter school because they already know much about the process of reading. In contrast, children who lack experience with books at home may still be gaining the skills other children mastered as preschoolers, as their classmates move ahead, learning to sound out words. Children with little exposure to books may also be less motivated to learn to read because they never had the experience of enjoying the stories that books contain.

The path to normal reading involves not only the practical skills involved with handling and appreciating books, but also a growing awareness of the function of print. Even children who are not read to, encounter print in their daily lives. Road signs, billboards, children's television programming, and toy boxes all offer exposure to print in the environment. One model for the progression from prereading to true reading (Frith, 1985) suggests that children first develop an awareness of whole printed words through repeated environmental exposure. For example, Abraham would point to a stop sign and say "stop" long before he had any notion that the word was made of individual letters that, when pronounced in combination, made up the word "stop." In some regards, the "stop" on a stop sign or the "Lego" label on a toy box functions more like a picture that has a specific name than a written word.

In order to differentiate between words like *stop* and *step* or *stop* and *top*, children must recognize that there is a difference in the individual letters that make up these words, and these letters make a difference. Increasing familiarity with the alphabet and the sounds made by the different letters assists children in this process. However, this knowledge does not simply come from environmental exposure alone; it must be taught. Many children learn to sing the alphabet song or are given alphabet books as preschoolers. Others may have limited opportunities to learn the alphabet and the corresponding sounds each letter can represent before they begin formal schooling. Regardless of when awareness of the alphabet arises, children must eventually learn that printed words are made up of individual letters, and changing these letters changes the words. The ability to pair sounds with letters is a key skill necessary for "sounding out" words in print. This requires children to associate sounds with the printed letter symbols, a skill known as **sound–symbol correspondence**.

As Abraham enters school, he learns that he can tell what a word is by "sounding it out." As he is taught to read, Abraham will learn that certain combinations of letters are not sounded out individually (e.g., "th" in "these") and that a vowel in one word can sound different than the same vowel in another word. These skills are critical for decoding words he has not encountered before. If Abraham knows the story being read, he finds he often just needs to sound out the first one or two sounds before he can guess what the word is. Most of the time, he guesses correctly. This demonstrates that he is using his comprehension of the prior text to predict what a new word should be. He also relies on the pictures that accompany the text to help his comprehension and to anticipate the text to come.

The child who is developing reading normally may sound out words the first few times they are encountered. However, if the same word is encountered repeatedly, the child will quickly begin to recognize the whole word. At this point, the word is said to be in their "sight vocabulary." Books geared to young children facilitate this process by presenting the same vocabulary items repeatedly within the context of the story. The more books the child reads, the more sight words he or she will accumulate, further speeding the reading process.

The early stages of reading demonstrate the importance of two skills for reading development: phonological decoding and language comprehension. For early readers, phonological decoding may be the most important skill. This allows readers to turn letters into sound sequences and sound sequences into words with meaning. Until the reader builds a corpus of words that are known by sight, he or she must rely on decoding as a primary strategy for accessing meaning. For later readers, comprehension becomes more critical. Readers not only have to track the meaning of the individual words, but also make sense of the sentences and the overall narrative of the text being read. As readers become more proficient, and are sounding out fewer words per page, their ability to follow the overall meaning of a story is more predictive of their success as a reader than their ability to decode individual words. This is also the point at which children are expected to use reading as a means for learning in school. Children transition from reading as an instructional objective to reading textbooks to gain information around third grade. After this point, children who have not mastered reading sufficiently to learn class material are at risk for academic failure. We will consider two such individuals in Chapter 8.

Literacy skills develop in parallel with spoken language skills. Abraham's earliest literacy skills emerged even before his first words were spoken. Early literacy experiences also provide a mechanism for language growth. The pictures in the book provide a context for learning new words. For example, words like *pair*, *zebra*, and *ark* may have little opportunity to arise in conversational language, but a child will be repeatedly exposed to these words if he or she is given a book on Noah's ark. The pictures and text provide a means of teaching the meaning of these words, as does the opportunity for the child and the reader to talk about these concepts. Books also contain language forms that may not occur frequently in conversational language as well. Books for young children

> Written language provides exposure to a host of concepts, expressions, and facts that are not otherwise encountered by a child.

may include rhyming text or use alliteration liberally. These literary devices cue children into similarities and differences in the sound sequences of words. Books for older children may include sentence structures that do not occur in oral language (e.g., "'Get the dog!' he said"). The stories read to children provide a framework for how information may be organized when they tell stories of their own. For these reasons, language and reading are considered reciprocal skills (e.g., Raikes et al., 2006). Reading builds a variety of language skills. In turn, children with stronger language skills are better able to understand the books they read.

By age 4, Abraham is interested in writing on his own. He can recognize his own name when his mother writes it. He also likes to copy his name onto the pictures that he draws. The letters are uneven in size, and often he needs to continue part of his name below the initial few letters if he runs out of room. Sometimes he misses a few of the letters despite having a model. By 5, he is interested in writing captions to pictures he draws. He will sometimes make up words by stringing random letters together. Other times, he asks his parents what letters he should use. He can form both uppercase and lowercase letters. However, he does not understand when each type of letter is used, so sometimes uppercase letters appear in the middle of words rather than just at the start of sentences. He commonly reverses letters as well. Often there is no space between words, or letters are spaced randomly on the page. However, he "reads" his written captions with pride to his parents.

By the time a child like Abraham begins school, he or she already has rudimentary writing skills. This may include being able to copy letter forms or even write letters that are named for him. Other children may lack the experience or even the basic motor skills to control a pencil or crayon to form letters. Early home or school experiences may include practice in forming letters. By kindergarten or first grade, children will be taught the sounds that go with each letter as a prerequisite to spelling words. Some words, like those the child recognizes consistently from stories or his environment, may be spelled correctly even before he or she can sound out the individual letters of the word.

Just as reading occurs in a variety of contexts, from environmental print to books, writing also develops in a variety of contexts. A child may see a parent noting appointments on a calendar or texting on the phone. Many children will produce scribbles for words before they can form individual letters. A child might begin developing more functional writing skills with simple activities like copying his or her name onto a birthday card or putting a label on a hand-drawn picture. School assignments may include more formal activities like practice with letter formation, written spelling practice, and writing worksheets. Many teachers may allow young children to spell words phonetically in order to facilitate the child's expression through print without the added burden of using the correct spelling conventions. However, as children become more proficient with the physical demands of writing, the expectations for correct spelling and grammar also increase. Advanced writing skills will eventually require integration of language form, content, and use to inform or persuade a reader — skills that refine over a lifetime of use.

Clinical Problem Solving

Here are two language samples obtained from Abraham at two different ages.

Twenty-eight Months

MOTHER: Is that a taco that you're making?

ABRAHAM: Yeah.

MOTHER: Where do you eat tacos?

ABRAHAM: With a mat.

MOTHER: On a placemat?

ABRAHAM: (Pours beans into a bowl) Put all in.

(The beans start to fall on the floor.)

MOTHER: Hey, honey, honey . . .

ABRAHAM: Oh no, mommy!

MOTHER: Do you want help with the beans?

ABRAHAM: It's a cooking beans!

Forty-four Months

ABRAHAM: I ate eggs for breakfast.

AUTHOR: Did mommy make it?

ABRAHAM: I got a gargoyle and I got a Casper today.

AUTHOR: What was the gargoyle on?

ABRAHAM: They're just on my underwear.

AUTHOR: Oh, you have gargoyle underwear on.

ABRAHAM: I have them not on today!

AUTHOR: You have Caspers on today?

ABRAHAM: Yeah.

Look at the transcripts above and consider them from the perspective of language form, content, and use:

1. How has Abraham's language changed from 28 to 44 months?
2. Do you think that his content is typical of other children at each age? Why or why not?
3. What evidence can you find that Abraham has not yet reached adultlike competence in form, content, and use at each age?

REFERENCES

Bates, E. (1976). Pragmatics and sociolinguistics in child language. In D. Morehead & A. Morehead (Eds.), *Normal and deficient child language.* Baltimore: University Park Press.

Bates, E. (1999). Language and the infant brain. *Journal of Communication Disorders, 32*(4), 195–205.

Bates, E., Benigni, L., Bretherton, I., Camaioni, L., & Volterra, V. (1977). From gesture to the first word: On cognitive and social prerequisites. In M. Lewis & L. Rosenblum (Eds.), *Interaction, conversation, and the development of language.* New York: Wiley.

Bloom, L. (1988). What is language? In M. Lahey (Ed.), *Language disorders and language development.* New York: Macmillan.

Brown, R. (1973). *A first language: The early stages*. Cambridge, MA: Harvard University Press.

Brown, R. (1976). *A first language*. New York: Penguin.

Bruner, J. S. (1975). The ontogenesis of speech acts. *Journal of Child Language, 2,* 1–19.

Chomsky, N. (1988). *Language and problems of knowledge: The Managua lectures*. Cambridge, MA: MIT Press.

Clark, E. (1979). What's in a word? On the child's acquisition of semantics in his first language. In V. Lee (Ed.), *Language development*. New York: Wiley.

Diessel, H. (2004). *The acquisition of complex sentences*. Cambridge, England: Cambridge University Press.

Demetras, M. J., Post, K. N., & Snow, C. E. (1986). Feedback to first language learners: The role of repetitions and clarification questions. *Journal of Child Language, 13,* 275–292.

Frith, U. (1985). Beneath the surface of developmental dyslexia. In K. E. Patterson, J. C. Marshall, & M. Coltheart (Eds.), *Surface dyslexia* (pp. 301–330). Mahwah, NJ: Lawrence Erlbaum Associates.

Gerken, LA., Wilson, R., & Lewis, W. (2005). Infants can use distributional cues to form syntactic categories. *Journal of Child Language, 32,* 249–268

Gómez, R., & Gerken, L. (2000). Infant artificial language learning and language acquisition. *Trends in Cognitive Sciences, 4*(5), 178–186.

Gómez, R.L. & Lakusta, L. (2004). A first step in form-based category abstraction by 12-month-old infants. *Developmental Science, 7,* 567–580.

Gómez, R.L. & Maye, J. (2005). The developmental trajectory of nonadjacent dependency learning. *Infancy, 7,* 183–206.

Hubbell, R. (1985). Language and linguistics. In P. Skinner & R. Shelton (Eds.), *Speech, language, and hearing* (2nd ed.). New York: Wiley.

Ingram, D. (1981). Transitivity in child language. *Language, 47,* 888–910.

Johnson, E. K., & Seidl, A. H. (2008). At 11 months, prosody still outranks statistics. *Developmental Science, 12,* 131–141.

Jusczyk, P. W., Houston, D. M., & Newsome, M. (1999). The beginning of word segmentation in English-learning infants. *Cognitive Psychology, 39,* 159–207.

Kail, M. (2004). On-line grammaticality judgments in French children and adults: A cross-linguistic perspective. *Journal of Child Language, 31,* 713–737.

Karmiloff-Smith, A., Plunket, K., Johnson, M., Elman, J., & Bates, E. (1998). What does it mean to claim that something is 'innate'? Response to Clark, Harris, Lightfoot and Samuels. *Mind & Language, 13*(4), 588–604.

Lahey, M. (1988). *Language disorders and language development*. New York: Macmillan.

Locke, J. (1990). Structure and stimulation in the ontogeny of spoken language. *Developmental Psychobiology, 23,* 621–643.

McNeill, D. (1970). *The acquisition of language*. New York: Harper & Row.

Mehler, J., Jusczyk, P., Lambertz, G., Halsted, N., Bertoncini, J., & Amiel-Tison, C. (1988). A precurser of language acquisition in young infants. *Cognition, 29,* 143–178.

Miller, J. (1981a). The relation between age and mean length of utterance in morphemes. *Journal of Speech and Hearing Research, 24,* 154–161.

Miller, J. (1981b). *Experimental procedures: Assessing language production in children*. Baltimore: University Park Press.

Nazzi, T., Jusczyk, P. W., & Johnson, E. K. (2000) Language discrimination by English-learning 5-month-olds: Effects of rhythm and familiarity. *Journal of Memory and Language, 43,* 1–19.

Nippold, M. A., Mansfield, T. C., & Billow, J. L. (2007). Peer conflict explanations in children, adolescents, and adults: Examining the development of complex syntax. *Language, Speech, and Hearing Services in Schools, 16,* 179–188.

Nippold, M. A., & Taylor, C. L. (1995). Idiom understanding in youth: Further examination of familiarity and transparency. *Journal of Speech and Hearing Research, 38*, 426–433.

Oller, D. (1980). The emergence of speech sounds in infancy. In G. Yeni-Komshian, J. Kavanaugh, & C. Ferguson (Eds.), *Child phonology. Vol. 1: Production.* New York: Academic Press.

Pelucchi, B., Hay, J. F., & Saffran, J. R. (2009). Statistical learning in a natural language by 8-month-old infants. *Child Development, 80*, 674–685.

Pinker, S. (1984). *Language learnability and language development.* Cambridge, MA: Harvard University Press.

Poeppel, D., & Wexler, K. (1993). The full competence hypothesis of clause structure in early German. *Language, 69*, 1–33.

Raikes, H., Luze, G., Brooks-Gunn, J., Raikes, A. H., Pan, B. A., Tamis-LeMonda, C. S., Constantine, J., Tarullo, L. B., & Rodriguez, E. T. (2006). Mother-child bookreading in low-income families: Correlates and outcomes during the first three years of life. *Child Development, 77*, 924–953.

Saffran, J. R., Aslin, R. N., & Newport, E. L. (1996). Statistical learning by 8-month-old infants. *Science, 274*, 1926–1928.

Searle, B. (1969). *Speech acts.* London: Cambridge University Press.

Thiessen, E. D. & Saffran, J. R. (2003). When cues collide: Use of stress and statistical cues to word boundaries by 7- to 9-month-old infants. *Developmental Psychology, 39*, 706–716.

Weigel, D. J., Martin, S. S., & Bennett, K. K. (2006). Mothers' literacy beliefs: Connections with the home literacy environment and pre-school children's literacy development. *Journal of Early Childhood Literacy, 6*, 191–211.

Whalen, J. M., Pexman, P. M., & Gill, A. J. (2009). Should be fun—Not!" : Incidence and marking of nonliteral language in e-mail. *Journal of Language and Social Psychology, 28*, 263.

CHAPTER 8

Disorders of Language in Children

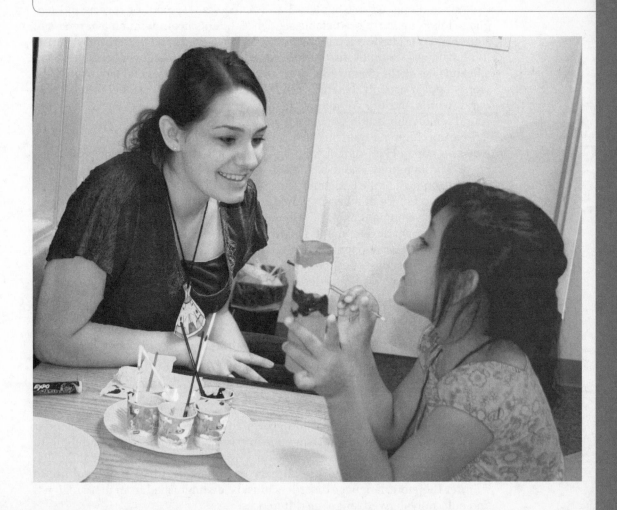

PREVIEW   When normal language acquisition is impeded because of a developmental disorder or childhood illness, it may become evident that language is impaired. Language disorders in children can occur secondary to illness or injury, but they often arise without an identifiable cause. For the young child, impaired oral language may interfere with the ability to express needs or understand what others say. As children progress through school, weak language skills may also impact reading, writing, and academic success. Because developmental language disorders result from a variety of causes and are associated with diverse skill profiles, assessment and intervention methods are tailored to the needs of the individual child.

As we discussed in Chapters 3 and 7, the development of speech and language follows a fairly predictable sequence. Infants begin with an awareness of sound and quickly develop a preference for the sounds and patterns of their native language(s). Sounds, first produced reflexively, are soon produced intentionally and take on the characteristics of speech. Across cultures and languages, first words appear around the child's first birthday. By age 2, most children know many words and are combining them into short phrases. By age 4, children sound remarkably adult-like in their spoken language.

Not all children experience normal language acquisition. Language disorders may affect up to 13 percent of children (Tomblin, Records, & Zhang, 1996). A variety of conditions may lead to a language disorder. Genetic conditions may disturb the development of the brain and alter its capacity for normal language development. The presence of a hearing impairment can have a profound effect on oral language development. Injury or illness can arrest language development after a period of normal development. Finally, there is a wide variety of developmental syndromes that include impaired language as part of the presenting signs.

Although many conditions can lead to a language disorder, the types of skills affected may vary considerably. A language disorder includes any impairment of the ability to understand or use language—when compared to same-age peers of the same community. Severity can vary widely among types of language disorders and even among children who are identified as having the same type of language disorder. Language disorders can affect language in any modality, spoken, written, or signed. In fact, it is often the case (although there are exceptions) that multiple modalities are affected when language is impaired. A language disorder is often first suspected because the child's language development lags behind the expected norms for children of the same age. Because age-expected language skills expand as the child grows, the nature of the language disorder may change too. For example, language impairment will not affect reading until the child has reached an age at which reading skills would be expected. Finally, language form, content, and use all vary from region to region and culture to culture. Therefore, language disorders must be distinguished from these regional and culturally derived language differences.

Language Differences

There are children from particular cultural and social groups whose speech may differ in some respect from Standard English. However, these differences do not, in themselves, constitute a language disorder. Such children have learned the language code of their community and may be quite competent in their use of their native language.

Some linguistic variation reflects regional differences in language, known as dialects. We recognize dialectal differences in the way certain sounds are produced in the Northeast and the Deep South and the Midwest. Other differences may affect the choices of words that are used within a region. Carbonated drinks may be "soda" in one region and "pop" in another. Large-scale sandwiches on long rolls are "submarines," "hoagies," or "po' boys" depending on the region. Dialects can vary with social or cultural groups within a particular region. Communities with strong Hispanic roots may use a variant of English that includes influences from Spanish. Residents of both inner cities and rural districts may speak one or more versions of a dialect known as Black English (sometimes called Ebonics). Although these dialects are culturally influenced, speakers do not necessarily have to be members of the particular minority group to speak the dialect. Furthermore, any given speaker of a dialect may not use it at all times. Social rules may dictate when a dialect, or even which variant of a dialect, is appropriate to the situation. Thus, an individual who uses one version of Black English among friends may use another with parents and switch to Standard American English when addressing a teacher. This situational shifting of speech and language patterns is referred to as **code switching**.

The variations in language *form* observed in dialects are rule governed, meaning that there are strict conventions that dictate correct use of these forms. However, for the listener who is unfamiliar with the conventions of a dialect, it may seem as if the speaker is making linguistic errors. For example, residents of Maryland may "go down the shore for the weekend," omitting the preposition "to" that speakers in other parts of the country would typically use. Forms of Black English may include omissions of certain grammatical forms (e.g., the contracted "is" or "are"; the infinitive "to") and changes in grammatical form (e.g., "hisself" for "himself"; "be" for "has been [continually]") in certain sentence contexts. These are normal forms within some versions of this dialect. However, not all speakers of Black English and other dialects use all the linguistic or pragmatic elements associated with the dialect. For example, Washington and Craig (1994) reported that young children within the same region may vary in the frequency and types of Black English forms in their speech. Speech-language pathologists must be able to distinguish between linguistic variation that reflects a dialect and variation that signals a disorder and to treat those aspects that are attributable to the disorder alone. However, if a dialect speaker who shows no sign of a language disorder wishes to improve his or her use of Standard American English, a speech-language pathologist may provide such assistance (ASHA, 1983).

A dialect is a variation of a mainstream language. It does not constitute a disorder. In fact, most of us use a dialect to some extent.

Children who speak more than one language may also show language content differences that may be mistaken for a disorder. For example, the Navajo child in northeastern Arizona may be bilingual, using Navajo at home and English at school. Vocabulary development in each language may be restricted to the environment in which it is used. For example, the child may know the Navajo word for *grasshopper* but not the English word. Likewise, the child may know a particular English word, but not its Navajo equivalent. These children may appear to have limited lexical knowledge, when tested in only one of their languages, but often have a large and rich vocabulary when both languages are considered. Furthermore, if a Navajo child moves to Los Angeles, his or her language use might be judged faulty by the non-Navajo listeners in the new city. Children in many parts of the world are multilingual, using a particular language for a specific situation. For most children, learning two or more languages (or dialects) is relatively easy, given adequate experience with those languages. Some children, however, are unable to use any of the languages of their community proficiently.

> Bilingual language proficiency is best characterized on a continuum with varying levels of competence for each language.

Early Signs of a Language Disorder

Infants at Risk

Some infants are born with genetic conditions, illnesses, or disabilities that interfere with their development (Clark, 1994; Sparks, 1984). In Chapter 11, we will see that a great many genetic and acquired conditions may affect hearing and consequently alter the course of language development. Many other conditions, such as drug exposure (Johnson, Seikel, Madison, Foose, & Rinard, 1997), infection (Bent & Beck, 1994), low birth weight, and premature birth (Byrne, Ellsworth, Bowering, & Vincer, 1993), increase the risk that a child will experience language and learning difficulties. In some cases, prolonged serious illness itself may interfere with language development. Infants who require hospitalization will not receive the same stimulation from their parents as healthy babies. Infants who are confined to a hospital nursery will have limited opportunities to explore and interact with the people and objects around them. Other infants have physical disabilities that interfere with normal development, including speech and language development.

A speech-language pathologist may work with an infant's family and the hospital staff to provide experiences that facilitate language development. In these cases, speech and language intervention often must be integrated with medical treatments, physical therapy, and occupational therapy. The speech-language pathologist and audiologist are members of a multidisciplinary team, which may also include medical staff, rehabilitation staff, and social services. The team works closely with the infant's family to ensure understanding of the child's needs and the best ways to address them. When a child is born with an obvious disability, parent counseling and intervention for the child can begin right away. However, the impact of prematurity on language and academic performance may appear years later as the child develops (e.g., Halsey, Collin, & Anderson, 1996). Therefore, parents and professionals may need to monitor progress throughout childhood.

Late Talkers

One group of children at risk for language disorders is toddlers who lag behind their peers in the ability to understand or produce words. These children have been referred to as "late talkers." In the research literature, late talkers are typically defined as young children (between approximately 16 and 30 months) whose language skills fall below 90 percent of their same-age peers. These children are slow to acquire their first 50 words and slow to combine words into phrases. For example, Rescorla, Roberts, and Dahlsgaard (1997) reported their group of late talkers had an average of 20 words at age 26 months, compared with their normal peers who had an average of 226 words. Furthermore, only one of thirty-four late talkers in this study was combining words into phrases. The parents of late-talking toddlers may also report that their children seem to understand fewer words than would be expected for their age. These children lack a history of hearing loss, cognitive impairment, or medical factors that would otherwise place them at risk for poor language development.

[handwritten margin note: late talkers have lak receptive + expressive lang behavios similar to peers but lack factos that would place them @ risk.]

Investigators who have followed the development of late-talking children have demonstrated that these children are at risk for continued language problems. Toddlers who are identified as late talkers tend to remain behind their peers over time (Rescorla et al., 1997; Thal, Bates, Goodman, & Jahn-Samilo, 1997). However, what is true for the group is not necessarily true for all its members. In fact, some late talkers do "catch up" with their peers (Ellis Weismer, Murray-Branch, & Miller, 1994; Rescorla et al., 1997; Thal et al., 1997). Some studies have suggested factors that may predict poor language outcome, including poor comprehension skills (Thal & Tobias, 1992), limited use of gestures for communication (Thal et al., 1997; Thal & Tobias, 1992), limited vocabulary (Fischel, Whitehurst, Caulfield, & Debaryshe, 1979; Thal et al., 1997), and initial overall severity (Rescorla et al., 1997; Rescorla & Schwartz, 1990). In addition, the age at which a child is identified as a late talker also appears to be predictive, with the young late talkers faring better than older ones (Paul, 1993; Rescorla & Schwartz, 1990; Thal et al., 1997). However, there is currently no foolproof means to predict which children prove to be "late bloomers" and which ones will continue to experience difficulty with language skills.

> Children who are "late talkers" are at risk for language impairment, but some children who are slow to begin talking proceed to develop language in a typical manner.

Late-talking toddlers are typically first identified by their impoverished vocabularies. For those late talkers who do not move into the normal range, a variety of signs of a language disorder emerge over time. Even those who do catch up with their peers in terms of vocabulary may continue to be at risk for other, later-appearing language impairments. As we saw in Chapter 7, normally developing children acquire a corpus of single-word utterances that they then begin to combine into two-word utterances. From this point, children lengthen their phrases and eventually begin to produce more complex sentences. By age 3 or 4, many children who were late-talking toddlers moved into the normal range for vocabulary skills (Rescorla et al., 1997). However, these same children produced much shorter and morphologically and syntactically simpler phrases than their normally developing peers (Paul & Alforde, 1993; Rescorla et al., 1997). They may also show subtle differences in comprehending certain syntactic forms as preschoolers (D'Ororico, Assanelli, Franco, & Jacob, 2007). Kindergarten children who were late talkers were less proficient in relating a story in logical order than their normally developing peers (Paul, Hernandez, Taylor, & Johnson, 1996). By second grade, these children appeared to have caught up in terms of narrative ability. However, there were still other differences in expressive language skills between this late-talking group and their peers (Paul, Murray, Clancy, & Andrews, 1997). Even many years later as teens, those who were late talkers can have weaker language skills compared to their peers, even when overall language skills are within normal limits (Rescorla, 2009).

These studies demonstrate that long-term difficulty with language can be associated with late-talking status as a toddler. We also saw that not all late-talking toddlers have a poor language outcome. However, despite our imperfect ability to predict outcome, status as a "late talker" is sufficient to indicate risk for language disorder. The long-term risk warrants close monitoring of late-talking children so that those who go on to show clear signs of a language disorder may receive the earliest possible intervention (Thal et al., 1997).

Developmental Language Disorders

For many children with language problems, there is no obvious cause for the impairment. These children do not have the physical characteristics that would signal the presence of a developmental syndrome. They hear normally and lack any sign of brain damage or disease that might lead to impaired language, but their language skills lag behind those of their peers. These children are said to have a **developmental language disorder**.

Developmental language disorder is actually an umbrella term that encompasses children with a wide range of language-related problems. Although the exact cause of these disorders is unknown, parents are often relieved to know that it does not appear to be related to child-rearing practices or the way they have talked to their child. Instead, the underlying cause appears to be biological. Current information suggests that the brains of language-disordered children develop differently than those of most people (Cohen, Campbell, & Yaghmai, 1989; Gauger, Lombardino, & Leonard, 1997; Plante, Swisher, Vance, & Rapcsak, 1991). This altered brain development may underlie altered language development. Evidence of altered brain anatomy can also be found among the parents and siblings of these children (Jackson & Plante, 1997; Plante, 1991). Likewise, when one member of the family has a developmental language disorder, it is common that others do also (Tallal, Ross, & Curtiss, 1989; Tomblin, 1989). The fact that both the

[handwritten margin note: no physical characteristics signaling the presence of a developmental syndrome.]

biological and behavioral aspects of this disorder tend to cluster in families is consistent with a genetic contribution to the disorder (Bishop, Laws, Adams, & Norbury, 2006; O'Brien, Zhang, Nishimura, & Tomblin, 2003; SLI Consortium, 2002).

Children may have problems with the development of receptive language, expressive language, or both. Language deficits may encompass any or all of the components of language *form, content,* or *use* (see Chapter 7 for a review), and an individual child's language difficulties may change over time. When language deficits occur in the absence of other handicapping conditions (e.g., cognitive, motor, sensory, emotional), the child is said to have a **specific language impairment**. To understand this disorder, let us look at the development of one child diagnosed with specific language impairment.

> *Troy* had difficulty with communication from a very early age. He was reportedly about 20 months of age before he used his first word. His parents became concerned when, at age 2, he used few words, communicating instead largely by grunting and pointing. Despite his limited expression, both parents felt that he understood speech well for his age. Troy's pediatrician also noticed his slow language development and arranged for him to be evaluated by a speech-language pathologist.

> During his initial evaluation, Troy passed a hearing screening. His parents completed a questionnaire that surveyed cognitive, motor, self-help, and social skills. Their responses placed him well within normal limits for each of these areas. Troy was then given a formal evaluation of language skills that involved a series of simple activities to test receptive and expressive skills. He correctly pointed to pictures and followed simple commands appropriate for his age. Test scores for receptive language confirmed relatively normal skills for his age. In contrast, his expressive score placed him in the first percentile, or below 99 percent of other children his age. He had great difficulty naming pictures and imitating words on request. He often used the same "word," /da/, to refer to a variety of pictures and objects. In addition, Troy had a limited number of sounds that he used spontaneously, relying mostly on stop consonant-vowel combinations in the words he attempted.

> Specific language impairment (SLI) occurs in the absence of any other disorder.

In Troy's case, early deficits involved vocabulary and phonology. These delayed communication skills were present despite the fact that he was developing normally in other areas. As we saw in our discussion of late talkers, such delay is a risk factor for a developmental language disorder. However, not all children with a developmental language disorder are noticeably different from other children at this young age. For some, the first words emerge right on schedule for normal development, and the disorder only becomes apparent as the child fails to progress from words to sentences.

> Troy was enrolled in a preschool program for children with specific language impairment at age 3. His parents reported remarkable improvement from that time forward. In addition to his preschool class, his parents implemented a home program of language stimulation. This involved techniques for introducing new vocabulary and encouraging him to produce longer utterances. Troy's vocabulary expanded rapidly from 14 words to well over 100 words in five months. His

phonological repertoire also expanded, so that he was producing many more of the sounds appropriate for his age. At age 3, he was occasionally combining words to form two-word utterances as well. His mother reported that Troy was showing fewer signs of frustration in his attempts to communicate and that people outside of the family were having much less difficulty understanding his speech.

At age 4, Troy was using many two- and three-word phrases, with an occasional four-word phrase in spontaneous speech. However, he used few grammatical morphemes (e.g., verb tense markers, prepositions), which is unusual for a child his age. At age 4 years, 7 months, the following conversation was recorded while he played with a toy fire station:

TROY: This the fireperson. This the bell. (Indicating the fire alarm)

MOTHER: Does the bell ring in an emergency?

TROY: No. The bell, it has . . . the car come out.

MOTHER: The cars come out when the bell rings?

TROY: (Nods) The telephone do that too!

Not surprisingly, formal tests documented below-normal expressive language skills at this time, including morphology and syntax. Although language form was still delayed, Troy showed marked improvement in language content and use. He spoke readily in a variety of contexts and was able to use language for a variety of purposes (e.g., requesting, explaining, directing).

This pattern of differential impairment across language domains is fairly common for children with specific language impairment during the preschool years. In Troy's case, we observed a shift from the initial vocabulary deficit, which was apparent at age 2, to a morphosyntactic deficit at age 4. This phenomenon is known as "growing into a deficit." We did not see the morphosyntactic deficit early on, simply because English-speaking children do not use syntax or morphology until words are combined into phrases. Therefore, we had to wait until Troy reached a developmental stage where these skills could be expected before determining whether they were impaired.

Children with early language disorders may ultimately achieve parity with their normally developing peers. For some, this marks the end of their language difficulties. However, for others, this period of normal language is temporary and is referred to as a period of "illusory recovery" (Scarborough & Dobrich, 1990). Children who appear to recover may once again fall behind their peers as they progress through grade school. Still other children with early language problems continue to show signs of language deficits as they enter the school years. We saw this pattern with Troy.

Troy's speech and language skills were reevaluated by the school speech-language pathologist when he entered first grade at 5 years, 9 months. At that time, his early problems with phonology were almost completely resolved. His speech could be easily understood. The only remaining speech errors were occasional mispronunciations in conversation, and these involved only the late-acquired sounds of speech (see Chapter 3). However, his conversations consisted primarily of short, simple sentences. He continued to have difficulty with grammatical morphemes, making substitutions like "the paint guy" for "pain*ter*" and "the more big one" for "big*ger*" or omissions like "He run" for "He run*s*." Once again, formal testing documented poor language expression despite good overall comprehension. Both receptive and expressive vocabulary remained strong.

The school speech-language pathologist continued to see Troy twice a week to work on morphology. She also coordinated activities with the classroom teacher and Troy's parents to reinforce correct use of the morphological items that Troy was learning. This intervention was quite successful, and by the middle of second grade Troy's conversational speech no longer contained obvious morphological errors. He was retested at this time because the school was considering his dismissal from therapy. His standardized test scores continued to indicate that his expressive language skills lagged behind his peers. However, because he was keeping up in the classroom and was doing well socially, it appeared that his weak expressive language skills were not a handicapping factor at this time. The school decided to monitor his progress but discontinued direct services.

The school staff's decision to discontinue services for Troy is consistent with their mandate to provide services to children with *educationally handicapping conditions*. The public law (P.L. 94–142) that first mandated services in 1975 guaranteed a free and appropriate education for all children with educationally handicapping conditions. Speech and language disorders are among the disorders covered under this law, and under subsequent versions of this law (e.g., Individuals With Disabilities Education Improvement Act of 2004). Because Troy was functioning well in the educational system, the school staff decided he was best served in the regular classroom with monitoring and consultative support by the speech-language pathologist. For Troy, this educational plan places him in the *least restrictive environment* in which he is capable of functioning.

Other children with more serious handicaps may require greater educational support. This may include "pullout" services, in which the child leaves the classroom for brief periods of direct therapy, placement in special classrooms within the regular school, or even placement in specialized schools for severely handicapped children. Each of these modes of intervention involves increasing restrictions on the child's environment, because less time is spent with normally developing peers. The type and frequency of service each child receives may change over the years as the degree to which the child's disorder impacts educational progress changes. Where and how the child receives services is determined by a multidisciplinary team that includes parents, teachers, therapists, and others who can provide insight into a particular child's learning difficulties. This team develops an *individualized educational plan* (IEP) that specifies the level of services, who will provide the services, and what the goals will be.

Three years later, at age 10, Troy's skills were reevaluated. This testing session revealed a further evolution in his language profile. Up to this time, his comprehension test scores had always been a relative strength compared with his

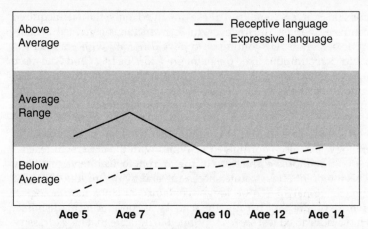

FIGURE 8.1 For children with developmental language disorders, the components of language can change over time. Here we can see receptive and expressive language skills shift over time in a single child (Troy) relative to typically developing peers.

expressive scores. However, at age 10, his comprehension scores now fell below average (see Figure 8.1). The appearance of comprehension deficits during the school years can be accounted for in part by the fact expectations for understanding language change between the ages of 7 and 10 years of age. For example, older children are expected to be able to follow complex and multistage directions and to be able to follow the plot of a story that may have multiple subplots. In school, children are expected to perform multiple language tasks simultaneously: listening to a lecture, extracting the principle concepts, and encoding them as written notes. Comprehension becomes a learning tool, not just in listening but also in reading. It is sometimes the case that a child's limitations in the receptive domain become apparent only when the demands increase to the point where the deficits emerge.

Troy's poor language comprehension was still apparent during his teen years. In fact, by age 14, his expressive language skills were slightly better than his receptive skills. However, he continued to show problems with expressive language as well. We no longer see the same types of expressive problems that characterized his spoken language at earlier ages. Troy no longer omits grammatical morphemes, for example, but the effectiveness of his oral communication remains compromised. Consider Troy's attempt to relate the plot of a movie during a conversation, recorded when he was 12 years old:

> It was hilarious. He didn't put the . . . um . . . "owies." He only put the best "owie." No, that was the second best "owie." The first was when the rope that he went down was soaked in some kind of thing . . . that it makes fire go on . . . makes it go faster and they were on the rope and say "Hey Harry, are you there?" No, that's Clorox, or something like that. (Speaks for a movie character.) "Oh guys." (Sound effect of guys falling). "Get up! Get up!" (Sound effect of guys yelling and hand gestures.) Then there's like a bridge and they fall right through and they get covered with all kinds of . . . sticky stuff.

We can see a number of problems in this short sample. First, the story he is telling lacks the structure of an identifiable beginning, middle, and end. Characters are referred to without first being introduced to the listener (e.g., He didn't put the . . . um . . . "owies"). We hear pauses and revisions throughout. In addition, the use of sound effects and gestures suggests that Troy may have been having difficulty retrieving specific words to communicate his thoughts.

The ability to organize and sequence verbal information becomes increasingly important as a child progresses through school. In fact, Troy's written work showed many of the same characteristics that we saw in the verbal sample above. In addition, he often made the same morphological errors in written language that we saw in his spoken language at age 5. For example, at age 12 he wrote the following sentences:

> Mom caned the riped vejedetables.
>
> I don't wan't any.
>
> But the two dog eat it.

At this point, Troy's language difficulties were still interfering with his academic progress. His reading was slow, and he did not always glean as much meaning from reading as he should. His writing was messy, with many spelling errors, and the flow of thoughts did not always follow a logical sequence. Because his weak language skills were having the greatest impact on educational skills, the school staff considered providing services for a **learning disability**. Children with learning disabilities typically have difficulties in listening, speaking, reading, or writing. Their poor language skills can hold them back in any academic subject in which language is used as a tool for learning or problem solving.

The long-term outcome of children with developmental language disorders is quite variable. Some will overcome the handicap of an early language disorder. Others may struggle with language in either the oral or written modalities for years. Even as adults, individuals with a history of language therapy may still show subtle, residual deficits on standardized measures (Fidler, Plante, & Vance, 2011; Poll, Betz, & Miller, 2010). However, these language difficulties may or may not prove handicapping in the individual's everyday life. In fact, adults with a childhood history of language disorders appear no less satisfied with their quality of life than those without such a childhood history (Records, Tomblin, & Freese, 1992).

Reading Impairments

Reading and writing require a child to transfer what he or she already understands about oral language to visual and manual modalities. In Chapter 7, we saw the importance of two skills, phonological decoding and language comprehension, for developing reading competence. Here we consider two boys, both in second grade, who are having difficulty learning to read.

Jimmy had been receiving services targeting language and phonology since he was 4 years old. He was now in second grade, and his mother had concerns about his reading ability. She had approached the school about her concerns when Jimmy was in first grade but had been assured that different children learn to read at different times and Jimmy would catch on in his own time. The speech-language pathologist, Therese, agreed to listen to Jimmy read. She selected some short stories written at different reading levels. When Jimmy came into her room, she passed the easiest story to him. He looked quickly at it and immediately announced he didn't want that one. He picked up another and put it down again, saying maybe they should read later. Jimmy's attempt to get the third story was abandoned when Therese pointed out that it was even longer, and had no pictures. Jimmy reluctantly took the easiest story and then announced he "didn't know any of those words." Therese offered to read the story with him. In the title, he read the word "the" without sounding it out, but then stopped immediately after this first word. Therese asked what the next word started with and Jimmy responded "B." Therese then asked what sound that made, and Jimmy responded that he didn't know. When Therese made the /b/ sound, Jimmy responded "oh yeah!" Therese then pointed to the picture to see if Jimmy could find something that might correspond to that sound. Jimmy guessed "dog." As they progressed through the title and first sentence, Jimmy never got past the first sound of any word. Furthermore, by the time he got to the last word, he had forgotten so much that he couldn't repeat the sentence they had "read together."

Jimmy demonstrates several traits that predict the occurrence of reading problems. First is his history of speech and language difficulties. Children with early language impairment are at increased risk for later reading problems (Botting, Simkin, & Conti-Ramsden, 2006; Snowling, Bishop, & Stothard, 2000). Next, Jimmy appears to know the names of letters, but has a weak grasp on what sounds the letters make. This undermines his ability to use phonological decoding as a reading strategy. Not only is he not sounding out the letters that make up words, but he is unable to link letter sounds to corresponding pictures (e.g., /b/ with the picture of a boy). Therefore, he is not able to use the pictures to support his decoding of the text. Furthermore, his reading is so labored because of his lack of decoding skills and the very few words he knows by sight, he does not build up any comprehension of the text already read. This breakdown of comprehension is a consequence of poor decoding. Poor comprehension is also a major predictor of reading proficiency. Even if decoding improves, his weak language skills may still interfere with comprehension.

> Children with early language impairment are at increased risk for reading problems later on.

We see that Jimmy is already actively trying to avoid reading. He is well aware of his problems at this point, and also knows that others in his class are not struggling as he is. Furthermore, he is only a year away of having to start reading to gain knowledge in classes like social studies or to solve word problems in math. Because of this, the speech-language pathologist recommended that reading goals be added to his education plan. Jimmy will work with the school's reading specialist and the classroom teacher to strengthen his decoding

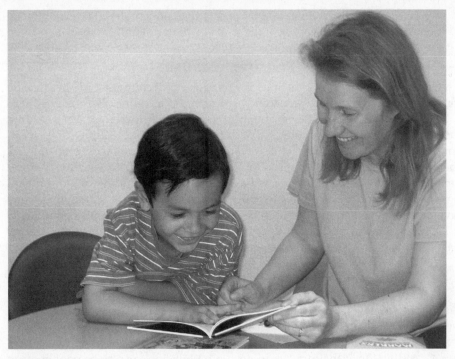

FIGURE 8.2 A speech-language pathologist may build oral skills through activities centered around books and reading.

skills, beginning with linking letters to the sounds they make rather than just to their letter names (see Figure 8.2). This skill is referred to as knowledge of **sound–symbol correspondence**. Along with this skill, intervention will include sounding out and blending the sounds in printed words along with building a core of "sight words" that occur frequently in text. These sight words provide a means of offering quick success for reading without having to sound out every word. Finally, Jimmy will be encouraged to use story pictures to help his comprehension of printed text.

Carlos was another child who was on Therese's caseload. He had been diagnosed with specific language impairment. Therese was working in Carlos's class one day when he was asked to read aloud to his reading group. He proceeded to read the story from the title to "The End." The only things Therese noted was that he read relatively fast, and his intonation was somewhat flat, possibly because of his rapid reading rate. He mispronounced only two words (*gray* was pronounced as "grew," *try* was pronounced as "tie"), and he pronounced two words as if he was working out the sound at first (e.g., *ssllled*). Otherwise, his oral reading was error free. But when Therese asked questions about the story, which involved a boy who found a way to sneak out of the house to go sledding, Carlos produced a plot that involved a boy who didn't want to go sledding along with other major deviations from the actual meaning of the text. It was almost as if Carlos remembered key vocabulary words (e.g., boy, sledding) and then reconstructed a story that worked for those words.

Carlos showed indications that he was actively decoding words because he paused to sound out words on occasion. His strong decoding skills allowed him to build an impressive sight vocabulary over time. However, Carlos's reading illustrates a case where phonological decoding is strong, but reading comprehension is poor nonetheless. Such children are referred to as "poor comprehenders." The speech-language pathologist's job then becomes to discover why comprehension is poor. Some children may have a poor understanding of word meanings such that they do not build comprehension as a story is read. Others may have more complex comprehension problems that involve multiple components of language content and form. Reading intervention must address the specific reasons for an individual child's comprehension difficulty. Intervention for a child like Carlos, therefore, would take an entirely different form than that for a child like Jimmy.

> Children who have problems learning to read often have difficulty with phonological decoding or language comprehension skills.

Reading disorders in children can take a variety of forms. Perhaps the most well known reading disorder is **dyslexia**, sometimes also called *specific reading disability*. Dyslexia is diagnosed when children's poor word reading appears to be caused by especially poor phonological decoding. As with Jimmy, reading comprehension can also be poor because poor decoding skills interfere with the child's ability to appreciate the meaning of what is eventually decoded. In contrast, comprehension of spoken language is relatively good for these children.

Dyslexia may be contrasted with other forms of reading disability. For example, a child may experience difficulty learning to read because he or she has another type of developmental disorder, such as mental retardation. One of the most commonly occurring conditions associated with reading problems is specific language impairment. Many, but not all, children with specific language impairment struggle with reading as well. However, dyslexia and specific language impairment are thought to constitute separate disorders, even though they sometimes co-occur (Bishop & Snowling, 2004; Catts, Adlof, Hogan, & Ellis Weismer, 2005). Children with dyslexia, with or without specific language impairment, appear to have worse phonological skills than children with specific language impairment alone (Catts et al., 2005), whereas children with specific language impairment appear to have language deficits that are broader in nature than those with specific reading impairment alone (Bishop & Snowling, 2004). For children with specific language impairment, these broader language skills, including oral language comprehension and early phonological skills, predict reading outcome by the end of grade school (Botting et al., 2006). Like Carlos, children with specific language impairment may evidence a lack of reading comprehension when they retell the stories they read (Gillam & Carlile, 1997). Although a phonological approach to reading remediation may be effective for improving reading for children with specific language impairment (Gillon, 2002), they may also require additional support to improve reading comprehension.

For some children, oral reading seems completely divorced from reading comprehension. These children can read aloud but show no understanding of what they have read. In these cases, children seem to "crack the phonological code" of written language without formal instruction. This phenomenon is known as **hyperlexia**. Hyperlexia often occurs in the context of a broader disorder such as autism or pervasive developmental disorder. Unfortunately, for the child with hyperlexia, what appears to be advanced reading ability is not actually functional for the child, because reading comprehension is very poor or absent.

> Hyperlexia, in which very young children can read out loud at levels that are far beyond their comprehension, is not necessarily a good thing.

Other Disorders That Impact Language

Children experience difficulty with language for a variety of reasons. In the 1950s, the audiologist and speech-language pathologist tended to emphasize the cause, or etiology, of the child's language disorder. With the growth of behavioral and operant psychology in the 1960s, however, emphasis switched from etiology *per se* to changing the child's behavior regardless of etiology. However, knowledge of etiology presents at least two primary advantages. The first is being able to address parents' desires to know why their child has a disorder (Aram, 1991). The second involves clinical management. The initial diagnosis can serve to orient the clinician to the likely behavioral strengths and weaknesses. Given a diagnosis of seizure disorder, for example, a clinician is alerted by the diagnostic category to examine receptive language skills. A diagnosis of dyslexia would signal a need to examine the impact of language on reading abilities. Although the diagnostic label does not predict with 100 percent accuracy an individual's language profile, it can alert the clinician to what the most salient problems may be. Let us take a look at a small selection of the many conditions associated with impaired language to see how language may vary with different developmental conditions.

Attention Deficit Disorder

For the general public, Attention Deficit/Hyperactivity Disorder, or ADHD, is one of the most familiar developmental disorders. The prevalence of this disorder is thought to be around 7 to 8 percent of the population, and this figure is relatively stable across different countries and cultures (Alloway, Elliott, & Holmes, 2010; Palili, Kolatis, Vassi, Veltsista, Bakoula, & Gika, 2011; Sánchez, Velarde, & Britton, 2011). Males are more frequently identified as having ADHD than females (Rösler, Casas, Konofal, & Buitelaar, 2010). The disorder is most frequently diagnosed in children, but there is growing awareness that this disorder does not always resolve and can persist into adulthood (Knutson & O'Malley, 2010; McArdle, 2004). However, the prevalence of the disorder tends to be lower for adults than children (Palili et al., 2011). An estimated one-half to two-thirds of individuals with ADHD continue to show signs of ADHD in late adolescence (Claude & Firestone, 1995; McGee, Partridge, Williams, & Silva, 1991).

It is not uncommon for many of us to feel we display characteristics of ADHD, even if we would not meet the full criteria for this disorder (Garnier-Dykstra, Pinchevsky, Caldeira, Vincent, & Arria, 2010). The criteria for a formal diagnosis of ADHD is provided by the *Diagnostic and Statistical Manual of Mental Disorders* (American Psychiatric Association, 2000). The current diagnostic criteria specify three subtypes of ADHD: Predominantly Inattentive Type, Predominantly Hyperactive/Impulsive Type, and Combined Type (DSM-IV-TR). The inattentive subtype involves behaviors that suggest difficulty establishing and maintaining attention. This might include signs like difficulty focusing on school work, difficulty staying on task when sustained mental effort is needed, a general disorganization, forgetfulness, and seeming to not listen when being spoken to. The Hyperactive/Impulsive Type describes individuals who have difficulty sitting still for long periods, may interrupt others, or may engage in risky behaviors because they fail to consider the potential consequences before acting. As the name implies, those with Combined Type experience a mixture of signs associated with both inattention and hyperactivity or impulsivity. The majority of children diagnosed with ADHD have hyperactive and impulsive components (Alloway et al., 2010; Palili et al., 2011; Sánchez et al., 2011).

Although all of us may occasionally experience any of these signs of ADHD, a diagnosis is only warranted when multiple signs are consistently present. They have to be sufficiently frequent and severe to interfere with the ability to function well in daily life. The signs must also be present in more than one setting (e.g., school and home). This prevents diagnosis of an individual who has difficulty functioning in one setting for any number of reasons (e.g., lack of rules at home, school activities the child finds boring), but otherwise behaves well. The diagnosis also assumes that the behaviors are not due to another disorder. For example, those with traumatic brain injury may show considerable impulsivity, but would not be considered to have ADHD. Finally, the signs of the disorder have to be present from childhood, even if it is not formally diagnosed until adulthood.

ADHD and language impairment are considered separate conditions, but ones that frequently co-occur. A survey of parents of ADHD children indicated that half had been referred to a speech-language pathologists because of concerns with speech and language development (Bruce Thernlund, & Nettelbladt, 2006). Some have reported that language deficits (McGrath, Hutaff-Lee, Scott, Boada, Shriberg, & Pennington, 2008) and reading deficits (Willcutt & Pennington, 2000) occur more frequently with the Predominantly Inattentive subtype than with the Predominantly Hyperactive/Inattentive subtype, even though the latter is more prevalent form of ADHD overall. Children with both ADHD and language disorders have the types of difficulties that we have described earlier in this chapter (McGrath et al, 2008). However, even those children with ADHD who do not have a language disorder may show subtle language difficulties. The inattention and impulsivity that defines ADHD subtypes can lead to social-pragmatic difficulties. Children with ADHD may not listen carefully or may interrupt others, making them socially unpopular.

Language tasks that require a good deal of attention seem to be particularly affected by ADHD even when language skills overall are relatively strong. These skills include following spoken directions or recalling sentences (Redmond, 2004, 2005; Wassenberg, Hendriksen, Hurks, Feron, Vles, & Jolles, 2010). Expressively, these children score somewhat lower than their non-ADHD peers on tasks requiring them to construct sentences using particular words or phrases (Oram, Fine, Okamoto, & Tannock, 1999). Although their narrative skills are generally good, children with ADHD may make more revisions and self corrections when providing information.

Given the high rate of language difficulties, or frank language disorders, in children with ADHD, it is not surprising that speech-language pathologists frequently serve these children. The American Speech-Language-Hearing Association (ASHA, 1997) recommended that speech-language pathologists (and audiologists) serve on multidisciplinary teams for the assessment of children with ADHD. The speech-language pathologist may perform a language assessment for children with ADHD to determine if a co-morbid language disorder is present. If a language disorder is diagnosed, the speech-language pathologist will develop an intervention plan and may work with the child to improve specific language skills. If no language disorder is diagnosed, the speech-language pathologist may still have a professional role to play (Hill, 2000). They may work with children on social communication skills, which may improve how these children interact with their peers. The speech-language pathologist may serve in a consultative role to assure that parents and teachers understand the how attentional problems, or even subtle language problems, may make learning to listen, speak, read, and write more difficult. Often simple modifications, including removing background distractions, or providing visual cues to help children remember instructions are enough to help children with ADHD succeed in the classroom. The speech-language pathologist may be able to help identify useful strategies that parents and teachers can employ to maximize success.

Autism

The term *autism* describes a developmental disorder that profoundly affects the child's interactions with other people and with the world. The earliest signs of the disorder include disturbed social interaction between the infant and its parents. Even as infants, these children do not seem to bond with or take comfort from others. They may seem content watching the movements of their hands or performing repetitive actions. Delayed development of language skills, as well as little use of language for play or social interactions, is typically noted. We can see the classic signs of autism in the following case:

> Ben was 4 years old when his pediatrician urged his parents to have him evaluated. The pediatrician noted that Ben used few words and seemed to interact with the world in an odd way. The pediatrician suspected Ben had autism. His parents took him to a university-affiliated center that specialized in the diagnosis and treatment of children with autism. The center used an integrated team approach to diagnosis, which involved a speech-language pathologist, a psychologist, and

a psychiatrist. Ben and his mother were met in the waiting room by all three of these individuals, who began by talking with the mother and observing Ben. Ben had taken a train engine from the play area, which he had turned over and was slowly rolling the wheels back and forth with his finger. His mother reported that he often "plays" with toys in this repetitive manner, without using them for their actual purpose or in an imaginative way. Moreover, she reported that she often has to "tear him away" from whatever he is interested in, which was also the case today when it was time to proceed back to an exam room. Ben became quite upset but did not attempt to communicate this in words. He also did not greet any of the other adults present or interact with them when spoken to or offered toys. He did not look at the adults except fleetingly and did not look at objects with them (known as maintaining joint attention). Instead he took toys he was interested in off to the side of the room. His sole interactions with his mother involved prompting her to do things for him or grabbing her hand to make her pick up objects he could easily reach himself. His only words were repetitions of single words spoken by others (called *echolalia*). The diagnostic team agreed that the lack of social interaction, very limited language, and repetitive and restricted play all indicated that he indeed had autism. They recommended enrolling him in a therapy program that would address communication, provide behavioral management of difficult behaviors (e.g., tantrums and eating problems reported by the mother), and provide opportunities to learn group play. The mother was also given information about a local support group for families with autism so that Ben's family could meet others who were raising an autistic child.

> Autism affects the ability to use language appropriately.

As children with autism grow older, other aspects of disturbed communication become apparent. Some of these children acquire some early language skills, only to lose them during the preschool years. For others, language development is disturbed from the start. Dunn (1997) reviewed the characteristics of autistic language, which can include deficits in language form, content, and use. Common characteristics include poor language comprehension and poor pragmatic skills. In more severe forms of the disorder, expressive language characteristics may become more apparent. A complete lack of speech, or mutism, is most likely to occur when the signs of autism are most severe (Miranda-Linne & Merlin, 1997).

The language signs most typical of this disorder involve disturbances of language *use*. Individuals with autism frequently have disturbed prosody in spoken language. They may repeat the words of others or use stereotyped speech routines rather than the context-appropriate, original utterances of normally developing children. For example, one child repeated the phrase "want juice please" over and over again as he spun in a circle. However, this was not an actual request for juice, but continued use of a phrase beyond the setting in which it was appropriate. The bizarre elements of communication in individuals with autism also extend to nonverbal pragmatics. For example, children with autism often have a flat facial affect, aberrant patterns of attention to people and objects, and abnormal gaze during conversations (Lord & Pickles, 1996; Shields, Varley, Broks, & Simpson, 1996).

A majority of children with autism fall into the mentally retarded range of intellectual functioning. However, not all cognitive domains are equally affected.

Minshew, Goldstein, and Siegel (1997) tested autistic individuals whose IQ scores fell within normal limits (although many were at the low end of average) and found that these individuals' greatest deficits involved the ability to handle complex information processing in many forms (e.g., high-level language tasks, complex memory). Simple information processing and visual-spatial memory were relatively spared.

The bizarre social interactions of these children led early investigators to hypothesize that autism was the product of uncaring parents who failed to provide the emotional support children require (Kanner & Eisenberg, 1955). Later, more biological explanations of the disorder were offered (e.g., Rimland, 1964). Today, we have evidence of abnormal brain development in autistic individuals (e.g., Courchesne, Yeung-Courchesne, Press, Hesselink, & Jernigan, 1988) and preliminary evidence of a genetic role in the disorder (Petit et al., 1995).

Intellectual Disability

Language is complex and depends, in part, on other cognitive and social skills. Children who are delayed in all aspects of development are frequently also delayed in the acquisition of language skills. These individuals are described as having an intellectual disability or **mental retardation**. The *Diagnostic and Statistical Manual of Mental Disorders-IV Test Revision* (DSM-IV-TR; American Psychiatric Association, 2000) defines *mental retardation* by an intelligence quotient (IQ) of less than 70 on a standardized IQ measure along with significant deficits in adaptive functioning. Even when IQ is low, an individual who shows no difficulty functioning in everyday life would not be considered to have mental retardation. The degree of intellectual disability can vary considerably. DSM-IV-TR recognizes four broad severity levels: mild, moderate, severe, and profound, which reflect a range from individuals considered "educable" to those few who require lifelong assistance.

> Intellectual disability is associated with language impairment. There is considerable variability in language skill for different developmental disorders that include an intellectual disability.

There are many developmental conditions associated with intellectual disability. Some of these are genetic (e.g., Down syndrome, Noonan syndrome, Fragile X syndrome), some are due to exposure to toxins (e.g., fetal alcohol syndrome, lead poisoning), and for others the cause is unknown (**idiopathic** mental retardation). Given the range of conditions associated with intellectual disability, it is not surprising that the language correlates can be quite variable. In general, however, these children are typically slow to acquire communication skills. Even at the prelinguistic stage, some toddlers with retardation are less interactive and use fewer nonverbal forms of communication than normally developing children at these ages. The onset of spoken words may occur at a later chronological age than seen for other children.

Language performance in children with intellectual disability is sometimes reported to be like that of younger, normally developing children. This general profile of language delay may not apply to all conditions associated with intellectual disability. Children with different disorders that involve intellectual

[handwritten margin notes: syntax morphology, Williams - good grammar but difficulties w/ multiple aspects of language, Fragile X - verbal + nonverbal pragmatic skills]

disability have more difficulty with certain areas of language development than others. For example, some children with Down syndrome appear to have particular problems with syntax and morphology (Roberts, Price, & Malkin, 2007). In contrast, children with Williams syndrome have relatively good grammar compared to children with Down syndrome (Bellugi, Lichtenberger, Jones, Lai, & St. George, 2000). Children with Williams syndrome do, however, have difficulties with multiple aspects language compared to children without retardation (Mervis & Becerra, 2007). Children with Fragile X syndrome tend to have particular problems with verbal and nonverbal pragmatic skills (Scharfenaker, 1990) and approximately 30 percent have other speech or language impairments (Burd, Cotsonas-Hassler, Martsolf & Kerbeshian, 2003). Within any group of children with intellectual disability, there is much individual variability in the acquisition of language skills. For example, some children with Williams syndrome have normal syntax and vocabulary skills, whereas others show significant impairment in these areas (Mervis & Becerra, 2007). Therefore, careful diagnosis of language skills is needed to determine the specific areas of language that may be impaired for individual children with mental retardation. With guidance, most children with mental retardation can learn to maximize their communication skills.

Childhood Aphasia

[handwritten margin note: Acquired language disorder caused by brain damage - left hem - caused by head injury, stroke, attack, tumors.]

Children who were developing normally can lose language skills because of brain damage. This acquired language disorder is known as childhood aphasia (Aram, Ekelman, Rose, & Whitaker, 1985; Cranberg, Filley, Hart, & Alexander, 1987). As in adults (see Chapter 9), aphasia typically results from damage to the left (rather than the right) hemisphere of the brain (Beharelle, Dick, Josse, Solodkin, Huttenlocher, Levine, & Small, 2010). The causes include head injury, stroke, infectious disease, and tumors. Stroke is certainly not a common occurrence in young people; however, between 4 and 18 children in 100,000 experience a stroke each year (Burkhard & Lütschg, 2010). When a child has a stroke, it is most likely to be related to a vascular abnormality that may have been present from birth, as opposed to vascular disease, which is a common underlying cause in adults. The characteristic features of aphasia in children are similar to the adult form of aphasia, as we see in the case of Daniel.

> *Daniel* was 4½ years old when he began having daily headaches, which were soon accompanied by behavioral problems and vomiting. He was taken to the hospital and received a brain scan. This revealed a large tumor in the temporo-parietal area of his left hemisphere. He was immediately scheduled for surgery to remove the tumor. On the morning following surgery, Daniel was unable to speak and showed signs of weakness on the right side of his body. A second brain scan showed that he had had a stroke, caused by bleeding of the middle cerebral artery, which damaged the language areas of the left hemisphere (see Chapter 2 for a review).

> Within days, Daniel began talking again, but his speech and language were not at the level they had been before he was hospitalized. Initially, his speech was slow and effortful, and he drooled intermittently. He had great difficulty attending to

what was said and could only follow simple directions. A preschool test of general language abilities indicated low language skills compared with others his age. He had difficulty naming pictures on a vocabulary test. Many times when speaking, he would substitute nonspecific terms or pronouns for specific nouns (e.g., "push thing" for wagon; "the one" for any object). In addition, Daniel had difficulty on a test that required him to produce grammatical sentences to describe pictures. The speech-language pathologist worked with him three times a week until Daniel was released from the hospital. She also arranged to have him enrolled in a preschool program for children with language disorders after he left the hospital.

> Aphasia is more commonly observed in adults than children, but this acquired language impairment occurs at any age when there is significant damage to the left hemisphere of the brain.

When a stroke leads to aphasia, children show difficulty comprehending or using spoken language, despite normal intelligence. As in Daniel's case, children may initially be mute following brain damage and, as they recover, begin to show signs of aphasia (we will look at specific aphasia types in Chapter 9). Childhood aphasia typically affects both receptive and expressive language skills (Ballantyne, Spilkin, Hesselink, & Trauner, 2008). Children may also have difficulty with reading and writing. Because reading, listening, and following directions are frequent school activities, it is not surprising that children with aphasia have academic difficulties (Cranberg et al., 1987). In contrast, appropriate language use is well preserved. Language difficulties may resolve with time, so that the casual listener may be unaware that the child had experienced aphasia. However, language problems can also persist and be documented with standardized testing years after the aphasia first appeared (Vargha-Khadem, O'Gorman, & Watters, 1985; Woods & Carey, 1979). This is particularly true if brain damage was sustained before the first birthday (Max, Bruce, Keatley, & Delis, 2010).

children have difficulty!
1) comprehending spoken lang
2) receptive + expressive issues
3) reading + writing
lang use ✓

Seizure Disorder

Childhood **seizures** can have many different underlying causes or have no known cause at all. For many, a childhood seizure episode may cause considerable concern at the time but have no long-lasting consequences. However, when seizures are severe and persistent, behavioral deficits, including impaired language, may follow. We saw one such case with Anita, who was diagnosed as having aphasia secondary to a seizure disorder:

> *Anita* had been having seizures since 6 months of age. Management of those seizures included drug therapy and periodic monitoring of brain electrical activity. However, this was only partially successful. Anita spoke her first words at 18 months, and speech-language development had been slow but steady since then. Following a particularly long generalized seizure at age 4, Anita lost her ability to speak, and communication was reduced to slurred sounds and gestures. Although she regained some language skills after that episode, her language remained markedly impaired.

> At age 5, Anita was evaluated at a university clinic. She failed to respond to sounds when her hearing was tested and seemed only somewhat aware that people were talking to her. A parent questionnaire revealed a significant delay in all areas of

development, including motor, social, and self-help skills. Formal language assessment was discontinued because Anita was unable to maintain attention to the tasks and became frustrated. However, during an hour-long session with her mother, Anita used fewer than 120 words total. Most of her utterances were one or two words in length, and she often used gestures in place of words. Speech was slow and effortful; words were sometimes slurred. Anita established attention very slowly and had difficulty maintaining it. This affected her comprehension, which was poor overall. Her mother used a number of techniques to facilitate attention and comprehension. She maintained close proximity to her daughter and touched her own lips before speaking to draw Anita's attention. The mother physically directed Anita's attention, first to her face as she spoke and then to the objects under discussion. She used short sentences and many repetitions to support the conversation. Occasionally, Anita echoed those repetitions back to her mother.

As we see in Anita's case, a prolonged period of seizure activity can lead to a deterioration of skills that were once evident. In fact, a change in language status, as seen here, is a leading sign of an underlying neurological disturbance. For Anita, the seizure activity affected both language comprehension and expression, as well as general functioning in nonverbal domains. In other cases of seizure disorder, receptive language abilities are far more impaired than expressive skills (Rapin, Mattis, Rowan, & Golden, 1977; Worster-Drought, 1971). Receptive abilities can be so severely impaired that the child behaves as if deaf. However, the child can have normal hearing acuity, as established by an audiometric evaluation. No longer able to understand his or her own speech, the child may stop talking altogether, or speech may become garbled. However, language expression can continue if the child is introduced to sign language or other modes of communication.

One subtype of seizure disorder is particularly associated with loss of language skills. Landau-Kleffner syndrome was first described as involving loss of language skills in children who had seizures (Landau & Kleffner, 1957). The seizure activity of these children typically involves both temporal lobes and, for some children, is managed with medication. However, the language disorder can persist even after their seizures are brought under control. Recovery of language is quite variable, ranging from a few weeks to many years (Mantovani & Landau, 1980).

Traumatic Brain Injury

Each year, between 100 and 300 of every 100,000 children experience a traumatic brain injury (TBI). TBI is most prevalent among teens and young adults, followed by preschool children (McKinlay, Grace, Horwood, Fergusson,. Ridder, & Macfarlane, 2008). TBI can be focal, due to a penetrating or "open-head" injury (e.g., a gunshot wound), or diffuse, as the result of force applied without penetration of the skull (i.e., a "closed-head" injury). Most commonly, it involves some combination of focal and diffuse injury. TBI can be caused by any number of events, including motor vehicle accidents, in which the injury includes both diffuse damage from the brain moving within the skull and focal contusions where the brain *nature + severity differ*

contacts the skull. Other events that can produce a combination of diffuse and focal injury include rough shaking (e.g., shaken baby syndrome), falls, sports injuries, assaults, and pedestrian–motor vehicle collisions.

There is considerable heterogeneity among individuals with TBI. Some of this can be accounted for by differences in the nature and severity of the injury (Chapman, 1997). Other sources of heterogeneity are related to pre-injury intelligence, health, and personality, as well as family and cultural factors. Because of the diffuse nature of the brain damage, the behavioral consequences range far beyond language skills. This is illustrated by the case of Gerard.

> *Gerard* was a 17-year-old high school junior when he had his car accident. He was ditching his afternoon classes with three friends when he lost control of his truck and it went off the road, flipping over several times. The two boys in the back were killed, and a third was paralyzed by the crash. Gerard was in a coma for two weeks with severe head injuries. When he emerged from his coma, cognitive and linguistic deficits were apparent. He was highly distractible and easily overwhelmed by new information or situations. Memory testing indicated that his post-injury abilities were in the fifth percentile, or below the performance of 95 percent of the normative sample for the test. He also had great difficulty understanding both written and spoken language, needing substantial amounts of time to process information and not always arriving at the correct interpretation. In contrast, his spoken language form and content appeared unaffected by his injury.

> Gerard's most noticeable communication deficit involved language use. His affect was flat, and he failed to use prosodic variation to convey emotion in his speech. Likewise, he did not seem to pick up on the nonverbal cues of others in conversations. His thinking had a concreteness that did not allow him to interpret jokes or sarcasm. This lack of abstract thinking had pervasive effects on his daily life as well. He was unable to conceptualize the future or plan for it effectively.

> Traumatic brain injury is a major cause of disability in young people, often affecting communication success and academic achievement.

Language difficulties after TBI are different from those associated with developmental language disorders. For example, many children with TBI perform relatively well on standardized tests of vocabulary, morphology, and syntax (Biddle, McCabe, & Bliss, 1996; Chapman et al., 1997; Ylvisaker, 1993). These tests tap knowledge gained prior to the injury. Communication breakdowns are more likely to occur in conversational or discourse contexts (Chapman et al., 1997; Chapman, Levin, Matejeka, Harward, & Kufera, 1995) or on language tasks that place particular demands on attention, information processing, and memory (Turkstra & Holland, 1988). Survivors also may have profoundly handicapping impairments in abilities referred to collectively as executive functions (Ylvisaker, Szekeres, & Feeney, 1998). These functions include the ability to plan and organize behavior, make decisions that take multiple factors into account, and regulate one's own behavior. An important difference between those with TBI and those with developmental language disorders is that individuals with TBI are likely to have had a period of normal development and must begin a new life with uncertainty about their post-injury skills and limitations (Ylvisaker, 1998). This may have a profound effect on their attitude toward therapy.

For Gerard, therapy began in the hospital as soon as he was conscious and medically stable. His treatment was a multidisciplinary effort, with a speech-language pathologist, physical therapist, and psychologist helping Gerard address the physical, cognitive, and emotional aftermath of his injuries. By the time he was well enough to resume school, he had missed most of his junior year. The school provided a full-time classroom aide who took notes for him in class, organized his program of study, and helped him with assignments. The school's speech-language pathologist focused on improving Gerard's basic reading comprehension and helped him learn strategies for working within the limits of his impaired memory. Other activities included role-playing practice for various social and vocational situations to improve his pragmatics in these communicative contexts. Therapy was a challenge, because Gerard did not acknowledge his language deficits and therefore did not see the point of the activities. Gerard also participated, although grudgingly, in a weekly meeting with other teens who had sustained brain injuries.

The long-term prognosis for individuals with TBI is dependent in part on which abilities were already acquired and which were still developing at the age when the injury occurred. The full effects of the injury may not be apparent until months or years later (Chapman, 1997). It has been said that after traumatic brain injury "time reveals all wounds" (DePompei, Blosser, Savage, & Lash, 1997). For example, we do not expect coherent, logical stories from 4-year-olds with or without TBI, but by 10 years of age incoherent storytelling would signal a deficit. When a brain injury is mild, the child may eventually return to normal or near-normal functioning. However, when injuries are severe, the long-term outlook may be less positive.

Two years after his injury, Gerard was finishing high school, although his graduation was uncertain. His involvement in the school's TBI program focused on vocational training to prepare him for post-graduation life. However, he had been through four jobs in as many months, quitting each time because he was bored or felt the job was beneath him in some way. He drifted away from the teens who were his friends before the injury, and his social and pragmatic problems made it difficult for him to make new social contacts.

Evaluation of Language Disorders

Evaluation of children with suspected language disorders takes many forms in order to accommodate the wide range of disorders that involve impaired language. The evaluation may address a number of questions of interest to the clinician and the parents. Does the child have a language disorder? Are there any factors that might account for the presence of a language disorder? How do the child's skills in various language domains compare to peers? If intervention is warranted, what aspects of language should be addressed? As we will see, components of the diagnostic process are tailored to address these types of questions.

[handwritten annotations: "goal determine whether language skills warrant a full eval — include normative sample"]

Language Screening

Language screenings are designed to determine whether a child's language skills warrant a full evaluation. Screenings are typically quick to administer and often sample a range of language skills that could potentially be impaired. Screenings may include formal measures that have been administered to large groups of children, who serve as a **normative sample**. Normative samples permit comparison of a single child's performance to a group of children who are of the same age. These children serve as a reference for the range of normal performance that can be expected. Other screenings may be informal in order to accommodate regional variations in language or dialect, or to target skills of particular interest for a certain setting (e.g., conversational speech, reading readiness). Frequently, language screening is used as a cost-effective method of evaluating large numbers of children, most of whom will not have any difficulties with language skills. For example, a school district may routinely screen the language of all of their incoming kindergarten children. Only those children who fail the screening are referred for a full evaluation.

The Case History

[handwritten annotation: "goal ↓"]

The case history is a way to gather background information that may be used for many purposes. A case history may be obtained through conversation with those who know the child best (usually the parents). In other cases, it may consist of a form that is completed prior to or during the initial evaluation. Many case histories include information concerning pregnancy, birth, and medical background. This information can be important for identifying potential causes for a language disorder. For example, if a mother reports having had rubella during her pregnancy, the clinician would be alerted to the possibility of hearing loss, which sometimes occurs under those conditions. The clinician can then plan a hearing screening during the evaluation or arrange a referral to an audiologist for a full hearing assessment, if the child's hearing has not already been tested. Information concerning developmental and family history can help determine the degree of risk for a language disorder. As we saw in earlier sections, children who have developmental language disorders are likely to have a family member who also has a language or learning disorder. In other cases, parental report of a change or cessation of language skills during the child's development would alert the clinician to explore the possibility of autism, seizure disorders, or disease processes that would impact previously normal development.

Sometimes a case history will probe for more subjective information. Parents may be asked what led them to become concerned about their child's language development. They may report what they see as their child's overall strengths and weaknesses. The parents' input may help identify those skills that, if remediated, would make the biggest improvement in their child's daily life. Parents may also be able to provide information on strategies that they have developed that seem to help their child. This type of information is invaluable for guiding subsequent therapy.

Observation

Important diagnostic information can be gathered simply through observation. Let us consider the following case:

> *Charise* was a speech-language pathologist who worked at a community clinic that handled referrals from the state's program for children with disabilities. She always made a point of meeting her clients in the lobby because, as she said, "I can always tell a lot about the way things are going to go on the walk from the front door to my office." One particular morning, she had a new referral for a child with a reported language delay. The child, a 2-year-old boy, came in hand-in-hand with his mother. He was a little overweight, and his belly peeked out beneath his T-shirt. When Charise dropped down to his eye level, he greeted her with a smile as she explained who she was. He had a round, pleasant face, with widespread, almond-shaped eyes, a broad nose, and full cheeks and lips. Overall, his face appeared soft, as if the underlying muscle tone might be low. He seemed social, and he pointed and made short one- or two-word comments about the children's paintings that hung along the hallway. There was one moment of difficulty when it came time to turn the corner and his eye caught something interesting in the opposite direction. He stamped his foot and sat down defiantly in the middle of the hallway. With a bit of cajoling, his mother got him back up and back on track. Once in the office, Charise confirmed the presence of a language delay with formal diagnostic measures. She also made a referral to a medical geneticist. The facial features, low tone, and high weight, combined with a general immaturity, made her think that a genetic syndrome might be playing a role in this child's language problems. In fact, two months later, a follow-up report was received that confirmed a diagnosis of Prader-Willi syndrome, which involves a genetic abnormality located on chromosome 15.

In this case, the speech-language pathologist's initial observations contributed to this child's diagnosis. Observation is important at all stages of the diagnostic process. The speech-language pathologist may visit the child's home in order to get an idea of typical communication style within the family. A gross assessment of language functioning can be obtained by listening to a child's conversations. How the child plays can provide insight into the level of cognitive and social functioning. Classroom observations can provide insight into the specific conditions that precipitate communication problems for the school-age child. Furthermore, the speech-language pathologist may notice simple things that can greatly enhance a child's chances of success.

> Speech-language pathologists typically become keen observers of human behavior.

Formal Measures

There are a multitude of commercially available, formal measures for assessing children's language. These tests vary remarkably in their focus, quality, and suitability for a specific diagnostic purpose. One method that clinicians use to select among formal measures is to consider the information that they hope to gain by administering the test. Different formal measures are developed for different purposes. For example, clinicians who wish to compare a child's performance to

child v other children @ same age

that of other children of the same age will select a **norm-referenced test**. If they wish to establish whether a child can use certain syntactic structures in various speaking tasks, a **criterion-referenced test** would be needed.

Norm-referenced tests allow comparisons between a child's performance and that of a group of children of similar age. Beyond this common feature, however, there is great variation among norm-referenced tests. Some measure narrow domains of language functioning. For example, one norm-referenced test may examine the number of words that a child recognizes; another will evaluate broader knowledge of word meanings. Some consist of several subtests compiled into a battery that examines various components of language functioning. These may sample across the language domains of phonology, morphology, syntax, and semantics in both receptive and expressive modalities.

Criterion-referenced tests are typically more narrowly focused than norm-referenced tests. These tests are used to compare a child's performance against a standard, or criterion, for behavior. Most college course examinations, for example, are criterion-referenced tests, in that the instructor compares each student's performance against a standard for knowledge of the course content. Criterion-referenced tests may be informal, as when a clinician develops a series of "probes" to assess whether a child is able to use structures trained in therapy. Others are commercially available measures that sample language skills to determine a child's proficiency.

Once the purpose for administering a test has been determined, the clinician will examine the test's qualities. Specifically, the clinician must determine whether administering a particular test will result in valid conclusions about the child's language. Let us consider an example of why this is important.

> *Brendon* was just 3½ when he was first enrolled in therapy for a language delay. At that point, his mean length of utterance (MLU) was moderately low for his age (see Chapter 7 for a review of MLU). A norm-referenced test of expressive language placed him below the first percentile for his age, which means that 99 out of 100 children his age could be expected to score higher than Brendon on that particular test. A single-word vocabulary test was also administered, and he did not pass enough items to show that he understood even the simplest words. By contrast, his hearing, motor, and cognitive development tested well within normal limits. Based on these results, he was enrolled in a preschool program for children with specific language impairment. A little over a year later (age 4 years, 10 months), his skills were retested using a different battery of tests. At that time, all skills were well within normal limits according to the test norms. It was concluded that Brendon had overcome his earlier difficulties, and he was dismissed from the preschool program.

> Two months later (age 5 years, 0 months), his mother, still concerned about Brendon's language skills, enrolled him in a university-based research project for children with specific language impairment. His language was retested with a third battery of tests. This time, Brendon received expressive language scores and receptive vocabulary scores that were once again below the first percentile for his age.

How could the appearing-disappearing-reappearing language deficits be explained? The lead researcher, a speech-language pathologist, consulted the normative tables for the tests Brendon received at age 4. She discovered that the test items were so difficult that most normal 4-year-old children could not pass them. Therefore, failure to pass *any* items on that test battery still placed a child within normal limits of performance!

The test given to Brendon at age 4 lacked **validity**. Validity refers to the degree to which test results lead to correct conclusions concerning the skills measured (Messick, 1989). Another technical feature that clinicians will consider is a test's **reliability**. This refers to the degree to which a test provides consistent information each time it is given. An unreliable test is never valid. However, high reliability does not ensure validity. A ruler whose inch markings are too closely spaced will provide the same mis-measurement every time—highly reliable, but not at all valid! Standards for the assessment of test reliability and validity have been detailed by the combined efforts of the American Educational Research Association, American Psychological Association, and National Council on Measurement in Education (AERA, APA, & NCME, 1999). Despite such standards, many tests of child language fall short of minimal criteria for validity and reliability (e.g., McCauley & Swisher, 1984; Plante & Vance, 1994; Spaulding, Plante, & Farinella, 2006). Unfortunately, use of a psychometrically weak test can lead to erroneous conclusions. In Brendon's case, the erroneous conclusions that were based on the test results obtained when he was 4 led to the discontinuation of services that he still needed.

A final consideration in test selection is the context in which the skill domains are tested. The same items can be passed on one test and failed on another, just based on the context in which those items appear (e.g., Merrell & Plante, 1997; Wiig, Jones, & Wiig, 1996). Sabers (1996) pointed out that "the way a test measures behavior may introduce measurement aspects not intended for the test." In fact, if the simplest linguistic elements are presented in strange or difficult contexts, children will fail those items long after they are able to use and understand the elements in everyday life. For example, a child who has been using "me" since the age of 2 years will not use it in the context of "You would have liked me to see the painting" until many years later. Test items designed to measure language may in fact be a stronger test of memory if the child is required to hold multiple words in memory before composing an answer using those words. Sometimes, the way test items are presented by a test is enough to influence the child's performance. Wiig and colleagues (1996) demonstrated this when they developed a computerized version of one of their tests. They found that teens' performance differed significantly on the traditional and computer-based versions of the test, even though the items were identical. For these reasons, test content and context influence how a clinician interprets the test results.

Response to Intervention (RTI)

Response to intervention (RTI) is a method of assessing children through intervention. RTI has emerged from the field of special education in part because of concerns that standardized intelligence and academic testing do not adequately

> A practicing speech-language pathologist must become familiar with standard testing procedures, but also should understand the statistical properties of tests that are used.

address what type of intervention is needed. Furthermore, standardized tests may not be able to differentiate between children whose poor learning is due to a learning disability and those whose poor learning may be due to inadequate instruction or lack of prerequisite knowledge on the part of the child. RTI typically utilizes a tiered system of instruction (Fuchs, Mock, Morgan, & Young, 2003). In the lowest tier, children receive the general instruction of the classroom. Children who struggle under those conditions are advanced to a second tier where more targeted instruction is provided. Children who continue to struggle under these conditions may be identified as having a learning disability, reading disability, or other educationally handicapping condition that warrants a third tier of instruction that is individualized and intensive. A speech-language pathologist may develop a response to intervention plan for a child, or serve on a team that implements such plans in school classrooms.

The current version of the Individuals with Disabilities Educational Improvement Act (IDEA, 2004) allows RTI as a method of identifying children eligible for special educational services. However, some have raised concerns about this practice (e.g., Mather & Kaufman, 2006). For example, decisions about how much improvement during a treatment phase is enough to rule out a learning disability can be highly subjective. Likewise, the RTI procedures may identify children who need alternative methods of instruction to succeed, but additional and more formal testing may be needed to identify the child's strengths and weaknesses that will inform individualized instruction at the highest tier of intervention (Willis & Dumont, 2006). However, RTI can be particularly valuable in difficult-to-diagnose cases, such as differentiating between children whose language and learning difficulties are attributable to learning English as a second language and those due to a language or learning disorder in children who are bilingual (e.g., Barrera, 2006; Linan-Thompson, Vaughn, Prater, & Cirino, 2006). Furthermore, implementing RTI procedures can assist children who are struggling before being identified as having a handicapping condition.

RTI is related to procedures speech-language pathologists have also used in the assessment of children with suspected language disorders. These procedures have been referred to as *dynamic assessment.* The term "dynamic" in dynamic assessment is intended to contrast with "static" measures of assessment that measure a child's skills at one point in time. Static measures include norm-referenced and criterion-referenced measures. Dynamic assessment is designed to determine a child's potential to learn under specific conditions (like RTI) or to determine whether better performance might be obtained if the testing situation were more appropriate to a child's background experiences, culture, or language (e.g., Gutiérrez-McClelland & Peña, 2001; Hwa-Froelich & Matsuo, 2005). For example, a young child who has never been read to at home may lack prerequisite skills for taking a vocabulary test. As in book-reading activities, a vocabulary test may require children to look at pictures on a test page, then point to a picture that is named. If a child is unfamiliar with this routine, he or she could fail the vocabulary test, not because the words are unknown, but because the task is unfamiliar. If the skills of joint attention to pictures and pointing to named pictures are trained outside of the context of the test, and the child is then retested, then a more accurate measure of vocabulary might be obtained. It is important to note that dynamic assessment should not include training with actual test materials or its exact format, because either would invalidate the test for future use with that child.

Hearing Evaluation

As we will see in Chapter 11, hearing impairment can be an underlying cause of poor language development. Therefore, a pure-tone hearing screening is typically part of a language evaluation. If a child fails to respond during the hearing screening, a full audiological evaluation should be scheduled to rule out hearing loss as a contributing factor in the child's language difficulties.

Language Intervention

Approaches to the treatment of language disorders are as diverse as the children who receive services. There is no "recipe book" of procedures or one-size-fits-all method that will work with all children. In fact, therapy methods that are successful with one child may not work well with another. As we saw above, children with different types of language disorders can vary considerably in terms of their language profiles. Furthermore, children's ages, cultural backgrounds, and family situations may greatly affect the types of intervention that are best for them. Therefore, language therapy tends to be highly individualized.

When we examine different intervention methods, we first consider what the treatment approach is intended to do for the child. Wilcox (1994) reviewed major approaches to intervention: prevention, remediation, and compensation. *Preventive* services may be provided to children at risk for language disorders. These children may be at risk because they are born with conditions associated with language disorders (e.g., mental retardation, genetic disorders). Other children may receive preventive services because they are showing early signs of communication delay (e.g., late talkers). In this case, services are intended to maximize the child's potential early in development so that the impact on language can be lessened or avoided. Examples of preventive services include preschool "head start" programs and other programs designed to enrich a child's early language and educational experiences.

Remediation involves correction of current deficits and is perhaps the most frequent form of therapy for children. When therapy is oriented toward remediation, the clinician typically has very specific goals (e.g., increase use of target syntactic structures, morphemes, vocabulary). The clinician then devises a program to teach these linguistic targets. Let us look at an example of a therapy program designed to remediate expressive language deficits in a young boy.

Davin is a 20-month-old boy who receives therapy in his home from Sue, a clinician in private practice. When therapy began recently, Davin had six "word approximations" that he used occasionally, although he understood about fifty words. Therefore, both his comprehension and expression were well below what is typical for a child his age. Sue decided that the top priority for Davin would be expressive language, specifically expanding the number of words he could use to express his needs. More words would help reduce the frustration Davin was displaying because of his poor ability to communicate. Furthermore, the fact that he had some word approximations suggested he was ready to communicate with words.

On her first visit to Davin's home, Sue taught him signs for "eat," "drink," "want," "more," and "help." Sue elected to incorporate signs into Davin's therapy because children can often produce the more gross hand movements for words before they are able to produce the very precise oral-motor movements needed for intelligible speech. For many children, successful use of signs provides an immediate means for successful communication and a bridge to spoken language. Sue modeled the signs, then demonstrated them to Davin by placing her hands over his while forming the signs with him. By the second visit, it was apparent that Davin was using these first signs on his own.

A critical part of Davin's therapy program is the involvement of his parents. Sue knows that it would be unrealistic to expect Davin to catch up with his peers in the hour a week she sees him at home. It is much more effective for language therapy to be continuous throughout the week. Therefore, a large part of the therapy program involves ensuring that both parents develop techniques that they can use to continue Davin's progress after Sue leaves. Davin's mother requested that Sue come when both parents were available to participate in the therapy sessions. They learn signs along with Davin and also learn how to create opportunities for Davin to use the words he has and learn new words as well. Sue thus teaches the parents how to teach their child and gets feedback on their efforts of the previous week.

It seems obvious that parental involvement in therapy programs can be a positive thing. However, successfully bringing parents into the therapy process can be one of the biggest challenges for the clinician. Sue points out that Davin's parents were eager to be involved in the therapy process. They were also both highly educated, with college degrees, and came from middle class backgrounds. Davin is their only child, and his mother is able to stay at home with him full-time. "I don't want to overwhelm parents, and parents need to be honest with me when I suggest something that is just not possible," says Sue. For example, Sue suggested to Davin's parents that they allow him to make some choices of his own at mealtimes as a way to encourage requests. This same suggestion would not work for a working mother trying to get five young children—one with a disability—dressed and off to school on time. Sue comments, "I can tell I have gone too far when I make a suggestion and their eyes glaze over."

Compensation involves the introduction of strategies that assist the child to manage the effects of the disorder, rather than eliminating its signs. Compensation is often used with conditions that are not completely correctable, such as brain injury or hearing loss. For example, in our case of seizure disorder, the mother's use of visual cues provided a strategy to aid comprehension. For older children and teens, the child may be responsible for use of the strategy. A child with a learning disability, for example, may be taught how to use diagrams to summarize information from his lecture notes. For a teen, compensation may involve strategies to support academic learning. Let's look at one such example.

> *Mary* works as a speech-language pathologist in a school system. Her role there is to support the children whose language deficits impact their educational progress. Jack is one of her students. In eighth grade, he still struggles with reading. It takes him a long time, and he doesn't always comprehend what he has read. Therefore, he does not learn as much from reading his textbooks as his peers do. Mary has worked with Jack on strategies that are designed to maximize his comprehension of text materials. She teaches him to recognize the cues that are used in textbooks to signal important information. These include strategies like reading the chapter and subheading titles to gain a broad idea about the content area that will be covered. Jack learns that bolded words are important, and if he doesn't fully understand them, he should look in the glossary found at the back of his book. Mary also has trained Jack to distinguish between a main point and the details that support it and on how to spot these in text. Finally, Mary has worked with Jack's teacher to modify his homework load so that he can keep up with the content without falling behind, because of the amount of time it takes him to complete assignments.

As we saw with the cases presented in this chapter, children with language disorders often have many areas of difficulty that could benefit from therapy. However, working on everything at once would be overwhelming for both the clinician and child. Therefore, the clinician may need to prioritize the areas of need and target these sequentially. Some goals receive priority because they offer the greatest potential for positive improvement in the child's quality of life. For example, a program that provides a nonverbal child with more communicative functions (e.g., requesting, commenting) can reduce frustration for parent and child. A school-age child may benefit most from therapy that allows him or her to participate more fully in classroom activities. Occasionally, the goal that would make the greatest difference in the child's language is not necessarily the one selected. For example, one mother of a severely handicapped child was interested in her child learning social routines (e.g., greetings, "please," and "thank you"), even though other more functional aspects of communication could have been targeted. Social communication was important to the mother because she saw it as a way for her child to have positive interactions with others.

Certain therapy goals may receive priority because they help the child progress to a higher developmental stage. Wilcox (1992) developed an intervention program designed to move infants and toddlers from preverbal gestures and vocalizations to the verbal stage of communication. For a late-talking toddler, increasing the number of vocabulary words is a prerequisite for acquiring phrases and sentences. For older children, the developmental sequence for morpheme acquisition may guide selection of therapy targets. A developmental focus can combine both remediation and preventive components. For example, Dale and colleagues described a treatment method that used storybook activities to facilitate language in preschoolers (Dale, Crain-Thoreson, Notari-Syverson, & Cole,

1996). The immediate goal of this program was language facilitation. However, the treatment context of reading introduced preliteracy skills that are thought to contribute to reading success in later years.

Once the language goals are selected, the speech-language pathologist must consider the structure used to train those goals. Naturalistic contexts have become very popular over the last decade. As a result, there has been an emphasis on home programs, classroom-based programs, and other intervention techniques that are incorporated into the child's daily life. For example, many programs have demonstrated that parents can be effectively trained to facilitate language development at home. Various programs have been used to teach parents to modify their speech and change how they respond to the child's attempts at communication (e.g., Eiserman, Weber, & McCoun, 1995; Gibbard, 1994; Girolametto, Pearce, & Weitzman, 1996). In fact, parent-administered programs can be as effective as clinician-administered programs, at least in the early stages of intervention (Eiserman, Weber, & McCoun, 1995; Fey, Cleave, & Long, 1997). Other programs emphasize remediation in naturalistic contexts (e.g., conversation, play) during which a clinician, parent, or teacher facilitates the learning of new linguistic forms as opportunities arise within the interaction (Figure 8.3). This technique is sometimes called "incidental teaching," because language

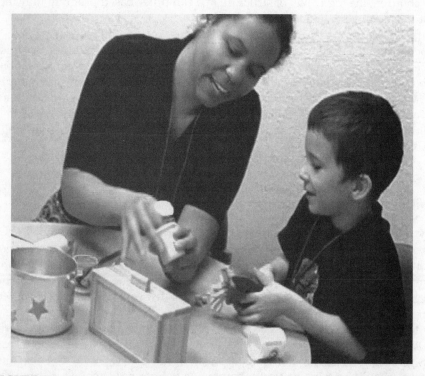

FIGURE 8.3 Language intervention with young children may make use of age-appropriate toys and activities that allow the child to practice language goals in a conversational context.

instruction follows from natural interactions with the child. For example, a child may learn to use questions by being prompted to request toys, food, and other items encountered in his or her daily life. The effectiveness of naturalistic intervention can vary depending on the specific techniques used to facilitate language (e.g., Kaiser & Hester, 1994; Leonard, Camarata, Pawtowska, Brown, & Camarata, 2008; Warren, Gazdag, Bambara, & Jones, 1994) and the characteristics of the child (Yoder, Kaiser, & Alpert, 1991).

Some children need more structure than is afforded by naturalistic contexts because of the nature of their disorder. For example, a child with attention deficit disorder may prove too distractible in a completely naturalistic context to benefit from incidental teaching techniques. A teenager with a traumatic brain injury may need increased structure relative to his or her peers in order to function in school or in a work setting. Students who need assistance with language skills in the academic domain may use strategies that are explicitly taught. Finally, what is "natural" to one child may be completely unfamiliar to another. For example, in some cultures, a conversation between a child and an adult who is not a close relative is not at all natural. A clinician who uses such a "natural" context may be confronted with a child who will not talk at all under those conditions. In contrast, the use of computers as a tool for therapy may be natural for children who have been interacting with educational software programs from early ages. For these children, the high level of structure in a computer-based program may feel as natural as conversationally based therapy.

Effective therapy takes into account all of these considerations and makes adjustments to fit the needs of each child. The clinician may use a highly structured, compensatory approach with one child and a parent-administered, conversationally based approach with another. For a third child, the clinician may simply serve as a consultant to a classroom teacher who assists the language-disordered child with modifications of teaching activities and materials. This kind of flexibility allows therapy approaches to be tailored to each child's developmental stage and communication needs.

Clinical Problem Solving

Becky is a 30-month-old girl who was brought to the clinic by her parents. They were concerned about her language development because she did not seem to use as many words as the other children at her preschool. Although Becky seemed quite interested in the toys and books in the clinic playroom, she said few words and often seemed to substitute gestures for words. All of her verbal utterances consisted of single words, with no multiword combinations. She was in good health, and other than language, the parents did not have any concerns about her development.

1. Is this child at risk for a language disorder? Why or why not?
2. What should be included in the initial evaluation of this child? What is the purpose for including each of these components?

3. Given the child's age and language level, what approach might therapy take?
4. What do we know about the long-term outlook for young children whose language lags behind their age-mates?

REFERENCES

Alloway, T., Elliott, J., & Holmes, J. (2010). The prevalence of ADHD-like symptoms in a community sample. *Journal of Attention Disorders*, 14(1), 52–56.

Alloway, T., Elliott, J., & Holmes, J. (2010). The prevalence of ADHD-like symptoms in a community sample. *Journal of Attention Disorders*, 14(1), 52–56.

American Educational Research Association, American Psychological Association, & National Council on Measurement in Education. (1999). *Standards for educational and psychological testing.* Washington, DC: Author.

American Psychiatric Association. (2000). *Diagnostic and statistical manual of mental disorders* (4th ed., text revision). Arlington, VA: Author.

American Speech-Language-Hearing Association (ASHA). (1983). Social dialects. *Asha, 25,* 23–27.

American Speech-Language-Hearing Association (ASHA). (1997). Position statement: Roles of audiologists and speech-language pathologists working with persons with attention deficit hyperactivity disorder. *Asha, 39,* 14.

Aram, D. (1991). Comments on specific language impairment as a clinical category. *Language, Speech, & Hearing Services in Schools, 22,* 84–87.

Aram, D. M., Ekelman, B. L., Rose, D. F., & Whitaker, H. A. (1985). Verbal and cognitive sequelae following unilateral lesions acquired in early childhood. *Journal of Clinical and Experimental Neuropsychology, 7,* 55–78.

Ballantyne, A. O., Spilkin, A. M., Hesselink, J., & Trauner, D. A. (2008). Plasticity in the developing brain: Intellectual, language and academic functions in children with ischaemic perinatal stroke. *Brain: A Journal of Neurology, 131,* 2975–2985.

Ballantyne, A. O., Spilkin, A. M., Hesselink, J., & Trauner, D. A. (2008). Plasticity in the developing brain: Intellectual, language and academic functions in children with ischaemic perinatal stroke. *Brain: A Journal of Neurology, 131,* 2975–2985.

Barrera, M. (2006). Roles of definitional and assessment models in the identification of new or second language learners of English for special education. *Journal of Learning Disabilities, 39,* 142–156.

Beharelle, A. J., Dick, A. S., Josse, G., Solodkin, A., Huttenlocher, P. R., Levine, S. C., & Small, S. L. (2010). Left hemisphere regions are critical for language in the face of early left focal brain injury. *Brain: A Journal of Neurlology, 133,* 1707–1716.

Bellugi, U., Lichtenberger, L., Jones, W., Lai, Z., & St. George, M. (2000). The neurocognitive profile of Williams Syndrome: A complex pattern of strengths and weaknesses. *Journal of Cognitive Neuroscience, 12 (supplement),* 7–29.

Bent, J. P., & Beck, R. A. (1994). Bacterial meningitis in the pediatric population: Paradigm shifts and ramifications for otolaryngology-head and neck surgery. *International Journal of Pediatric Otorhinolaryngology, 30,* 41–49.

Biddle, K. R., McCabe, A., & Bliss, L. S. (1996). Narrative skills following traumatic brain injury in children and adults. *Journal of Communication Disorders, 29,* 447–470.

Bishop, D. V. M., Laws, G., Adams, C., & Norbury, C. F. (2006). High heritability of speech and language impairments in 6-year-old twins demonstrated using parent and teacher report. *Behavior Genetics, 36,* 173–184.

Bishop, D. V. M., & Snowling, M. J. (2004). Developmental dyslexia and specific language impairment: Same or different? *Psychological Bulletin, 130,* 858–886.

Botting, N., Simkin, Z., & Conti-Ramsden, G. (2006). Associated reading skills in children with a history of specific language impairment (SLI). *Reading and Writing, 19,* 77–98.

Bruce, B., Thernlund, G., Nettelbladt, U., (2006). ADHD and language impairment: A study of the parent questionnaire FTF (Five to Fifteen). *European Child & Adolescent Psychiatry, 15,* 52–60.

Burd, L., Cotsonas-Hassler, T. M., Martsolf, J. T., & Kerbeshian, J. (2003). Recognition and management of fetal alcohol syndrome. *Neurotoxicology and Teratology, 25,* 681–688.

Burkhard, S., & Lütschg, J. (2010). Epidemiology and etiology of pediatric stroke. *Journal of Pediatric Neurology, 8,* 245–249.

Byrne, J., Ellsworth, C., Bowering, E., & Vincer, M. (1993). Language development in low birth weight infants: The first two years of life. *Journal of Developmental and Behavioral Pediatrics, 14,* 21–27.

Catts, H. W., Adlof, S. M., Hogan, T. P., & Ellis Weismer, S. (2005). Are specific language impairment and dyslexia distinct disorders? *Journal of Speech, Language, and Hearing Research, 48,* 1378–1396.

Chapman, S. B. (1997). Cognitive-communication abilities in children with closed head injury. *American Journal of Speech Language Pathology, 6,* 50–58.

Chapman, S. B., Levin, H. S., Matejka, J., Harward, H. N., & Kufera, J. (1995). Discourse ability in head injured children: Consideration of linguistic, psychosocial, and cognitive factors. *Journal of Head Trauma Rehabilitation, 10,* 36–54.

Chapman, S. B., Watkins, R., Gustafson, C., Moore, S., Levin, H. S., & Kufera, J. A. (1997). Narrative discourse in children with closed head injury, children with language impairment, and typically developing children. *American Journal of Speech Language Pathology, 6,* 66–76.

Clark, D. A. (1994). Neonates and infants at risk for hearing and language disorders. In K. G. Butler (Ed.), *Early intervention I: Working with infants and toddlers.* Gaithersburg, MD: Aspen Publishers.

Claude, D., & Firestone, P. (1995). The development of ADHD boys: A 12-year follow-up. *Canadian Journal of Behavioral Science, 27,* 226–249.

Cohen, M., Campbell, R., & Yaghmai, F. (1989). Neuropathological abnormalities in developmental dysphasia. *Annals of Neurology, 25,* 567–570.

Courchesne, E., Yeung-Courchesne, R., Press, G., Hesselink, J. R., & Jernigan, T. L. (1988). Hypoplasia of the cerebellar vermal lobes VI and VII in infantile autism. *New England Journal of Medicine, 318,* 1349–1354.

Cranberg, L. D., Filley, C. M., Hart, E. J., & Alexander, M. P. (1987). Acquired aphasia in childhood: Clinical and CT investigations. *Neurology, 37,* 1165–1172.

Dale, P. S., Crain-Thoreson, C., Notari-Syverson, A., & Cole, K. (1996). Parent-child book reading as an intervention technique for young children with language delays. *Topics in Early Childhood Special Education, 16,* 213–235.

DePompei, R., Blosser, J. L., Savage, R., & Lash, M. (1997, November). *Effective long-term management for youths with TBI.* Miniseminar presented at the annual conference of the American Speech-Language-Hearing Association, Boston, MA.

D'Odorico, L., Assanelli, A., Franco, F., & Jacob, V. (2007). A follow-up study on Italian late talkers: Development of language, short-term memory, phonological awareness, impulsiveness, and attention. *Applied Psycholinguistics, 28*(1), 157–169.

Dunn, M. (1997). Language disorders in children with autism. *Seminars in Pediatric Neurology, 4,* 86–92.

Eiserman, W. D., Weber, C., & McCoun, M. (1995). Parent and professional roles in early intervention: A longitudinal comparison of the effects of two intervention configurations. *Journal of Special Education, 29,* 20–44.

Ellis Weismer, S., Murray-Branch, J., & Miller, J. F. (1994). A prospective longitudinal study of language development in late talkers. *Journal of Speech and Hearing Research, 37,* 852–867.

Fey, M. E., Cleave, P. L., & Long, S. H. (1997). Two models of grammar facilitation in children with language impairments. *Journal of Speech and Hearing Research, 40,* 5–19.

Fidler, L. J., Plante, E., & Vance, R. (2011). Identification of adults with developmental language impairments. *American Journal of Speech-Language Pathology, 20,* 2–13.

Fischel, J. E., Whitehurst, G. J., Caulfield, M. B., & Debaryshe, B. (1989). Language growth in children with expressive language delay. *Pediatrics, 82,* 218–227.

Fuchs, D., Mock, D., Morgan, P., & Young, C. (2003). Responsiveness-to-intervention: Definitions, evidence, and implications for the learning disabilities construct. *Learning Disabilities Research & Practice, 18,* 157–171.

Garnier-Dykstra, L. M., Pinchevsky, G. M., Caldeira, K. M., Vincent, K. B., & Arria, A. M. (2010). Self-reported adult attention-deficit/hyperactivity disorder symptoms among college students. *Journal of American College Health, 59*(2), 133–136.

Gauger, L. M., Lombardino, L. J., & Leonard, C. M. (1997). Brain morphology in children with specific language impairment. *Journal of Speech, Language, and Hearing Research, 40,* 1272–1284.

Gibbard, D. (1994). Parental-based intervention with pre-school language-delayed children. *European Journal of Disorders of Communication, 29*(2), 131–150.

Gillam, R. B., & Carlile, R. M. (1997). Oral reading and story retelling of students with specific language impairment. *Language, Speech, and Hearing Services in Schools, 28,* 30–42.

Gillon, G. T. (2002). Follow-up study investigating the benefits of phonological awareness intervention for children with spoken language impairment. International *Journal of Language & Communication Disorders, 37,* 381–400.

Girolametto, L., Pearce, P., & Weitzman, E. (1996). Interactive focused stimulation for toddlers with expressive vocabulary delays. *Journal of Speech & Hearing Research, 39*(6), 1274–1283.

Gutiérrez-Clellen, V. F., & Peña, E. (2001). Dynamic assessment of diverse children: A tutorial. *Language, Speech, and Hearing Services in Schools, 32,* 212–224.

Halsey, C. L., Collin, M. F., & Anderson, C. L. (1996). Extremely low-birth-weight children and their peers. A comparison of school-age outcomes. *Archives of Pediatrics and Adolescent Medicine, 150,* 790–794.

Hill, G. P. (2000). A role for the speech-language pathologist in multidisciplinary assessment and treatment of attention-deficit/hyperactivity disorder. *Journal of Attention Disorders, 4,* 69–79.

Hwa-Froelich, D. A., & Matsuo, H. (2005). Vietnamese children and language-based processing tasks. *Language, Speech, and Hearing Services in Schools, 36,* 230–243.

Jackson, T., & Plante, E. (1997). Gyral morphology in the posterior sylvian region in families affected by developmental language disorder. *Neuropsychology Review, 6,* 81–94.

Johnson, J. M., Seikel, J. A., Madison, C. L., Foose, S. M., & Rinard, K. D. (1997). Standardized test performance of children with a history of prenatal exposure to multiple drugs/cocaine. *Journal of Communication Disorders, 30,* 45–72.

Kaiser, A. B., & Hester, P. P. (1994). Generalized effects of enhanced milieu teaching. *Journal of Speech and Hearing Research, 37,* 1320–1340.

Kanner, L., & Eisenberg, L. (1955). Notes on the followup studies of autistic children. In P. H. Hoch & J. Zubin (Eds.), *Psychotherapy of childhood.* New York: Grune & Stratton.

Knutson, K. C., & O'Malley, M. (2010). Adult attention-deficit/hyperactivity disorder: A survey of diagnosis and treatment practices. *Journal of the American Academy of Nurse Practitioners, 22*(11), 593–601.

Landau, W. M., & Kleffner, F. R. (1957). Syndrome of acquired aphasia with convulsive disorder in children. *Neurology, 7*, 523–530.

Leonard, L. B., Camarata, S. M., Pawtowska, M., Brown, B., & Camarata M. N. (2008). The acquisition of tense and agreement morphemes by children with specific language impairment during intervention: Phase 3. *Journal of Speech and Hearing Research, 51*, 120–125.

Linan-Thompson, S., Vaughn, S., Prater, K., & Cirino, P. T. (2006). The response to intervention of English language learners at risk for reading problems. *Journal of Learning Disabilities, 39*, 390–398.

Lord, C., & Pickles, A. (1996). Language level and nonverbal social-communicative behaviors in autistic and language-delayed children. *Journal of the American Academy of Child and Adolescent Psychiatry, 35*, 1542–1550.

Mantovani, J. F., & Landau, W. M. (1980). Acquired aphasia with convulsive disorder: Course and prognosis. *Neurology, 30*, 524–529.

Mather, N., & Kaufman, N. (2006). Introduction to the special issue, part one: It's about the what, the how well, and the why. *Psychology in the Schools, 43*, 747–752.

Max, J. E., Bruce, M., Keatley, E., & Delis, D. (2010). Pediatric stroke: Plasticity, vulnerability, and age of lesion onset. *The Journal of Neuropsychiatry and Clinical Neurosciences, 22*(1), 30–39.

McArdle, P. (2004). Attention-deficit hyperactivity disorder and life-span development. *British Journal of Psychiatry, 184*, 468–469.

McCauley, R. J., & Swisher, L. (1984). Psychometric review of language and articulation tests for preschool children. *Journal of Speech and Hearing Disorders, 49*, 34–42.

McGee, R., Partridge, F., Williams, S., & Silva, P. A. (1991). A twelve-year follow-up of preschool hyperactive children. *Journal of the American Academy of Child and Adolescent Psychiatry, 30*, 224–232.

McGrath, L. M., Hutaff-Lee, C., Scott, A., Boada, R., Shriberg, L. D., & Pennington, B. F. (2008). Children with co-morbid speech sound disorder and specific language impairment are at increased risk for attention-deficit/hyperactivity disorder. *Journal of Abnormal Child Psychology, 36*, 151–163.

McKinlay, A., Grace, R. C., Horwood, L. J., Fergusson, D. M., Ridder, E. M., MacFarlane, M. R. (2008). Prevalence of traumatic brain injury among children, adolescents, and young adults: Prospective evidence from a birth cohort. *Brain Injury, 22*, 175–181.

Merrell, A. W., & Plante, E. (1997). Norm-referenced test interpretation in the diagnostic process. *Language, Speech, & Hearing Services in Schools, 28*, 50–58.

Mervis, C. B., & Becerra, A. M. (2007). Language and communication in Williams syndrome. *Mental Retardation and Developmental Disabilities Research Reviews 13*, 3–15.

Messick, S. (1989). Meaning and values in test validation: The science and ethics of assessment. *Educational Researcher, 18*, 5–11.

Minshew, N. J., Goldstein, G., & Siegel, D. J. (1997). Neuropsychologic functioning in autism: Profile of a complex information processing disorder. *Journal of the International Neuropsychological Society, 3*, 303–316.

Miranda-Linne, F. M., & Merlin, L. (1997). A comparison of speaking and mute individuals with autism and autistic-like conditions on the Autism Behavior Checklist. *Journal of Autism and Developmental Disorders, 27*, 245–264.

O'Brien, E. K., Zhang, X., Nishimura, C., Tomblin, J. B., & Murray, J. C. (2003). Association of Specific Language Impairment (SLI) to the Region of 7q31. *American Journal of Human Genetics, 72,* 1536–1543.

Oram, J., Fine, J., Okamoto, C. & Tannock, R., (1999). Assessing the language of children with attention deficit hyperactivity disorder. *American Journal of Speech-Language Pathology, 8,* 72–80.

Palili, A., Kolaitis, G., Vassi, I., Veltsista, A., Bakoula, C., & Gika, A. (2011). Inattention, hyperactivity, impulsivity—Epidemiology and correlations: A nationwide Greek study from birth to 18 years. *Journal of Child Neurology, 26*(2), 199–204.

Paul, R. (1993). Patterns of development in late talkers: Preschool years. *Journal of Childhood Communication Disorders, 15,* 7–14.

Paul, R., & Alforde, S. (1993). Grammatical morpheme acquisition in 4-year-olds with normal, impaired, and late-developing language. *Journal of Speech and Hearing Research, 36,* 1271–1275.

Paul, R., Hernandez, R., Taylor, L., & Johnson, K. (1996). Narrative development in late talkers: Early school age. *Journal of Speech and Hearing Research, 39,* 1295–1303.

Paul, R., Murray, C., Clancy, K., & Andrews, D. (1997). Reading and metaphonological outcomes in late talkers. *Journal of Speech and Hearing Research, 40,* 1037–1047.

Petit, E., Herlault, J., Martineau, J., Perrot, A., Barthelemy, C., Hameury, L., Sauvage, D., Lelord, G., Muh, J. P. (1995). Association study with two markers of a human homeogene in infantile autism. *Journal of Medical Genetics, 32,* 269–274.

Plante, E. (1991). MRI findings in the parents and siblings of specifically language-impaired boys. *Brain and Language, 41,* 52–66.

Plante, E., Swisher, L., Vance, R., & Rapcsak, S. (1991). MRI findings in boys with specific language impairment. *Brain and Language, 41,* 52–66.

Plante, E., & Vance, R. (1994). Selection of preschool language tests: A data based approach. *Language, Speech, & Hearing Services in Schools, 25,* 15–23.

Poll, G., Betz, S., & Miller, C. (2010). Identification of clinical markers of specific language impairment in adults. *Journal of Speech, Language, and Hearing Research, 53,* 414–429.

Rapin, I., Mattis, S., Rowan, A. J., & Golden, G. G. (1977). Verbal auditory agnosia in children. *Developmental Medicine and Child Neurology, 19,* 192–207.

Records, N. L., Tomblin, J. B., & Freese, P. R. (1992). The quality of life of young adults with histories of specific language impairment. *American Journal of Speech-Language Pathology, 1,* 44–53.

Redmond, S. M. (2004). Conversational profiles of children with ADHD, SLI and typical development. *Clinical Linguistics & Phonetics, 18,* 107–125.

Redmond, S. M. (2005). Differentiating SLI from ADHD using children's sentence recall and production of past tense morphology. *Clinical Linguistics & Phonetics, 19,* 109–127.

Rescorla, L. (2009). Age 17 language and reading outcomes in late-talking toddlers: Support for a dimensional perspective on language delay. *Journal of Speech, Language, and Hearing Research, 52,* 16–30.

Rescorla, L., Roberts, J., & Dahlsgaard, K. (1997). Late talkers at 2: Outcome at age 3. *Journal of Speech and Hearing Research, 40,* 555–566.

Rescorla, L., & Schwartz, E. (1990). Outcome of toddlers with expressive language delay. *Applied Psycholinguistics, 11,* 393–407.

Rimland, B. (1964). *Infantile autism.* New York: Appleton-Century-Crofts.

Roberts, J. E., Price, J., & Malkin, C. (2007). Language and communication development in Down syndrome. *Mental Retardation and Developmental Disabilities, 13,* 26–35.

Rösler, M., Casas, M., Konofal, E., & Buitelaar, J. (2010). Attention deficit hyperactivity disorder in adults. *The World Journal of Biological Psychiatry, 11*(5–6), 684–698.

Sabers, D. L. (1996). By their tests we will know them. *Language, Speech, and Hearing Services in Schools, 27,* 102–108.

Sánchez, E. Y., Velarde, S., & Britton, G. B. (2011). Estimated prevalence of attention-deficit/hyperactivity disorder in a sample of Panamanian school-aged children. *Child Psychiatry and Human Development, 42*(2), 243–255.

Scarborough, H. S., & Dobrich, W. (1990). Development of children with early language delay. *Journal of Speech and Hearing Research, 33,* 70–83.

Scharfenaker, S. K. (1990). The fragile X syndrome. *ASHA, 32,* 45–47.

Shields, J., Varley, R., Broks, P., & Simpson, A. (1996). Social cognition in developmental language disorders and high-level autism. *Developmental Medicine and Child Neurology, 38,* 487–495.

SLI Consortium. (2002). A genomewide scan identifies two novel loci involved in specific language impairment. *American Journal of Human Genetics, 70,* 384–398.

Snowling, M. J., Bishop, D. V. M., Stothard, S. E. (2000). Is preschool language impairment a risk factor for dyslexia in adolescence? *Journal of Child Psychology and Psychiatry, 41,* 587–600.

Sparks, S. N. (1984). *Birth defects and speech-language disorders.* Boston: College Hill.

Spaulding, T. J., Plante, E., & Farinella, K. A. (2006). Do children with impaired language score at the low end of the normative distribution? *Language, Speech, and Hearing Services in Schools, 37,* 61–72.

Tallal, P., Ross, R., & Curtiss, S. (1989). Familial aggregation in specific language impairment. *Journal of Speech and Hearing Disorders, 54,* 287–295.

Thal, D. J., Bates, E., Goodman, J., & Jahn-Samilo, J. (1997). Continuity of language abilities: An exploratory study of late- and early-talking toddlers. *Developmental Neuropsychology, 13,* 239–274.

Thal, D. J., & Tobias, S. (1992). Communicative gestures in children with delayed onset of oral expressive vocabulary. *Journal of Speech and Hearing Research, 35,* 1281–1289.

Tomblin, J. B. (1989). Familial concentration of developmental language impairment. *Journal of Speech and Hearing Disorders, 54,* 287–295.

Tomblin, J. B., Records, N. L., & Zhang, X. (1996). A system for the diagnosis of specific language impairment in kindergarten children. *Journal of Speech and Hearing Research, 39,* 1284–1294.

Turkstra, L. S., & Holland, A. L. (1998). Working memory and syntax comprehension after adolescent traumatic brain injury. *Journal of Speech, Language, and Hearing Research, 41.*

Vargha-Khadem, F., O'Gorman, A. M., & Watters, G. V. (1985). Aphasia and handedness in relation to hemisphere side, age at injury, and severity of cerebral lesion in childhood. *Brain, 108,* 677–695.

Warren, S. F., Gazdag, G. E., Bambara, L. M., & Jones, H. A. (1994). Changes in the generativity and use of semantic relations concurrent with milieu language intervention. *Journal of Speech and Hearing Research, 37,* 924–934.

Washington, J. A., & Craig, H. K. (1994). Dialectal forms during discourse of poor, urban, African American preschoolers. *Journal of Speech and Hearing Research, 37,* 816–823.

Wassenberg, R., Hendriksen, J. M., Hurks, P. M., Feron, F. M., Vles, J. H., & Jolles, J. (2010). Speed of language comprehension is impaired in ADHD. *Journal of Attention Disorders, 13*(4), 374–385.

Wiig, E. H., Jones, S. S., & Wiig, E. D. (1996). Computer-based assessment of word knowledge in teens with learning disabilities. *Language, Speech, and Hearing Services in Schools, 27,* 21–28.

Wilcox, M. J. (1992). Enhancing initial communication skills in young children with developmental disabilities through partner programming. *Seminars in Speech and Hearing, 13,* 194–212.

Wilcox, M. J. (1994). Delivering communication-based services to infants, toddlers, and their families: Approaches and models. In K. G. Butler (Ed.), *Early intervention I: Working with infants and toddlers.* Gaithersburg, MD: Aspen Publications.

Willcutt, E. G., & Pennington, B. F. (2000). Comorbidity of reading disability and attention-deficit/hyperactivity disorder: Differences by gender and subtype. *Journal of Learning Disabilities, 33,* 179–191.

Willis, J. O., & Dumont, R. (2006). And never the twain shall meet: Can response to intervention and cognitive assessment be reconciled? *Psychology in the Schools, 43,* 901–908.

Woods, B. T., & Carey, S. (1979). Language deficits after apparent clinical recovery from childhood aphasia. *Annals of Neurology, 6,* 405–409.

Worster-Drought, C. (1971). An unusual form of acquired aphasia in children. *Developmental Medicine and Child Neurology, 13,* 563–571.

Ylvisaker, M. (1993). Communication outcome in children and adolescents with traumatic brain injury. *Neuropsychological Rehabilitation, 3,* 321–340.

Ylvisaker, M. (1998). Traumatic brain injury in children and adolescents: Introduction. In M. Ylvisaker (Ed.), *Traumatic brain injury rehabilitation in children* (2nd ed., pp. 1–10.). Boston: Butterworth-Heinemann.

Ylvisaker, M., Szekeres, S. F., & Feeney, T. J. (1998). Cognitive rehabilitation: Executive functions. In M. Ylvisaker (Ed.), *Traumatic brain injury rehabilitation in children* (2nd ed., pp. 221–270). Boston: Butterworth-Heinemann.

Yoder, P. J., Kaiser, A. P., & Alpert, C. L. (1991). An exploratory study of the interactions between language teaching methods and child characteristics. *Journal of Speech and Hearing Research, 34,* 155–167.

READINGS FROM THE POPULAR LITERATURE

Brenna, B. (2005). *Wild orchid.* Calgary, Alberta: Red Deer Press. (Asperger's syndrome)

Dorris, M. (1996). *Broken cord.* Boston: G. K. Hall. (fetal alcohol syndrome)

Geraldi, C. (1996). *Camille's children.* Kansas City, KS: Andrews and McMeel. (foster mother of multiply handicapped children)

Gerlach, E. (1999). *Just this side of normal: Glimpses into life with autism.* Eugene, OR: Four Leaf Press. (family and autism)

Grandin, T., & Scariano, M. M. (1996). *Emergence: Labeled autistic.* New York: Warner Books. (personal account of autism)

Greenfield, J. (1980). *A place for Noah.* New York: Holt, Rinehart and Winston. (family with autistic child)

Haddon, M. (2005). *The curious incident of the dog in the night-time.* New York: Vintage Books. (fictional story of child with autism)

Jablow, M. (1982). *Cara: Growing up with a retarded child.* Philadelphia: Temple University Press. (intellectual disability)

Kaufmann, B. (1976). *Son-rise.* New York: Warner Books. (autism)

Kaufmann, S. (1995). *Retarded isn't stupid, Mom!* Baltimore: Paul H. Brookes. (intellectual disability)

Lane, G., & Sagmiller, G. (1996). *Dyslexia my life.* Waverly, IA: Doubting Thomas. (dyslexia)

Maurice, C. (1994). *Let me hear your voice: A family's triumph over autism.* New York: Fawcett Columbine. (autism)

Moody, J. (2007). *The short bus: A journey beyond normal.* New York: Henry Holt & Company, LLC. (dyslexia)

Papazian, S. (1997). *Growing up with Joey: A mother's story of her son's disability and her family's triumph.* Santa Barbara, CA: Fithian Press. (cerebral palsy and the family)

Robison, J. E. (2007). *Look me in the eye: My life with Asperger's.* New York: Crown.

Rogers, D. E. (1992). *Angel unaware:* Westwood, NJ: Fleming Revell Press. (Down syndrome)

Stallings, G., & Cook, S. (1998). *Another season: A coach's story of raising an exceptional son.* New York: Broadway Books. (Down syndrome)

Tammet, D. (2007). *Born on a blue day: Inside the extraordinary mind of an autistic savant.* New York: Free Press. (Asperger's syndrome, autistic savant)

Williams, D. (1994). *Nobody nowhere.* New York: Perennial. (personal account of autism)

Williams, D. (1995). *Somebody somewhere: Breaking free from the world of autism.* New York: Times Books. (sequel to *Nobody Nowhere,* a personal account of life with autism).

Williams, D. (1996). *Like color to the blind: Soul searching and soul finding.* New York: Times Books. (personal account of life with autism)

CHAPTER 9

Disorders of Language in Adults

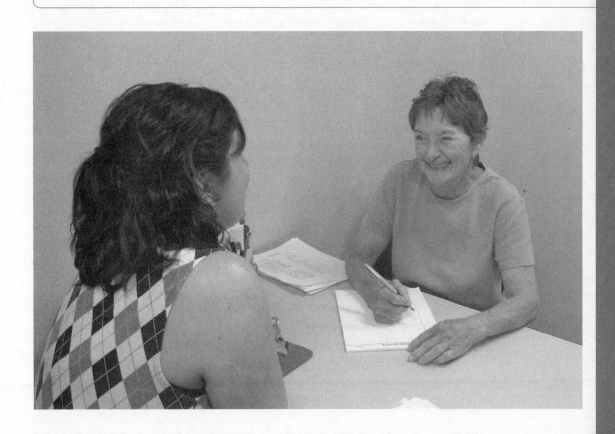

PREVIEW Language skills are well established by adolescence, so that spoken and written communication are accomplished with relatively little effort. Vocabularies continue to grow as life experience is gained, and adults typically become more adept at the subtleties of language use. With advanced age, language knowledge and use remain relatively stable, with the exception of some minor difficulty in retrieving specific words from time to time. In some adults, however, sudden or progressive damage to portions of the brain important for language and thought can disturb the ability to communicate. The extent and the location of brain damage influence the resulting behavior, such that various syndromes are associated with certain patterns of brain damage. In fact, much of what is known about the organization of the brain has come from the study of individuals with acquired impairments of language. The rehabilitation of language disorders in adults is the professional focus for speech-language pathologists in a variety of settings. It is challenging and rewarding work, typically accomplished in partnership with the affected individual, their family/caregivers, and other professionals.

Normal language and cognition are dependent upon a healthy nervous system, and damage to the brain can disrupt those processes. When the damage specifically affects the portions of the brain that support language, the resulting impairment is referred to as **aphasia**. Because language centers are in the left hemisphere in most people, aphasia typically is associated with left hemisphere damage. Acquired language impairments may occur in children, as reviewed in Chapter 8, but aphasia is most often observed in adults. When the right hemisphere is damaged (rather than the left), the resulting syndrome of cognitive and communication impairment is quite different from aphasia. Right hemisphere damage typically affects the social aspects of communication, or the *use* of language, rather than the skills required to produce well-formed sentences. Other cognitive and communication difficulties arise when there is widespread or diffuse brain damage affecting both hemispheres, as is frequently observed following traumatic brain injury (TBI). As discussed in Chapter 8, teenagers and young adults are at greatest risk for TBI, but older adults may suffer the cognitive and behavioral consequences of head injury as well. With advanced age, there is increased likelihood of progressive intellectual and linguistic decline associated with various types of dementia.

Aphasia

Aphasia is an acquired impairment of language. It results from damage to the language centers of the brain, which are typically located in the left hemisphere, as reviewed in Chapter 2. In the case of aphasia, an individual who had normal language suddenly finds those abilities impaired or degraded. The term *dysphasia* is used interchangeably with *aphasia* to refer to the acquired language impairment, but the latter is more common in the United States. Speech-language pathologists in medical settings frequently participate in the evaluation and rehabilitation of individuals with aphasia.

> *Mr. Wallace* was a right-handed man who had a bachelor's degree in engineering and retired after a distinguished career in the army. At age 67, he had a stroke in the left cerebral hemisphere. He did not suffer any physical impairment after the stroke, but his ability to communicate was markedly impaired due to aphasia. A conversational exchange with Mr. Wallace went as follows:
>
> **AUTHOR:** Tell me about the work that you did.
>
> **MR. WALLACE:** When I grew up in the army, this was my whole *fife, lar . . . light.* I was in the army, the army, and the war and everything else under the sun. Everything. And various *coun, coun, coun,* countries, and things in different places we went and in the armies. I was a colonel in the infantry. And I liked it. I was very fond of . . . I knew everybody in West Point. We all grown in our lives, grown up, and we were children. And we knew a lot of people and I think we were useful. And the people we work with. And so we did.

Mr. Wallace was having difficulty coming up with the words he needed to express his thoughts. For example, it was obvious that he intended to say, "When I grew up in the army, this was my whole *life.*" But he did not say the word *life.* He first said the word *fife,* then he said a nonword *lar,* and finally he said an incorrect word, *light.* Mr. Wallace retained his lifelong memories and did not have an impairment of his intellect, but he had an impairment specific to language—he had aphasia.

> People with aphasia often indicate that they know what they want to say, but they just can't say it.

It is important to appreciate that aphasia is an impairment of language, not simply a problem with speech production. Recall from Chapter 3 and 7 that language is a symbol system used to convey thoughts, whereas speech refers to the meaningful sounds produced by articulatory movements. Language includes the words we speak and the rules that govern how words are combined to make utterances. Mr. Wallace had trouble coming up with the appropriate words and also had difficulty combining them into meaningful sentences. Although some of Mr. Wallace's words were pronounced incorrectly, this was not due to a speech problem; it was part of his language impairment. Some individuals with aphasia *do* have difficulty articulating words because they have speech problems that coexist with their aphasia. Such acquired speech disorders include *dysarthria* and *apraxia of speech,* which were discussed in Chapter 4.

Language is distinguished not only from speech but also from thought. People with severe aphasia often demonstrate that they have relatively well-preserved thought processes. They retain their world knowledge, remember their life histories, and learn new things about what is going on in the world. Therefore, aphasia is not an impairment of general intellect as is observed in dementing diseases. It would be an oversimplification to suggest that individuals with aphasia possess all the cognitive abilities they had before the onset of their aphasia (see, e.g., Beeson, Bayles, Rubens, & Kaszniak, 1993; Murray, 2002), but it is the language impairment that is central to their communication problems.

Characteristics

The difficulty coming up with words that was evident in Mr. Wallace's conversation is called **anomia**, which refers to a failure to retrieve a word (or, literally, the name of something). Anomia is the hallmark of aphasia in that all people with aphasia complain of difficulty coming up with the names of things. The rambling emptiness of Mr. Wallace's conversation resulted from his anomia. He overused pronouns such as *we, thing*, and *it*, rather than giving specific names of people, places, or things. Individuals with aphasia may identify instances of anomia by saying something like, "oh, I can't think of the word for it," or they may describe the item that they cannot name. For example, to refer to the Veteran's Affairs hospital, a patient said, "you know, the place where I met you . . . with all the soldiers and where we did those thing with the tests." This sort of "talking around the word" is called **circumlocution**. Although circumlocution is an indicator of word retrieval problems, it is also a very useful communication strategy to compensate for anomia.

> A paraphasia is the production of an incorrect or unintended word. Do you ever produce paraphasias?

Sometimes incorrect words or nonwords are produced in place of the desired word. Such errors are called **paraphasias**. Mr. Wallace's attempts to produce the word *light* resulted in several paraphasias. They can be whole-word substitutions, such as *world* for *life*, single-sound substitutions such as *fife* for *life*, or nonwords that are either closely related or totally unrelated to the target word, such as *lar* for *life*. Such nonwords are also called **neologisms**, meaning "new words," but they have no meaning to the listener. Individuals with aphasia vary as to whether they are able to detect such errors in their spoken language.

Fluent versus Nonfluent Aphasia Profiles

Mr. Wallace's speech output was considered "fluent." It had relatively normal prosodic variations of pitch, loudness, and stress, and although there were some hesitations due to word-finding difficulties, the words flowed in a manner that sounded fairly normal. Other characteristics of **fluent aphasia** include articulation without excessive effort, utterances that are of normal length in terms of the number of words, and the presence of some grammatical structure, such as the use of articles, prepositional phrases, and appropriate word endings, such as *-ed*.

Not all individuals with aphasia speak fluently. Those with **nonfluent aphasia** produce utterances characterized by effortful, hesitant speech that may be poorly articulated. Mr. Brown provides an example of nonfluent aphasia. He was a 36-year-old man who had a congenital malformation of his vascular system that required surgery when he was 31. The surgery was complicated by a hemorrhage that occurred in the region of the left middle cerebral artery and caused extensive damage to the language areas of his left hemisphere. He had weakness on the right side of his body and a significant nonfluent aphasia. Two years after his stroke we had the following conversation.

AUTHOR: What can you tell me about the stroke?

MR. BROWN: Um . . . (Sighs) . . . um . . . (Sighs) . . . left . . . (Gestures to right side of body) . . . right side . . . (Shakes his head and sighs)

AUTHOR: And before your stroke, what did you do?

MR. BROWN: Um . . . resale sales (Holds up six fingers).

AUTHOR: Six years?

MR. BROWN: No. Six . . . store . . . chain . . . California.

AUTHOR: Did you do sales?

MR. BROWN: No. No. This time . . . general . . . manager.

Mr. Brown's utterances were quite different from those of Mr. Wallace. He spoke mostly in single words and short phrases. Whereas Mr. Wallace had an excess of vague, empty words, Mr. Brown's words were almost all meaningful content words. This type of output has been called **telegraphic speech**, so called because of the omission of the little words, such as *is* or *the*, that were typically dropped in the days when telegrams were sent. Today, such utterances with reduced grammatical complexity are more akin to the content of electronic text messages composed with economy of time and effort. The pauses and interjection of "um" give the impression that Mr. Brown was struggling to find and produce the words he wanted to say, and he had difficulty constructing complete sentences with appropriate grammatical structure. The overall speech pattern is lacking normal prosody, in that there is not the normal melodic variation of pitch, loudness, and stress. The term nonfluent is used to capture the essence of this effortful, telegraphic speech pattern. It should not be confused with the term *disfluent*, which refers to the disruption of speech fluency observed in stuttering (see Chapter 5).

The differences in fluency noted between Mr. Wallace and Mr. Brown are consistent with differences in the location of brain damage that caused their respective aphasias. To understand the relationship between fluency and lesion location, we need to briefly review brain anatomy relevant to aphasia. Aphasia typically results from damage to the left hemisphere in an area that surrounds the major horizontal fissure called the Sylvian fissure. This region, shaded in Figure 9.1, is called the perisylvian region (*peri* = around). Figure 9.2 shows a brain scan of an individual who had a stroke in this area resulting in persistent aphasia. The damaged region of the brain is referred to as a **lesion**. The scan was taken several years following the stroke, and the dark regions of brain damage are clearly visible in the two images. It should be apparent from image (A) that the damage falls within the left perisylvian region, shown schematically in Figure 9.1.

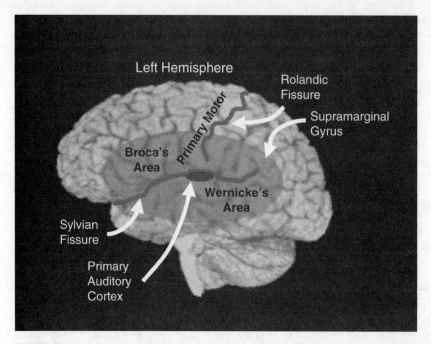

FIGURE 9.1   A schematic drawing of the left hemisphere indicates the language centers in the perisylvian region. Note that the primary auditory area is actually hidden from view inside the Sylvian fissure; the arcuate fasciculus is a white matter pathway that is deep within the hemisphere.

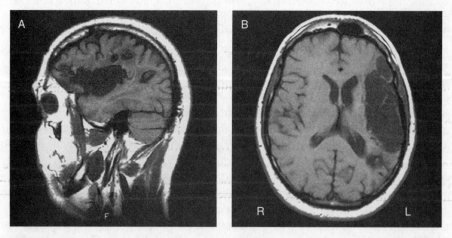

FIGURE 9.2   An MRI (magnetic resonance imaging) scan of the head showing a large perisylvian lesion in the left hemisphere that resulted in significant aphasia. Image A shows the dark region of damage from a lateral perspective (in a vertical plane), with the patient looking to the left. Image B shows an image in a horizontal plane near the sylvian fissure. Note that the lesion is on the right side in image B because radiologic films are often flipped so that right and left are reversed.

The relatively large perisylvian region is often divided into anterior and posterior regions relative to another major fissure, the Rolandic fissure (also called the central sulcus) that runs roughly perpendicular to the Sylvian fissure, as seen in Figure 9.1. The primary motor area and the areas important for motor planning are located in the frontal lobe, which is anterior to the Rolandic fissure. Broca's area is a frontal lobe region important for the motor planning of speech movements. It makes sense that brain damage to those anterior regions of the left hemisphere are likely to affect motor control and planning, and thus contribute to a disruption of speech production like that observed in nonfluent aphasias. As noted with Mr. Brown, anterior lesions often damage the neighboring motor areas for the right arm and leg as well, such that individuals with nonfluent aphasia often have right-sided weakness or paralysis, which is called right **hemiparesis**. Conversely, lesions that spare the motor regions of the brain are typically associated with fluent aphasia and no hemiparesis, as observed in Mr. Wallace. In general, anterior lesions are associated with nonfluent aphasia, and posterior lesions are associated with fluent aphasia. Large lesions that encompass both anterior and posterior regions would result in nonfluent aphasia because damage includes the critical anterior motor regions.

> Individuals with right hemiparesis are more likely to have nonfluent aphasia, rather than fluent aphasia. Why is that true?

Beyond the distinction between fluent and nonfluent aphasias, classification systems have been used over the past century to distinguish identifiable aphasia subtypes. The most commonly used aphasia classification system in North America emerged from the work of prominent aphasiologists in Boston in the 1960s and reflected a modern extension of the work initiated by Carl Wernicke in the 1870s (Goodglass, 1993; Helm-Estabooks & Albert, 2004; Kertesz, 2006). In general, the aphasia types reflect performance profiles that indicate (1) whether the aphasia is fluent or nonfluent, (2) whether auditory comprehension is relatively good or impaired, and (3) whether the ability to repeat sentences is preserved or impaired (Beeson & Rapcsak, 2006). Just as fluency characteristics offer some insight regarding lesion location, some inferences can be drawn from the status of auditory comprehension and verbal repetition abilities. An understanding of those processes is helpful before examining some aphasia types in more detail.

Auditory Comprehension

Auditory comprehension requires the extraction of meaning from spoken words and the processing of grammatical structures in connected utterances. The degree of impairment to auditory comprehension can vary considerably among individuals with aphasia. Some individuals have relatively good understanding of most spoken utterances, while others have trouble understanding the meaning of single words and simple commands, such as when they are instructed, "Show me the table." Others can respond to simple requests but have trouble when understanding depends on careful processing of each word in relation to other words in an utterance. For example, the following verbal request would challenge most individuals with aphasia: "Do you want chicken or steak for dinner? Because if you want chicken, you need to get it out of the freezer."

Auditory comprehension is dependent upon information processing in the superior temporal lobe in the region called Wernicke's area, which is adjacent to the primary auditory region (Figure 9.1). Damage to Wernicke's area does not impair the ability to hear but interferes with the understanding of spoken language. Lesions to Wernicke's area are considered "posterior" because they are posterior to the Rolandic fissure and do not include the frontal motor regions. Mr. Wallace's stroke damaged Wernicke's area, and he had trouble understanding what was said in conversation. He also made errors on yes/no questions such as "Do you eat a banana before you peel it?" Mr. Wallace's comprehension was assessed using a variety of tasks that included pointing to items in response to their name, simple and complex commands, yes/no questions, and more difficult tasks such as comprehending a paragraph read aloud.

Repetition

Although the ability to repeat what other people say is not a particularly important or meaningful use of language, it is a useful diagnostic task when examining for aphasia. The ability to repeat words, phrases, and sentences requires auditory processing by posterior regions of the left hemisphere as well as verbal formulation by the anterior regions of the left hemisphere. So, the ability to repeat sentences is a good test of the integrity of the entire left perisylvian region. Difficulty with verbal repetition can arise for several reasons. There might be difficulty with auditory processing of the spoken utterance, holding the information in short-term memory as one formulates the same utterance, or in aspects of speech production. The attempts by Mr. Wallace (with fluent aphasia) to repeat sentences resulted in errors because of his auditory comprehension problems and his many paraphasic errors. Mr. Brown (with nonfluent aphasia) had trouble repeating sentences because he omitted the little grammatical words, just like he did in his conversational speech. Repetition can also be disrupted by damage to nerve fibers that connect the posterior and anterior perisylvian regions (see Figure 9.1). Damage to these fibers, as well as to other posterior regions in the left hemisphere, disrupts repetition abilities even when Broca's and Wernicke's areas are spared (Damasio & Damasio, 1980). Such lesions appear to disconnect the posterior and anterior language regions, such that auditory input processed in Wernicke's area is not conveyed to Broca's area for speech production. Sometimes it is clear that the individual understands a sentence, but cannot hold the exact words in memory, even when the meaning is understood. For example, when asked to repeat the sentence, "She is not coming back," the individual replied, "She's gone!"

> Sentence repetition is a good diagnostic task because it requires adequate function of both anterior and posterior components of the left perisylvian language region.

Relatively good verbal repetition is observed in some aphasias that result from lesions on the periphery of the left perisylvian region, or from isolated lesions within the perisylvian region that do not disturb the input and output processes necessary for repetition. In such cases, it is somewhat surprising to observe a patient who can repeat full sentences but cannot formulate a sentence on his or her own. It also surprising to note that sometimes an individual can repeat a sentence, but not actually understand what it means. This is evident, for example, when the person repeats the question precisely, "Are you wearing red pajamas?" and then replies, "Yes, it is."

Summary of Neuroanatomical Principles Related to Aphasia

Several neuroanatomical principles have been introduced that highlight the relation between brain regions and language behaviors. Before summarizing those principles, it is important to remember that successful communication requires participation of many parts of the brain and that damage to a particular area does not mean that *only* the damaged area is responsible for the impaired function. The study of the consequences of brain damage, as well as functional brain imaging in healthy individuals, confirms that people vary in terms of their precise brain organization. With those caveats in mind, the following generalizations can be made:

[handwritten note: posterior lesions → fluent; anterior → non fluent]

1. Large anterior lesions interfere with fluent speech production, so nonfluent aphasias are associated with anterior lesions and fluent aphasias are associated with posterior lesions.
2. Lesions in and around Wernicke's area tend to interfere with auditory comprehension, so anterior lesions that spare posterior brain regions may leave auditory comprehension relatively well preserved.
3. Lesions within the perisylvian region disrupt the ability to repeat sentences, but lesions outside of the perisylvian region result in relatively preserved ability to repeat.
4. Lesions throughout the left hemisphere can disrupt naming abilities, resulting in anomia, so the presence of anomia is not predictive of lesion location.

Aphasia Types

We have noted the general predictability of language performance based on lesion location and have suggested that patients with similar lesions tend to have similar language characteristics. Aphasia classification systems are useful for identifying such clusters of language behaviors. We will review some of the more common aphasia types. The syndromes are labeled according to the Boston classification system, which characterizes aphasia type on the basis of fluency, auditory comprehension, and repetition abilities. Such classification systems are clinically useful, but not all individuals with aphasia will fit a specific type. In a large aphasia recovery study, Wertz and colleagues (1981) found that about 75 percent of the individuals with aphasia were classifiable by aphasia type, leaving 25 percent who were considered unclassifiable. In those cases, it is still useful to characterize the aphasia in terms of fluency, auditory comprehension, and repetition.

Figure 9.3 shows the decision process for classifying four of the more common aphasia types: Broca's, global, conduction, and Wernicke's. This simplified classification is based on the observed fluency of spontaneous speech (fluent

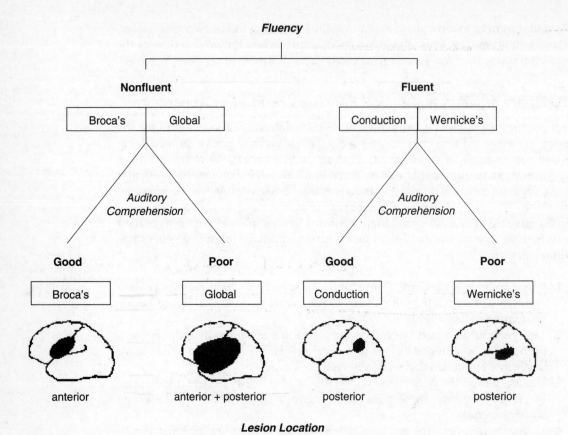

FIGURE 9.3 A decision tree used to guide the classification of four common aphasia types based upon fluency of spontaneous speech (fluent vs. nonfluent) and auditory comprehension (good vs. poor). Schematic drawings depict typical brain lesions associated with each aphasia type and indicate whether the lesion extends anteriorly or posteriorly relative to the Rolandic fissure.

versus nonfluent) and the status of auditory comprehension (good or poor). The figure also includes schematic drawings intended to depict a typical lesion location for each aphasia type. As indicated in Figure 9.3, the aphasia types differ with regard to observable language characteristics and likely lesion location. The nonfluent aphasias include damage to anterior portions of the brain, and the fluent aphasias are more often associated with posterior lesions. As mentioned, however, there is considerable variation from person to person, so the predicted relations between lesion location and language behavior are not without many exceptions. Fortunately, language performance typically improves over time, so there can be some change in aphasia profile associated with natural recovery and in response to language treatment. Presented below are the most typical behavioral profiles and associated lesion locations for four aphasia types that result from damage to the left perisylvian region, and anomic aphasia that often results from left hemisphere damage outside the perisylvian zone.

Broca's Aphasia.   Broca's aphasia is a nonfluent aphasia characterized by slow, hesitant, telegraphic speech. We saw an example of **Broca's aphasia** in Mr. Brown, the 36-year-old with nonfluent aphasia. As apparent in his conversational sample, utterances are of reduced length, typically fewer than four words, and have little syntactic complexity. The utterances are mostly isolated productions of nouns with some adjectives and verbs, and they are notably lacking in articles, prepositions, and other grammatical function words (called *functors*). Broca's aphasia is sometimes referred to as "motor aphasia" or "expressive aphasia," terms that highlight the observed production problems. Auditory comprehension is relatively good in individuals with Broca's aphasia, although they may have trouble understanding sentences with complex grammar. Repetition ability is limited to a few words. When asked to repeat full sentences, individuals with Broca's aphasia may simply repeat the content words, such as the nouns. Reading and writing are also impaired in individuals with Broca's aphasia, because the aphasia affects all language modalities.

→ telegraphic content wordy expressive

  Broca's aphasia results from lesions affecting the posterior portion of the left inferior frontal lobe. These are considered anterior lesions because they extend anteriorly relative to the Rolandic fissure (see Figure 9.3). When a lesion is small and restricted to Broca's area, the individual may have Broca's aphasia for only a short time following the brain damage and then recover to a more fluent aphasia. Persistent Broca's aphasia typically results from larger lesions that not only affect Broca's area but also extend posteriorly to the anterior parietal lobe. An extensive anterior lesion often results in right hemiparesis due to damage to the primary motor cortex in the frontal lobe, as noted with Mr. Brown.

> Broca's aphasia is the most common nonfluent aphasia type. How does it differ from Wernicke's aphasia?

Wernicke's Aphasia.   In contrast to Broca's aphasia, **Wernicke's aphasia** is characterized by fluent speech that is difficult to understand because it contains numerous paraphasias (i.e., incorrect words or nonwords) and is relatively devoid of content. Mr. Wallace, the man who was introduced as an example of fluent aphasia, has Wernicke's aphasia. Immediately following his stroke, his utterances were heavily sprinkled with paraphasias in place of meaningful words, such that he made comments like "Oh, and there is a *kusbit* and a *wuzman*." Other individuals with more severe Wernicke's aphasia produce strings of *neologisms* (nonwords), so they may sound like they are speaking a foreign language. They have a normal flow of speech with variations in prosody but few real words. This type of output is sometimes called **jargon aphasia**, and it sounds similar in some ways to the jargon of a young child learning a language.

receptive

  In addition to their fluent, paraphasic speech, individuals with Wernicke's aphasia have significant impairment of auditory comprehension (Figure 9.3). They have difficulty understanding spoken sentences and even have trouble comprehending many single words. This was the case for Mr. Wallace. When asked to point to the table, he blankly repeated, "table, table, I should know what that is." Another patient with more severe Wernicke's aphasia responded to the task by pointing to the door and saying something that sounded like "*illotime.*"

An additional sign of impaired auditory processing is the failure of individuals with Wernicke's aphasia to recognize their production errors. When asked to repeat words or sentences spoken by the clinician, their performance is no better. Repetition abilities are impaired due to the poor auditory processing and production problems. Reading and writing are also typically impaired in individuals with Wernicke's aphasia.

As might be expected, Wernicke's aphasia is associated with lesions in what is known as Wernicke's area (Figure 9.1). This region in the posterior, superior portion of the left temporal lobe is adjacent to the primary auditory cortex and is thought to be critical for auditory comprehension of language. Such posterior lesions typically spare the cortical areas important for motor control of the body, so individuals with Wernicke's aphasia rarely have hemiparesis.

Conduction Aphasia.   **Conduction aphasia** is somewhat similar to Wernicke's aphasia in that the verbal output is fluent, paraphasias are common, and repetition is impaired. However, individuals with conduction aphasia have better auditory comprehension than those with Wernicke's aphasia, presumably because much of Wernicke's area is spared (Figure 9.3). It is not uncommon for these individuals to attempt to self-correct their own errors, and frequently they are successful after several attempts. The self-corrections and hesitations associated with word-finding problems cause some disruption of the flow of speech, but the verbal output retains a sense of fluency in that articulation is accomplished with relative ease. Because the lesion spares the anterior motor regions, conduction aphasia typically is not associated with hemiparesis.

Conduction aphasia is associated with lesions in the left temporo-parietal region, particularly in an area immediately posterior to the Sylvian fissure called the supramarginal gyrus. As mentioned earlier, such a lesion disrupts the communication between the anterior and posterior language regions, resulting in the poor repetition of spoken utterances that is a hallmark of this aphasia type. Damage in this region also appears to disrupt the ability to hold verbal information in short-term memory, something that we typically do with relative ease.

Global Aphasia.   **Global aphasia** refers to severe language impairment affecting all domains. It is associated with large left-hemisphere lesions that essentially damage the entire perisylvian region (Figure 9.3). In global aphasia, meaningful verbal output is typically extremely limited. In some cases, it is limited to repetitive utterances, such as "one, two, three" or "I can see." In other cases, the utterances are repetitive jargon such as "nanna nanna nanna." Utterances that are repeated are called **perseverations**. It is worth noting that even individuals with global aphasia are capable of communicating wants, needs, and opinions if the listener provides a supportive communication environment.

Anomic Aphasia.   A common aphasia type not shown in Figure 9.3 is **anomic aphasia**. This syndrome is characterized by word retrieval difficulty in conversation and in the context of naming tasks, with relative preservation of fluency, auditory comprehension, and repetition abilities. Although all aphasia types exhibit word-finding difficulty, in the case of anomic aphasia, it is the primary deficit. Anomic aphasia can result from relatively isolated left hemisphere lesions that are outside of the perisylvian language zone. Some of the other aphasia types may evolve to anomic aphasia after a period of recovery if the brain damage is not extensive. Therefore, the presence of anomic aphasia does not provide information about the location of the aphasia-producing lesion.

Incidence, Prevalence, and Causes of Aphasia

There are about one million Americans with aphasia and about 100,000 new cases of aphasia every year (National Aphasia Association, 2011). It is a disorder most often associated with older age, with the highest incidence in people over the age of 65 (Hier et al., 1994). Stroke is the most common cause of brain damage resulting in aphasia. A **stroke**, also called a cerebrovascular accident (CVA), is an interruption of blood flow to the brain caused by blockage of an artery or the bursting of an artery (hemorrhage). When blood flow to brain cells is interrupted, they are deprived of oxygen, which ultimately results in cell death. Those brain cells do not regenerate, so the functions served by the damaged cells are impaired. Other causes of brain damage, such as traumatic accident, brain tumor, or infection, can also result in aphasia.

> Although *aphasia* is not a well-known term, there are about one million Americans who have this persistent language disorder.

It has long been known that in right-handed people (and most left-handed people) language problems tend to occur after damage to the left hemisphere. It is damage to the left perisylvian region that typically results in aphasia. The major blood vessel that serves the perisylvian region is the middle cerebral artery; therefore, stroke affecting the left middle cerebral artery is the most common cause of aphasia (Benson & Ardila, 1996).

The onset of aphasia is typically abrupt, but some etiologies may be associated with a slowly progressive onset. Brain tumors can cause slow onset of aphasia as they either infiltrate or compress critical language areas. **Primary progressive aphasia** is a relatively rare syndrome in which aphasia develops in the absence of an associated neurological event (McNeil & Duffy, 2001; Mesulam, 1982). In other words, the aphasia is not caused by a stroke or head injury, but rather by a progressive loss of brain cells in the cortical areas important for language. Progressive aphasia is caused by a number of different underlying disease processes, with the common feature that the language regions of the brain become disturbed before other cognitive functions (Gorno-Tempini et al., 2001). Unfortunately, progressive aphasia worsens over time as more brain cells die, and ultimately the problems extend to more general cognitive processes in addition to language.

Assessment

The initial evaluation of a person with aphasia may take place at his or her bedside in an acute care hospital. Informal interaction with the patient allows observation of conversational speech skills to provide a general impression of the adequacy of their sentence formulation, word retrieval, and ability to understand. A few structured tasks can further inform the speech-language pathologist of the patient's ability to comprehend spoken and written language, to name objects in the environment, to repeat sentences, and to communicate by writing. The initial assessment goals are typically to characterize the nature of the impairment and to appraise the functional abilities of the patient. A more comprehensive language assessment is usually deferred until a few days or weeks later, when the patient is able to sit at a table and tolerate the demands of sustained, structured interaction. However, the speech-language pathologist can be of considerable assistance to the patient and family during the first few days after the onset of aphasia as they seek to understand this strange disorder. Most important, the speech-language pathologist can facilitate successful communication with the patient and begin the process of training strategies to compensate for their language difficulties.

Mrs. Victor awoke one morning and fell as she tried to get out of bed. She realized that her right side was weak and that she felt odd. After dragging herself to the nightstand, she telephoned her daughter using her left hand. As she tried to respond to her daughter's "hello," Mrs. Victor realized that she could not speak. Her daughter saw her mother's phone number on her caller ID and was alarmed by her unintelligible speech. She assured her that she would call for help and come right over. After a trip to the emergency room and admission to the medical center, Mrs. Victor lay in a hospital bed with her daughter at her side. It had been a hectic five hours of medical examinations, a brain scan, and admission paperwork. When the hospital speech-language pathologist arrived for her first bedside visit, she found Mrs. Victor's daughter upset and confused about her mother's condition.

After ten minutes of informal interaction with Mrs. Victor, it was apparent to the speech-language pathologist that Mrs. Victor had global aphasia: She produced very little meaningful speech and appeared to have difficulty understanding much of what was said to her. In order to support Mrs. Victor in her attempts to communicate, the speech-language pathologist provided a pad of paper and began to write single words as possible responses to questions she was asking. For example, to help Mrs. Victor respond to the question, "Where are you from?" the speech-language pathologist wrote (and said) *Tucson?* When Mrs. Victor shook her head no, the speech-language pathologist offered *Green Valley?* To which Mrs. Victor smiled and said, "yes." After several successful exchanges of information using the written support, Mrs. Victor and her daughter were obviously showing some relief. This initial visit ended with the speech-language pathologist explaining to the daughter about aphasia and providing some written information about the nature of the communication impairment. Over the next several days, the daughter and nursing staff became adept at supporting Mrs. Victor's communication by offering written words, pictures, and objects as needed to clarify her intentions. Mrs. Victor was then transferred to a rehabilitation facility where she would receive aphasia treatment for several months. During her initial session with the speech-language pathologist at the rehab facility, she received a more extensive evaluation of her language abilities.

Comprehensive language assessment is frequently accomplished by the use of standardized tests of aphasia. Most of the tests require an hour or less to administer. They sample language behaviors of varying complexity and allow the examiner to determine the nature and severity of the aphasia. There are many supplemental tests that may also be used to characterize patient performance, as well as informal measures constructed by the speech-language pathologist. Some protocols are specifically designed to examine the impact of the language impairment on everyday communication situations and are considered functional communication measures. The overall goal of assessment is to understand and document the current strengths and weaknesses of the individual and to provide direction for the treatment plan.

Treatment

Individual Therapy. The goals of aphasia treatment are to maximize the recovery of impaired language functions, to assist in the development of alternative and compensatory communication strategies, and to help the patient adjust to the residual deficits. There are countless approaches to achieving such goals. It is the responsibility of the speech-language pathologist to either select an existing treatment approach or design a unique approach that is appropriate for the specific patient. The treatment plan should take into consideration the nature and extent of the language impairment as well as the residual language and cognitive abilities. Treatment plans are influenced by additional factors such as the time since the onset of aphasia and the patient's functional needs, motivation, and desires. Although the classification by aphasia type is useful to characterize the overall aphasia profile, it does not offer specific direction for treatment, because individuals with the same aphasia type may differ in many ways.

There is a large body of literature to guide speech-language pathologists toward appropriate treatment approaches for a particular set of symptoms (see, e.g., Chapey, 2008; Helm-Estabrooks & Albert, 2004; Holland & Forbes, 1993; Robey, 1998). Clinicians update their knowledge of the evidence-based treatment approaches by reading professional journals and attending continuing education presentations.

When planning treatment, the speech-language pathologist is guided by knowledge of the cognitive processes that support language in healthy adults, and how those processes are impaired in a specific individual following brain damage. However, the experienced clinician also knows that even people with similar impairments can have very different responses to the same treatment approach. Conversely, the same treatment can be effective for individuals whose impairments are dissimilar (Hillis & Caramazza, 1994). Therefore, each person's response to treatment should be carefully monitored and documented in order to evaluate its therapeutic effect and to make adjustments as needed.

When selecting or designing a treatment plan, the speech-language pathologist may approach treatment from several different perspectives. One approach is to stimulate the return of language abilities that are impaired but appear to have potential to improve or be restored. Many treatment protocols are designed to stimulate language by following a task hierarchy that requires progressively more difficult responses (some protocols are reviewed in Helm-Estabrooks & Alberts, 2004). The speech-language pathologist may determine what support or cues are necessarily to help the patient respond correctly and then systematically withdraw the support as the patient progresses. This approach incrementally shifts the burden from the clinician to the patient in order to achieve the desired response.

Some treatment approaches take advantage of residual abilities that can be used to substitute or compensate for impaired abilities. For example, a patient may be able to write a word, or part of a word, that he or she is unable to say. The use of writing to supplement spoken output may be an effective strategy. However, another possibility is that the written word may facilitate the spoken production of the word.

> After several months of language therapy, Mrs. Victor showed significant improvement of her comprehension of spoken and written language. Her spoken language remained severely impaired, however. She had several words and phrases that she typically uttered, such as "yes, but I don't know" and "oh my, oh my." The speech-language pathologist implemented treatment to improve Mrs. Victor's ability to write meaningful single words to communicate her thoughts. Mrs. Victor was able to relearn the spelling of many words, such that after several months of treatment she was able to write more than fifty words that were particularly relevant to her life. Most important was the fact that she was able to use these single written words as a means to communicate specific thoughts. It was noteworthy that on occasion Mrs. Victor was able to say the word that she was writing, despite the fact that she rarely spoke meaningful words in other contexts.

Individual treatment plans may include several goals that variously address aspects of spoken language production, auditory comprehension, reading, writing, and gestural communication. The treatment for Mrs. Victor focused on written rather than spoken language, due to the severity of her aphasia. Figure 9.4 shows another patient who responded well to a writing treatment (Beeson, 1999; Beeson, Rising, & Volk, 2003).

Obviously, the return of spoken language is the primary treatment goal whenever possible. A variety of treatment approaches to improve spoken language have been shown to be effective (e.g., see Chapey, 2008; Helm-Estabrooks & Albert, 2004). Many individuals with aphasia are able to say a word if they hear the first sound or syllable of the word. This responsiveness to phonemic cueing (as it is called) can be particularly useful if the patient can learn to provide his or her own phonemic cue for the word (Nickels, 1992). Therapy goals are selected so that they are appropriate for the particular patient and have immediate or eventual impact on their functional communication abilities.

Group Therapy.   It is not surprising that aphasia may result in social isolation and reduced opportunity to engage in conversation. Group therapy for individuals

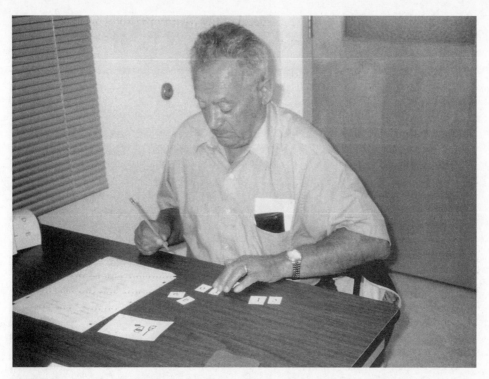

FIGURE 9.4 Individual therapy to improve writing for single words that includes arranging of letters to spell the word and copying the word.

with aphasia provides a setting where conversation is facilitated and supported by the clinician, and patients can learn to maximize their communication skills (see Figure 9.5). In a small group of three to five individuals with aphasia, the speech-language pathologist can work with the patients to (1) facilitate successful communication despite their residual language impairment, (2) encourage communication using all modalities, and (3) teach and elaborate specific communication strategies (Beeson & Holland, 2007). In the small group setting, patients can learn from the clinician and from each other how to compensate for language difficulties. When appropriate, group members are encouraged to use alternative communication strategies, including gestures, drawing, and writing to supplement the spoken utterances. Groups also can offer considerable psychological and social support for members as they adjust to their impairment. Many examples of structured and informal conversational activities have been reported in recent literature regarding group therapy (Elman, 2007), and there is evidence that many individuals with aphasia can continue to improve language abilities long after the time of their strokes (Beeson & Holland, 2007).

Aphasia is typically accompanied by reading and writing problems, but sometimes reading and writing problems occur when spoken language is relatively preserved.

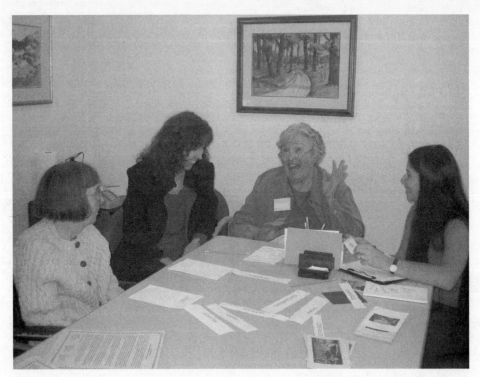

FIGURE 9.5   Group therapy for aphasia focuses on conversational language supplemented by writing and gestures.

Acquired Reading and Writing Impairments

As previously noted, most individuals with aphasia have difficulty reading and writing as well as listening and speaking, so aphasia treatment frequently includes intervention for all language modalities. On relatively rare occasions, damage to specific regions of the brain results in isolated impairments of reading and writing in the absence of significant aphasia. The speech-language pathologist is involved in the assessment and treatment of written language disorders. *Alexia* refers to an acquired impairment of reading, and *agraphia* refers to an acquired impairment of writing. **Pure alexia**, also known as *alexia without agraphia*, is an unusual syndrome wherein the patient is unable to read, but can still write. The syndrome is typically associated with left hemisphere damage affecting the left occipital lobe and the posterior regions of the temporal lobe. The damage may also affect the ability to see things in the right portion of the visual field, but the reading difficulty is not due to blindness; individuals can still receive visual information from the left visual field. The problem lies in the ability to make sense of written words. The individual with pure alexia can see the words and is often able to identify the letters of the word, but fails to recognize the word

alexia =
reading
agraphia =
writing

as a whole. Many individuals with pure alexia compensate for their lack of word recognition by reading the individual letters aloud; when they hear the word spelled aloud, they can recognize it. This letter-by-letter reading approach is useful, but painfully slow.

> One day *Mr. Lincoln* answered the telephone and wrote down a message from the caller for his wife. Later, when his wife called home, Mr. Lincoln picked up the note to read her the message. To his surprise, the letters made no sense to him; he could not read his own handwriting! He told his wife that there was something wrong with his eyes and that he thought he should go see his eye doctor. The eye doctor found nothing wrong with Mr. Lincoln's eyes but recognized that a stroke had affected his ability to recognize written words.

> Within a week, Mr. Lincoln was in treatment with a speech-language pathologist to improve his reading. He could recognize single letters and figure out most words by spelling them letter by letter, but he had great difficulty recognizing written words as whole units. The speech-language pathologist implemented a treatment that involved reading written passages multiple times in order to increase his rate for the practiced text (Beeson & Henry, 2008). Over the course of treatment, Mr. Lincoln showed improved reading rate for the practiced text, and, more important, his reading rate and accuracy improved for new reading material. In other words, the treatment appeared to improve his ability to recognize written words. Ultimately, Mr. Lincoln was able to read with adequate accuracy and speed to meet his daily needs.

Some individuals with acquired alexia also have difficulty spelling. In other words, they have *alexia with agraphia*. The term **agraphia** refers to an acquired impairment of spelling. Individuals with acquired agraphia vary with regard to their residual writing abilities (Rapcsak & Beeson, 2002). Some may be able to sound out words they cannot recall how to spell, relying on their preserved knowledge of the relations between sounds and letters. In such cases, it is not uncommon to make errors on irregularly spelled words. For example, "school" might be spelled *skool.* Given that individuals vary with regard to the nature of their reading or writing difficulties, treatment approaches for acquired alexia and acquired agraphia are tailored to the specific nature of the impairment (Beeson & Henry, 2008).

Right-Hemisphere Communication Disorders

Damage to the right hemisphere may result in some word retrieval difficulties similar to that observed in left-hemisphere damage. However, the prominent features of right-hemisphere damage tend to be quite different from those associated with left-hemisphere damage. Individuals with right-hemisphere damage may have a host of subtle impairments in their thought organization, mental flexibility, and use of language that affect their ability to understand and communicate effectively (Lehman Blake, Duffy, Myers, & Tompkins, 2002). Although individuals with right-hemisphere damage typically understand the content of individual sentences, they often fail to understand the gist of the conversation or appreciate humor or figures of speech. For example, when a patient with right-hemisphere damage was asked to explain what it means when someone says, "You can't have your cake and eat it too," he responded, "It means you have to share it, I guess. You can't eat the whole thing." These difficulties with the abstract use of language are accompanied by reduced use of facial expression and prosody to convey emotion while speaking, so that individuals with right-hemisphere damage appear to be disinterested during conversational exchange. They are also less perceptive of the nonverbal communication cues provided by other speakers and often fail to keep up with the natural give-and-take and shift of topic in conversation. These functions are referred to as extralinguistic aspects of communication, meaning that they are features other than the actual words used to speak. These problems sound rather vague, and, in fact, individuals with right-hemisphere damage simply may be perceived as odd, rude, or inattentive, rather than brain-damaged. However, their change in cognitive and communication abilities is clearly evident to friends and family who know them well. One of the patients at our clinic, Mr. Rice, explained his perception of one of the effects of his right-hemisphere stroke as follows:

> Taking turns in talking conversation was very difficult . . . because I would interrupt and have something to say in the middle of the conversation and interrupt everything. Train of thought and everything else. I thought I had to jump in otherwise I'd lose what I was trying to say.

Mr. Rice was 66 years old when he experienced a right-hemisphere stroke. One year after his stroke he still had weakness of his left arm and leg, but he could walk without assistance and communicate effectively. His speech was easy to understand, but the prosody sounded somewhat flat, as if lacking emotion; even when he joked, his voice and facial expression were difficult to interpret. It was notable that Mr. Rice was able to provide some insight into the nature of his problem, because many individuals with right-hemisphere damage do not recognize their deficits.

Mr. Rice also experienced **left neglect**, in that he tended to orient his gaze away from the left and was relatively unaware of sensory input on the left side of his body and the left side of his visual field. Left neglect is relatively common following right-hemisphere damage, and it occurs even when there is no loss of sensory or motor function on the left side and no loss of vision on the left (Heilman, Watson, & Valenstein, 2003). In other words, the visual images are getting to the brain, but they are essentially ignored.

These effects of brain damage have shown that the right hemisphere plays a special role in maintaining attention to the space around us, and our intrapersonal space, as well. Left neglect may interfere with communication, in that people to the patient's left are ignored and the left half of the page may be ignored when reading and writing. It is likely that the attentional problems associated with left neglect also relate to the impaired ability to attend to the extralinguistic information (e.g., prosody) provided during conversation (Myers, 1999). Future research may help to clarify the relation between neglect and the cognitive-communication impairment associated with right-hemisphere damage.

Incidence of Right-Hemisphere Damage

Given the relatively subtle nature of the cognitive-communication problems associated with right-hemisphere damage, it is not surprising that the incidence and prevalence are not well documented. The American Heart Association (2006) reported that there were about 500,000 new strokes each year in the United States, with about half affecting the right hemisphere. About half of those adults with right-hemisphere damage will have communication impairments, so we would estimate 125,000 new cases of right-hemisphere-related communication impairments caused by stroke per year (Benton & Bryan, 1996; Tompkins, 1995). Stroke is the most common cause of damage isolated to the right hemisphere, but other causes include traumatic injury or tumor.

Assessment and Treatment

Assessment of the patient with right-hemisphere damage typically includes sampling language in conversation and picture description tasks, assessing the extralinguistic aspects of communication, and examining for evidence of neglect or attentional problems (Myers, 1999; Tompkins, 1995). Examination of extralinguistic deficits includes tasks such as interpretation of a story or a pictured scene that requires integration of the component parts into one main idea. Patients may be asked to explain the meaning of figures of speech or to produce the certain expressions with appropriate prosodic variation to convey different emotions. They may also be asked to produce or understand narrative stories. All of these tasks share the common goal of probing comprehension and use of language in a flexible, abstract manner that comes naturally to most adults but may be problematic for those with right-hemisphere damage. Numerous tasks can be used to examine for neglect, including a very simple request for patients to put a mark on a line to divide it in half. Individuals with left neglect often bisect the line to the right of the midline because they do not perceive the leftmost part of the line. The ability to sustain attention is also assessed using tasks that increase from focused attention on one stimulus to divided attention on two stimuli. Some standardized tests are available to examine the patient with right-hemisphere damage.

Treatment for individuals with right hemisphere damage is challenging because they often fail to recognize that they have any problems.

In contrast to individuals with aphasia due to left-hemisphere damage, who are often highly motivated to improve their language skills, it is common for individuals with right-hemisphere damage to deny that they have had a change in their communication abilities. Treatment for right-hemisphere damage may be directed toward facilitating recovery of the underlying impairment or toward the development of compensatory strategies to overcome the problems. Greater understanding of the underlying causes of the communication deficits observed with right-hemisphere damage is needed, but it is currently assumed that the extralinguistic deficits are related to the features of neglect and inattention (Myers, 1999). For that reason, some treatment tasks are directed toward improving performance on attention tasks. For example, patients may be asked to listen or look for specific stimuli such as a particular number or word in the midst of other numbers or words (Sohlberg & Mateer, 2001). These types of attention tasks are also used with individuals with traumatic head injury because they often have problems with attention as well. Tasks that are directed toward improving extralinguistic abilities may be similar to those used for assessment. After observing the patient's deficits, the speech-language pathologist may structure the language tasks in such a way that a hierarchy of cues provides support for the patients. As discussed in aphasia therapy, the clinician's goal is to assist the patient to make small sequential gains in the direction of normal performance. This may require providing feedback when the patient fails to produce or comprehend the extralinguistic features, such as prosodic variation to mark emotion, followed by a model (example) of the appropriate response. The treatment goals are directed toward improved performance in a variety of settings and communication environments, not simply in the therapy room. This is true for all treatments for speech, language, and hearing disorders, but is especially relevant for the problems associated with right-hemisphere damage, because these problems often affect the social aspects of communication.

Dementia

An intermediate stage between the expected cognitive decline associated with aging and the full onset of dementia is called mild cognitive impairment (MCI).

Dementia refers to an acquired, progressive impairment of intellectual function that is chronic and affects several aspects of mental activity, including memory, cognition, language, and the processing of visual-spatial information (Cummings & Benson, 1992; Kaszniak, 2002). Dementia may also result in changes in emotion or personality. It is distinguishable from temporary conditions that impair mental function such as confusional states that may last for a few hours or a few days. The progressive intellectual decline in dementia is distinct from isolated, specific impairments such as aphasia due to focal brain damage. Numerous diseases can cause the diffuse brain damage that results in dementia, and the characteristics of the dementia vary to some extent depending on the disease process.

Types of Dementia

The most common type of dementia is **Alzheimer's disease**. This disease affects about 5.4 million Americans, and it accounts for more than half of all dementias (Alzheimer's Association, 2011). It is characterized by language, memory, and

cognitive impairments that include poor judgment and difficulty with calculation, reasoning, and higher-level thinking. Caregivers note that the early signs
of dementia include memory and concentration problems, such as forgetting
the location of things, poor recall for recent events, and trouble handling fi-
nances and performing complex tasks. Speech is typically well articulated and
fluent and may have good grammatical structure, but the content is increasingly empty as the disease progresses. In the early stages, the language impairment may appear similar to anomic aphasia in that there are many instances of
word-finding difficulties. In later stages, it may resemble the empty ramblings
observed in some individuals with Wernicke's aphasia. At the end stages, there
may be little verbal output at all.

word finding

Alzheimer's disease can be confirmed after death, by the presence of specific
brain changes observable if an autopsy is performed. For that reason, the diagnosis of Alzheimer's disease prior to death is typically tentative, referring to it
as "probable" AD, based on the presenting symptoms and the exclusion of other
causes of dementia. The criteria for the behavioral diagnosis of Alzheimer's disease and other types of dementia are described in detail in a manual published
by the American Psychiatric Association (2000).

In addition to Alzheimer's disease, there are some forty or fifty other
causes of dementia. After Alzheimer's disease, the second most common cause
of early onset dementia is a group of diseases that cause fronto-temporal dementia (Hodges, 2011). As indicated by the name, these dementias are associated with atrophy of brain tissue in the frontal and temporal lobes. When
language areas of the brain are affected, then a progressive onset of aphasia
is noted (Gorno-Tempini et al., 2010). Another common cause of dementia is
vascular disease resulting in multiple strokes that produce diffuse brain damage. Whereas Alzheimer's disease and the fronto-temporal dementias tend to
have a steadily progressive course, the cognitive decline associated with vascular, or **multi-infarct,** dementia may cause a stair-step decline as subsequent
strokes occur.

Memory impairment is often the initial symptom of dementia; however, in
some cases the language decline may be the first sign. At our clinic, Mr. Dean
brought his 67-year-old wife for an evaluation because, as he explained, her language "was becoming more and more confused." Her speech was well articulated
and easy to understand, but it was devoid of meaningful content and contained
many perseverative thoughts. A report of a head scan indicated a generalized loss
of brain substance but no evidence of a stroke.

When shown a toy gun and asked to name it, Mrs. Dean said:

MRS. DEAN: This is to put. Um, you can put a thing inside the . . .

AUTHOR: Can you tell me the name of it?

MRS. DEAN: Well, it's supposed to be, to do. But that, that's musty. It's hard,
    when you're on the table and the table is dirty, I take the longer thing, like
    this, and get the end. I don't, don't go by this thing. No, this I, see it always
    in my house. Oh, here I can do this, I can do this. It goes if you go.

Mrs. Dean's verbal output sounded in many ways like an individual with aphasia. However, there were some features of her behavior that were unlike those observed in aphasia. She showed anxiety and perseverative thoughts as she repeatedly asked where her husband had gone and how she was going to get home. Mr. Dean indicated during a private interview that his wife had become paranoid about her money. She no longer used the bank but had begun stuffing money under the mattress at home. Six months following the interview, Mrs. Dean's neurologist observed that her behavior had become increasingly bizarre, showing signs associated with frontal lobe damage, such as lack of inhibition and modesty (Miller & Cummings, 2007). The neurologist rejected a diagnosis of Alzheimer's disease in favor of a working diagnosis of Pick's disease. Like Alzheimer's disease, Pick's disease is a cortical dementia, meaning that there is a progressive loss of neurons in the cortex. In Pick's disease, brain changes occur primarily in the frontal and temporal lobes, resulting in changes in personality that accompany the decline in intellect, memory, and language. As with Alzheimer's disease, the diagnosis of Pick's disease is not actually confirmed unless the brain is studied after death.

Prevalence

Although the exact prevalence of dementia is not known, there is a clear increase with age. It has been estimated that Alzheimer's disease affects approximately 13 percent of individuals 65 years and older, and nearly half (43%) of those over 80 years have the disease (Alzheimer's Association, 2011). The prevalence of dementia is expected to increase as the older segment of our population continues to grow in number.

Assessment and Intervention

A comprehensive examination of cognitive function is critical to the diagnosis of dementia and may be performed by a neuropsychologist. Several standardized rating scales are used to screen for dementia. These scales include tasks that look at general knowledge, memory, communication, and visual-spatial skills (such as drawing). Other scales rate the severity of dementia using observational criteria, rather than direct testing. Comprehensive tests of cognitive function evaluate attention, initiation, visual-spatial construction, conceptualization, language, and memory. In many settings, a speech-language pathologist is involved in the assessment of language and communication abilities and contributes to the understanding of language function relative to other cognitive abilities. Individuals with dementia may also have concomitant hearing impairment that interferes with daily function and performance on cognitive assessments, so an audiologic evaluation is an important component of the diagnostic process.

Speech-language pathologists are taking an increasingly active role in the care of individuals with dementia. Although dementia is an irreversible process, therapeutic approaches may be employed that maximize communication and cognitive performance (Bayles & Kim, 2003). There are numerous sources of information regarding environmental and linguistic manipulations that positively influence the behavior of individuals with dementia (Bayles & Tomoeda, 1995; Davis, 2005; Hopper, 2001; Small & Perry, 2005). For example, communication performance can be improved by minimizing distractions and using familiar objects or pictures to stimulate recollections. Auditory comprehension may be improved with the use of simplified syntax and vocabulary. Memory demands can be minimized by making use of a memory book that contains biographical information, pictures of family and friends, and schedule information (Bourgeois, 1992).

The patient's performance profile on a test battery can be examined to determine his or her relative strengths and weaknesses. This information, combined with observation and experimentation, may help clinicians discover the cognitive, language, and environmental manipulations that minimize the effects of the dementia (Tomoeda, 2001). It is often the role of the speech-language pathologist to develop a program that outlines strategies for communicating with specific dementia patients. The speech-language pathologist works with caregivers, including family members and nursing home staff, to implement the plan and thus provide consistent support to maximize the performance of the dementia patient. In the case of Mrs. Dean, it was apparent that her husband was exhausted by his failure to communicate successfully with his wife. He stated, "She can't even tell me what she wants to eat for dinner." One easy solution to that problem was discovered: If Mr. Dean wrote down three choices for dinner and asked his wife which one she would like, she was able to respond by pointing to one of the options. Other suggestions were made to Mr. Dean to adapt his communication style in such a way as to maximize his wife's ability to communicate.

In closing this chapter, we want to emphasize that acquired impairments of language and cognition may have profound implications for the lives of the affected individuals and their families. Patients may experience significant limitations in their daily activities and restrictions on their participation in society. Thus, speech-language pathologists who work with adults with acquired language disorders are concerned not only with the acquired impairment but also with the consequences of that impairment. Evaluation and treatment approaches are sensitive to the specific needs of a given individual in his or her unique life situation.

Clinical Problem Solving

Mrs. Anderson was a 55-year-old woman who suffered a left-hemisphere stroke that resulted in aphasia. She was administrated the *Western Aphasia Battery* (Kertesz, 1982) to sample her language abilities. As part of the test, she was asked to describe what was happening in a pictured scene of a man and a woman having a picnic near a lake. Her spoken response follows:

Is family, um, picnic. And fish, and man is, um, oh, um reading, and, and, um lady, is pouring and set, um, son is, is, ha . . . is, um, is, um flying kite. And neighbor is dishing and neighbor is um, sailing, and boy, um, playing in water, and man, and lady in, listen to radio. And daughter, I mean, dog, oh . . . oh . . . stave, is lady, is man, is stave, oh, stay. I don't know.

1. Would you classify Mrs. Anderson's aphasia as fluent or nonfluent?
2. In what lobe of the brain is the lesion most likely to be located? Why?
3. Mrs. Anderson had trouble repeating sentences longer than four words. Would you expect her lesion to be in the perisylvian region or outside the perisylvian region? Why?
4. Would you guess that Mrs. Anderson had right hemiparesis? Why or why not?

REFERENCES

Alzheimer's Association. (2011). Alzheimer's disease facts and figures. Alzheimer's & Dementia, 7 (2). Retrieved September 7, 2011, from www.alz.org/alzheimers_disease_facts_and_figures.asp

American Heart Association. (2006). Heart disease and stroke statistics—2006 update: A report from the American Heart Association Statistics Committee and Stroke Statistics Subcommittee. *Circulation, 113*, e85–e151.

American Psychiatric Association. (2000). *Diagnostic and statistical manual of mental disorders*. (DSM-IV-TR). Washington, DC: Author.

Bayles, K. A., & Kim, E. S. (2003). Improving the functioning of individuals with Alzheimer's disease: Emergence of behavioral interventions. *Journal of Communication Disorders, 36*(5), 327–344.

Bayles, K., & Tomoeda, C. (1995). *The ABCs of dementia*. Tucson, AZ: Canyonlands Publishing.

Beeson, P. M. (1999). Treating acquired writing impairment: Strengthening graphemic representations. *Aphasiology, 13*, 367–386.

Beeson, P. M., Bayles, K. A., Rubens, A. B., & Kaszniak, A. W. (1993). Memory impairment and executive control in individuals with stroke-induced aphasia. *Brain and Language, 45*, 253–275.

Beeson, P. M., & Henry, M. L. (2008). Comprehension and production of written words. In. R. Chapey (Ed.), *Language intervention strategies in adult aphasia, Fifth Edition* (pp. 654–688). Baltimore, MD: Wolters Kluwer/Lippincott, Williams & Wilkins.

Beeson, P. M., & Holland, A. L. (2007). Aphasia groups in a university setting. In R. Elman (Ed.), *Group treatment of neurogenic communication disorders: The expert clinician's approach* (2nd ed.) San Diego: Plural Publishing.

Beeson, P. M., & Rapcsak, S. Z. (2006). The aphasias. In P. J. Snyder & P. D. Nussbaum (Eds.), *Clinical neuropsychology: A pocket handbook for assessment* (2nd ed., pp. 436–459). Washington, DC: American Psychological Association.

Beeson, P. M., Rising, K., & Volk, J. (2003). Writing treatment for severe aphasia. *Journal of Speech, Language, and Hearing Research, 46*, 1038–1060.

Benson, D. F., & Ardila, A. (1996). *Aphasia: A clinical perspective*. New York: Oxford University Press.

Benton, E., & Bryan, K. (1996). Right cerebral hemisphere damage: incidence of language problems. *International Journal of Rehabilitation Research, 19*(1), 47–54.

Bourgeois, M. S. (1992). *Conversing with memory impaired individuals using memory aids: A memory aid workbook.* Gaylord, MI: Northern Speech Services.

Chapey, R. (Ed.). (2008). *Language intervention strategies in adult aphasia* (5th ed.). Baltimore: Lippincott, William & Wilkins.

Cummings, J. L., & Benson, D. F. (1992). *Dementia: A clinical approach.* Boston: Butterworth.

Damasio, H., & Damasio, A. (1980). The anatomical basis of conduction aphasia. *Brain, 103,* 337–350.

Davis, L. A. (2005). Educating individuals with dementia: Perspectives for rehabilitation professionals. *Topics in Geriatric Rehabilitation, 21*(4), 304–314.

Elman, R.J. (2007). *Group treatment for neurogenic communication disorders: The expert clinician's approach* (2nd ed.). San Diego, CA: Plural Publishing.

Goodglass, H. (1993). *Understanding aphasia.* San Diego: Academic Press.

Gorno-Tempini, M. L., Hillis, A. E., Weintraub, S., Kertesz, A., Mendez, M., Cappa, S. F., Ogar, J. M., et al. (2011). Classification of primary progressive aphasia and its variants, *Neurology, 76*(11), 1006–1014.

Heilman, K. M., Watson, R. T., & Valenstein, E. (2003). Neglect and related disorders. In K. Heilman & E. Valenstein (Eds.), *Clinical neuropsychology* (4th ed., pp. 296–346). New York: Oxford University Press.

Helm-Estabrooks, N., & Albert, M. L. (2004). *Manual of aphasia and aphasia therapy* (2nd ed.). Austin, TX: Pro-Ed.

Hier, D. B., Yoon, W. B., Mohr, J. P., Price, T. R., & Wolf, P. A. (1994). Gender and aphasia in the stroke data bank. *Brain and Language, 47,* 155–167.

Hillis, A. E., & Caramazza, A. (1994). Theories of lexical processing and rehabilitation of lexical deficits. In M. J. Riddoch & G. W. Humphries (Eds.), *Cognitive neuropsychology and cognitive rehabilitation* (pp. 449–484). Hillsdale, NJ: Lawrence Erlbaum Associates.

Hodges, J. (2011). *Frontotemporal dementia syndromes.* Cambridge, UK: Cambridge University Press.

Holland, A. L., & Forbes, M. (Eds.). (1993). *Aphasia treatment: World perspectives.* San Diego: Singular Publishing.

Hopper, T. (2001). Indirect interventions to facilitate communication in Alzheimer's disease. *Seminars in Speech and Language, 22,* 290–304.

Kaszniak, A. W. (2002). Dementia. In V. S. Ramachandran (Ed.), *Encyclopedia of the human brain* (pp. 89–100). San Diego: Elsevier Science.

Kertesz, K. (2006). *Western Aphasia Battery–Revised.* San Antonio, TX: Harcourt Assessment.

Lehman Blake, M., Duffy, J. R., Myers, P. S., & Tompkins, C. A. (2002). Prevalence and patterns of right hemisphere cognitive/communicative deficits: Retrospective data from an inpatient rehabilitation unit. *Aphasiology, 16,* 537–547.

McNeil, M.R., & Duffy, J.R. (2001). Primary progressive aphasia. In R. Chapey, *Language Intervention Strategies for Aphasia.* 4th ed., pp. 472–486. Baltimore: Williams and Wilkins.

Mesulam, M-M. (1982). Slowly progressive aphasia without generalized dementia. *Annals of Neurology, 11,* 592–598.

Miller, B. L., & Cummings, J. L. (Eds.). (2007). *The human frontal lobes: Functions and disorders.* New York: Guilford Press.

Murray, L. L. (2002). Attention deficits in aphasia: Presence, nature, assessment, and treatment. *Seminars in Speech and Language, 23,* 107–116.

Myers, P. (1999). *Right hemisphere damage: Disorders of communication and cognition.* San Diego: Singular.

National Aphasia Association. Retrieved September 7, 2011, from www.aphasia.org/Aphasia%20Facts/aphasia_faq.html.

Nickels, L. (1992). The autocue? Self-generated phonemic cues in the treatment of a disorder of reading and naming. *Cognitive Neuropsychology, 9,* 155–182.

Rapcsak, S. Z., & Beeson, P. M. (2002). Neuroanatomical correlates of spelling and writing. In A. E. Hillis (Ed.). *Handbook on adult language disorders: Integrating cognitive neuropsychology, neurology, and rehabilitation* (pp. 71–99). Philadelphia: Psychology Press.

Robey, R. R. (1998). A meta-analysis of clinical outcomes in the treatment of aphasia. *Journal of Speech, Language, and Hearing Research, 41,* 172–187.

Small, J. A., & Perry, J. (2005). Do you remember? How caregivers question their spouses who have Alzheimer's disease and the impact on communication. *Journal of Speech, Language, and Hearing Research, 48*(1), 125–136.

Sohlberg, M. M., & Mateer, C. A. (2001). *Cognitive rehabilitation: An integrative approach.* New York: Guilford.

Tomoeda, C. K. (2001). Comprehensive assessment for dementia: A necessity for differential diagnosis and management. *Seminars in Speech and Language, 22*(4), 275–290.

Tompkins, C. A. (1995). *Right hemisphere communication disorders: Theory and management.* San Diego: Singular Publishing Group.

Wertz, R. T., Collins, M. J., Weiss, D., Kurtzke, J. F., Friden, T., Brookshire, R. H., Pierce, J., Holzapple, P., Hubbard, D. J., Proch, B. E., West, H. A., Davis, L., Matlvitch, V., Morley, G. K., & Resurreccion, E. (1981). Veteran's Administration cooperative study on aphasia: A comparison of individual and group treatment. *Journal of Speech and Hearing Research, 24,* 580–594.

READINGS FROM THE POPULAR LITERATURE

Bauby, J-D. (1997). *The diving bell and the butterfly.* New York: Random House. (locked-in syndrome)

Bayley, J. (2000). *Elegy for Iris.* New York: St. Martin's Press. (Alzheimer disease)

Bolte-Taylor, J. (2008). *My stroke of insight: A brain scientist's personal journey.* New York: Penguin Group. (a neuroscientist's account of stroke and her recovery)

Bryant, B. (1992). *In search of wings: A journey back from traumatic brain injury.* South Paris, ME: Wings Press. (traumatic brain injury)

Crimmins, C. (2000). *Where is the mango princess?* New York: Random House. (traumatic brain injury)

Davidson, A. (1997). *Alzheimers, a love story. One year in my husband's journey.* Secaucus, NJ: Carol Pub. Group. (Alzheimer's disease)

DeMille, A. (1981). *Reprieve.* New York: Doubleday. (famous dancer's account of her stroke)

Douglas, K. (2001). *My stroke of luck.* New York: W. Morrow. (actor's experience with stroke, aphasia, and dysarthria)

Edsall, S. (2004). *Into the blue: A father's flight and a daughter's return.* New York: St. Martin's Press. (a daughter's story about her father, who had a stroke)

Ellison, B., & Ellison, J. (2001). *Miracles happen: One mother, one daughter, one journey.* New York: Hyperion. (spinal cord injury)

Fishman, S. (1988). *A bomb in the brain: A heroic tale of science, surgery and survival.* New York: Scribner. (brain hemorrhage, subsequent epilepsy)

Harper, M. S. (2001). *The worst day of my life, so far.* Athens, GA: Hill Street Press. (Alzheimer's disease)

Kessler, L. (2007). *Dancing with Rose: Finding life in the land of Alzheimer's* (Alzheimer's disease)

Klein, B. S. (1998). *Slow dance: A story of stroke, love and disability*. Berkeley, CA: Page Mill Press. (stroke and aphasia)

McCrum, R. (1999). *My year off: Recovery from stroke*. Canada: Random House. (stroke and aphasia)

McEwen, M. (2008). *Change in the weather: Life after stroke*. New York: Gotham Books. (*Early Show* weatherman's account of stroke)

McGowin, D. F. (1994). *Living in the labyrinth: A personal journey through the maze of Alzheimer's disease*. New York: Dell Publishing. (early Alzheimer's disease from patient's perspective)

Newborn, B. (1997). *Return to Ithaca*. Rockport, MA: Element. (young woman with aphasia)

Osborne, C. (1998). *Over my head: A doctor's own story of head injury from the inside looking out*. Kansas City, MO: Andrews McMeel Pub. (traumatic brain injury)

Quinn, D. (1998). *Conquering the dark: One woman's story of recovering from a brain injury*. St. Paul, MN: Paragon House. (traumatic brain injury)

Rife, J. M. (1994). *Injured mind, shattered dreams: Journey from severe head injury to a dream*. Cambridge, MA: Brookline Books. (traumatic brain injury)

Shiplett, J. L. (1996). *A glass full of tears*. Aurora, OH: Writer's World Press. (dementia)

Swanson, K., & Chrunkra, M. (1999). *I'll carry the fork*. Los Altos, CA: Rising Star Press. (traumatic brain injury)

Talalvero, J. (1998). *Look up for yes*. New York: Kodansha International. (locked-in syndrome)

Timothy, M. (2006). *Let me die laughing!: Waking from the nightmare of a brain explosion* (aphasia)

Wulf, H. (1973). *Aphasia, my world alone*. Detroit, MI: Wayne State University.

The Biological Foundations of Hearing

Theodore J. Glattke

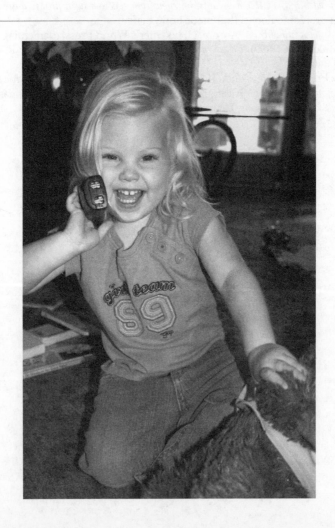

PREVIEW

Sound is a form of energy that is present everywhere in our environment. In Chapter 3, we learned that sound can be described in terms of frequency and intensity, and we were introduced to the characteristics of the sounds associated with speech. In this chapter, we consider how the sounds around us are received and processed by the auditory system. We will see how the structures of the outer and middle ear transmit sound to the inner ear. We will learn how the structure of the inner ear contributes to our ability to hear sounds of different pitches and how the nervous system further shapes sound perception.

Structure and Function of the Ear

The Outer Ear

The ear usually is described as having three distinct divisions: outer, middle, and inner. As illustrated in Figure 10.1, the outer ear consists of a visible portion, the **auricle**, or **pinna**, and a canal that leads from the pinna to the eardrum, or tympanic membrane. The canal between the pinna and tympanic membrane is the **external ear canal**.

The shape of the pinna is created by pieces of cartilage that form ridges and depressions that are peculiar to each person. In fact, pinna configurations are so unique that we could identify people using "pinna prints" instead of fingerprints. In adults, the pinna is about 3.5 inches in height and about 1.5 inches wide. It is a sound collector and also serves to enhance the sound pressure of certain frequencies. You can exaggerate this effect by cupping your hand behind your pinna and thus increasing the dimension of the sound collector. For most people, the pinna acts to increase high-frequency sounds by about 5 dB SPL. It also helps us to locate the sources of high-frequency sounds that are overhead, such as those produced by flying insects.

The external ear canal is about 1 inch long and about 0.4 inch in diameter. Cartilage forms the foundation of the canal near the pinna. The inner portion of the canal is framed by hard bone. The canal protects the tympanic membrane from physical trauma due to nearly everything except for cotton swabs pushed into the canal by the owner! Specialized cells in the floor of the ear canal produce a waxy substance called **cerumen** that helps to keep the skin of the canal moist and traps debris that might normally fall against the tympanic membrane. Like the pinna, the length and shape of the ear canal also serve to enhance sound pressure. The canal produces a boost in SPL of about 15 dB for sounds in the frequency region of 2500 to 3500 Hz and for multiples of those frequencies. Taken together, the effects of the pinna and external ear canal provide a helpful boost in the mid- and high-frequency region of the sound spectrum. Without those structures, we would have a slight loss of hearing.

If you place your finger slightly into your external ear canal, and then move your jaw, you can feel your jawbone moving against the flexible portion of the external ear canal. The inner part of the canal does not move, because it is embedded in bone.

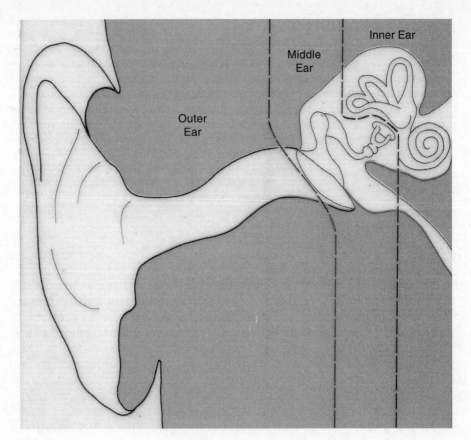

FIGURE 10.1 A schematic drawing of the divisions of the hearing mechanism.

The structure of the outer ear and tympanic membrane can be evaluated with an **otoscope**. An otoscope includes a light source to illuminate the ear canal and a magnifying lens to enhance visualization of the structures within the ear canal. An otoscopic exam may be used to determine whether the ear canal is clear and open from the pinna to the tympanic membrane (see Figure 10.2). The light from the otoscope will illuminate the translucent tympanic membrane, so that its physical condition can be determined. Some otoscopes are connected to a video monitor and computer so that images can be displayed, stored, and printed. An exam with this type of an otoscope is referred to as **video otoscopy**. A video otoscope is particularly useful for documenting conditions that that may change over time. For example, video otoscopy might provide an initial image of an infection in the external ear, or indicate a problem in the middle ear, and subsequent images may be used to document whether treatment to resolve the infection is effective.

The Middle Ear

The **middle ear** consists of a cavity, a ventilating tube that connects the cavity to the pharynx, and several moving parts that work together to boost the pressure

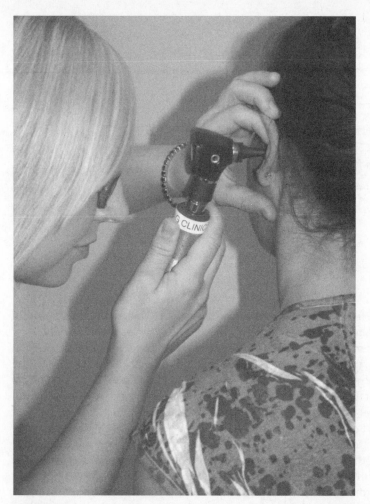

FIGURE 10.2   An otoscopic is used to view the ear canal and tympanic membrane.

created by the sound energy that arrives at the eardrum, or tympanic membrane. The middle ear apparatus is called a **transformer** because of the change in pressure that it creates. You probably use transformers every day: The small adapters that are found on the electrical cords of CD players, computer accessories, and video cameras are transformers that change the voltage supplied by the power company to a value that is required by the device. By analogy, the middle ear provides a boost in pressure to drive the inner ear system.

The principal parts of the middle ear are illustrated in Figure 10.3. The middle ear cavity is formed of bone that is covered by thin mucosa similar to the lining of the nasal cavities. The volume of the cavity is small, less than about 2 cc. The eardrum, or **tympanic membrane**, is stretched across the opening of the external canal so that nearly all of the sound energy entering the canal pushes on the eardrum. It is thin, flexible, and yet strong enough not to burst when humans

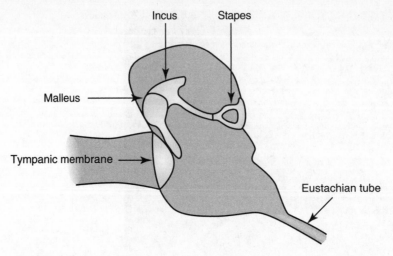

FIGURE 10.3 The middle ear.

dive 100 or more feet below the surface of the ocean. The eardrum is roughly circular in shape and has a diameter of about 1 cm, a little less than ½ inch.

The tympanic membrane is connected to three bones, or **ossicles**, that span the middle ear cavity between the eardrum and the inner ear. The names of the ossicles were inspired by their shapes. The hammer, or **malleus**, is the first of the ossicles. It is about 9 mm long, and its long arm is attached firmly to the eardrum. The anvil, or **incus**, is the second ossicle and is about 7 mm in size. The head of the incus and head of the malleus are covered by tissue that holds them together so that they move together. In this way, they form two arms of a lever. The difference in the length of the two bones helps to create the transformer effect of the middle ear. The third ossicle is the stirrup, or **stapes**. The footplate of the stapes looks like the bottom of a stirrup. The footplate is oval, and it is about 3 mm in length and about 1 mm in width. It fits into an opening called the oval window of the inner ear system.

The principles by which the middle ear transformer works are illustrated in Figure 10.4. The transformer boosts the pressure by a significant amount. The largest boost is due to the differences in the areas of the eardrum and stapes footplate. The part of the eardrum that moves in response to the incident sound has an area that is about twenty times the area of the stapes footplate. The force that collects on the eardrum is transmitted directly to the footplate, and so the force per square mm of area at the stapes is boosted by a factor of about 20 to 1. This boost in pressure, or *force per unit of area*, is the same effect that occurs when a thumbtack is used. The force applied to the large head is sufficient to enable the tack to penetrate a piece of wood because the area of the point of the tack is much smaller than the area of the head.

The second mechanism that helps to boost the pressure is found in the lever action resulting from the difference between the lengths of the malleus and incus.

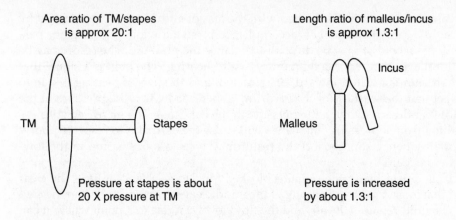

Area ratio of TM/stapes is approx 20:1

Length ratio of malleus/incus is approx 1.3:1

TM

Stapes

Incus

Malleus

Pressure at stapes is about 20 X pressure at TM

Pressure is increased by about 1.3:1

Combination of area ratio and lever system = pressure boost of 26:1

FIGURE 10.4 Mechanisms that create the transformer effect of the middle ear.

The ratio of 9 mm (malleus) to 7 mm (incus) is equivalent to about 1.3 to 1. Force applied to the long arm of the lever is increased by an amount equal to the ratio of the lengths of the long and short arms, or about 1.3 to 1. The combination of the ratio of the areas of the eardrum and stapes (20:1) and the lever action of the ossicles (1.3:1) provides a boost of about 26 to 1, or about 28 dB. The combined effects of the outer and middle ear systems allow us to hear sounds that are about 30 to 60 dB below the intensities that would be needed if our outer and middle ear apparatus did not exist or was destroyed. Individuals born without an external ear canal or middle ear apparatus, or persons who have an ear infection that leaves the middle ear full of thick fluid, will experience a loss of hearing of about 60 dB for airborne sounds.

This middle ear transformer will work properly only *when the eardrum is intact* and when the *cavity is filled with air*. The **Eustachian tube** connects the middle ear cavity with the pharynx, and it opens each time a swallow occurs. When the tube opens, air passes from the back of the throat into the middle ear, and fluid that is secreted by the lining of the middle ear is allowed to drain into the throat. If the tube is blocked, the exchange of air and drainage of fluid will be affected. The tube may become blocked due to upper respiratory allergies, a cold, or another condition that causes an increase in secretion or swelling of the tissue that lines the middle ear, Eustachian tube, or pharynx. If the air is not refreshed, the air in the middle ear cavity will be absorbed by the tissue, and the eardrum will be pushed inward by the difference in air pressure between the atmosphere and the middle ear cavity. A clinician looking at the eardrum with an otoscope will say that it is "retracted." Many people experience a temporary retraction of the eardrum when they are passengers in an airplane that descends rapidly for a landing. The

When your ears "pop" on an airplane, it is simply your Eustachian tube opening to allow the air pressure in your middle ear to match the changes in the atmospheric pressure as you ascend and descend on your flight.

increase in air pressure associated with the loss of altitude must be matched by the middle ear—this usually is accomplished by swallowing. If an airplane passenger has a cold, it may be difficult to balance the pressure. The result may be a painful experience and a temporary loss of hearing. The pain is a signal that the eardrum is pushed inward, or retracted, and the loss of hearing is due to the fact that the stiffness of the eardrum is increased when the pressure in the middle ear does not match the pressure in the ear canal. The increased stiffness resulting from a pressure imbalance will cause the eardrum to respond poorly to low-frequency sounds and the result may be a loss of hearing in the low-frequency region.

If the Eustachian tube remains blocked for a long period of time, the clear fluid that is secreted by the lining of the middle ear cavity will collect in the cavity. The fluid replaces the air, and the fluid level can rise to a point where it can be seen by a clinician using an otoscope to examine the eardrum. The addition of the fluid increases the stiffness of the eardrum considerably because of the reduction of the volume of air in the middle ear cavity and the incompressibility of the fluid. This produces a greater hearing loss that may eventually include both low- and high-frequency sounds if the cavity fills completely. The disorder caused by fluid in the ear is called *otitis media* (see also Chapter 11). It not only creates a hearing problem but it also is a serious medical problem that requires attention. If the fluid remains for a long period of time, it serves as a fertile medium for infection that can lead to serious consequences, including spontaneous rupture or perforation of the eardrum. A middle ear that is filled with fluid combined with a perforated tympanic membrane loses its ability to work as a transformer.

The function of the tympanic membrane can be assessed using a procedure known as tympanometry (Figure 10.5). In tympanometry, a probe that is covered with soft plastic is inserted at the edge of the external ear canal to create a sealed cavity. Puffs of air from this probe vary the air pressure in the ear canal while a tone is presented through the probe tip. Recall that high pressure in the ear canal will cause the tympanic membrane to retract into the middle ear until the action of the Eustachian tube equalizes the pressure. Conversely, low pressure in the ear canal will cause the tympanic membrane to bulge outward. The tympanic membrane will move back and forth in response to the change in air pressure created by the tympanometer. This in turn creates a change in the sound pressure

> The status of the middle ear can be tested using tympanometry with very young children because it does not require them to make a response.

within the ear canal that is detected by the probe. If anything prevents the normal movement of the tympanic membrane, the abnormal movement will be detected during tympanometry. For example, a tear in the tympanic membrane will prevent air pressure build up in front of or behind the membrane. Sound from the probe will "leak" into the middle ear cavity and the tympanometer will detect larger than normal volume of air. Conditions that impede movement of the tympanic membrane, such as fluid in the ear or fused ossicles, will result in additional stiffness in the system. This will also cause an abnormal pattern of movement of the tympanic membrane during tympanometry, helping to diagnose disorders of the middle ear.

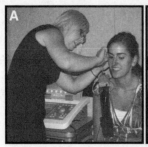
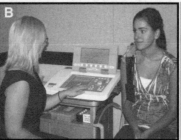
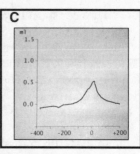

FIGURE 10.5 Tympanometry. (A) A probe is inserted into the ear. (B) The response of the typmpanic membrane is measured. (C) Results showing the response of the tympanic membrane are graphed.

The middle ear ossicles are attached to two small muscles. The tensor tympani muscle pulls the malleus inward, toward the center of the head. The muscle is named because it tenses or stiffens the eardrum or tympanum. The tensor tympani muscle is innervated by the Vth cranial nerve (trigeminal), which is the principal sensory nerve of the face and controls the muscles that are involved in chewing. The tensor tympani contracts when we swallow, yawn, and chew, and it also responds to tactile stimulation of the skin of the face. The second muscle is the stapedius. When it contracts, it pulls the stapes outward. The stapedius muscle is innervated by the VIIth cranial nerve (facial), which controls the muscles of facial expression. The stapedius muscle contracts in response to broadband sounds that are about 60 to 80 dB SPL in persons with normal hearing thresholds.

When the stapedius muscle contracts in response to sound, it adds stiffness to the middle ear transformer system. The change in stiffness can be measured by using a clinical instrument known as a tympanometer, along with the same probe system used to test the status of the tympanic membrane. The change in stiffness resulting from contraction of the stapedius is known as the *acoustic reflex*. The reflex is bilateral, which is to say that it appears on both sides during stimulation of either ear. In this way it is like the change in pupil diameter that occurs when a bright light is presented to either eye. Traditionally, the acoustic reflex was thought to serve to protect the ear from intense sound. However, few sounds found in nature (such as thunder, the roar of waterfalls, rockslides, an imminent predator) are of sufficient intensity to activate the acoustic reflex. It is noteworthy that our world became very noisy long after middle ear muscles were created. Therefore, it is unlikely that these muscles were designed to protect against the industrial noises of gunpowder, steam, internal combustion, and jet engines.

A modern view of the action of the acoustic reflex is that, although it may help to protect the ear from intense sounds, its principal role is to alter the transmission characteristics of the middle ear to enable us to hear important sounds, such as speech, in noisy situations. The tensor tympani muscle may serve the same role when we are generating noise by eating, swallowing, or talking. Neither muscle can react with sufficient speed to protect us from the most dangerous sounds in our world: the explosive reports of firearms.

The acoustic reflex can be tested by introducing a loud sound into either ear, which will normally result in a contraction of the stapedius muscle in both ears. The test involves monitoring the change in stiffness of the tympanic membrane in response to the loud sound in either the same ear as the tone is presented, or in the opposite ear. The softest sound that can cause the stapedius muscle to contract is known as the acoustic reflex threshold. As noted above, this is typically between 65 and 80 dB SPL for an individual with a normal hearing system. However, this threshold may be elevated or the reflex may be absent if there is damage to the VIIth cranial nerve (which would keep the muscle from contracting), any condition that interferes with the mobility of the ossicular chain (e.g., fluid in the middle ear), or hearing loss involving other parts of the auditory system. The acoustic reflex is usually tested along with tympanometry. Together, these two tests are known as **immittance audiometry**.

In Chapter 2, we considered how the biological systems that support speech and language were affected in a child with Down syndrome. This genetic disorder also affects the hearing mechanism as well. We can see how the outer and middle ear mechanisms are affected in the case of Alicia.

Alicia underwent a full audiologic evaluation to determine hearing function. Like most children with Down syndrome, she has small and irregular pinnas. The audiologist used an otoscope in order to examine the appearance of the ear canal and tympanic membrane. For some children with Down syndrome, the ear canal is narrower than usual. In the case of Alicia, the ear canals have a normal appearance and are open and clear. However, she appears to have some fluid in the middle ear. This is common in children with Down syndrome, who have a high rate of middle ear infections. Alicia's mother reports that her child has been plagued by these infections. On this day, an otoscopic exam suggested the presence of middle ear fluid. This was accompanied by abnormal results for tympanometry. The fluid changed the mechanical workings of the tympanic membrane and ossicles, resulting in a mild hearing loss. The fluid caused an increase in the stiffness of the moving parts of the middle ear apparatus.

The Inner Ear

The inner ear converts energy to a code that can be interpreted by the brain for hearing and balance. In this way, it serves the same role as the retina of the eye, touch receptors in the skin, and olfactory receptors in the nose and taste buds. The process of conversion is called *transduction*. The inner ear has three separate transduction systems: (a) the vestibule, (b) the semicircular canals, and (c) the cochlea. Transducers in the vestibule help us to maintain our orientation with respect to gravity, or the center of the earth. The semicircular canal systems provide us with information about head position and help us to maintain a fix on visual targets when we are moving. The cochlea contains the transducers for hearing. The three parts of the inner ear share important features. The first is that the inner ear is filled with fluid. Forces acting on the inner ear due to gravity, acceleration of the head or body, or sound ultimately create motion of the fluid in the inner ear system. The fluid couples the energy of the stimulus to the transducers that convert the stimulus to responses of neurons. The second shared feature is that the transducer mechanisms are similar in all three parts of the inner ear. They consist of a mechanical receptor, called a *hair cell*, and a *covering membrane* that causes or otherwise enhances the motion of the hairlike cilia found on the top of the hair cells. The remainder of the chapter will focus on how these principles apply in the cochlea—the end organ for hearing.

> Whereas a healthy middle ear is an air-filled cavity, the inner ear is filled with fluid.

Cochlear Structure and Function

The fundamental arrangement of several important parts of the cochlea is illustrated in the series of drawings in Figure 10.6 (after Kiang, 1975). The cochlea is a hard-walled chamber that is filled with fluid (Figure 10.6A). There are two flexible "windows." The **oval window** is the location at which the stapes footplate connects to the inner ear. The **round window** is a second opening on the body of the cochlea, and it is also covered with a flexible membrane. When the stapes forces the oval window inward, the round window is forced outward by the pressure of the fluid in the chamber. In Figure 10.6B the stapes has been added, and a "basilar" (basement), or supporting, membrane is stretched across the cavity. The inward motion of the stapes causes the **basilar membrane** to move in response to fluid displacement because it lies in the pathway of the fluid.

Sensory cells are added in Figure 10.6C. These are hair cells that sit on the basilar membrane. An opening called the helicotrema allows the fluid in the top channel to flow directly into the bottom channel. (Note that the helicotrema is located at the top, or apex, of the cochlea in its true, coiled shape.) Fluid will flow through this channel only when the stapes moves very slowly, such as in the case in which a change in air pressure within the middle ear causes the oval window to be pushed inward or pulled outward (laterally). When stapes vibrations occur rapidly enough, such as at the lower limit of our range of hearing, then it is the basilar membrane that responds to the forces applied by the stapes. The rate of stapes vibrations determines the location where the basilar membrane will flex and activate the hair cells. The location of stimulation along the basilar membrane provides information about the sound's frequency.

> Hair cells in the inner ear are critical for hearing. You protect them by wearing ear protection (such as earplugs) when you are in noisy environments.

There are about 16,000 hair cells in the cochlea of humans with healthy ears. The structure is designed to accommodate the hair cells along a length of about 36 mm (from the base close to the stapes to the opposite end, called the apex). To illustrate this point, Figure 10.6D extends the length of the fluid chamber. Figure 10.6E shows the fluid chamber coiled into a shell shape, approximating the true configuration of the cochlea. Sitting on the basilar membrane is the **organ of Corti**, named for the anatomist who provided an early description of its structure.

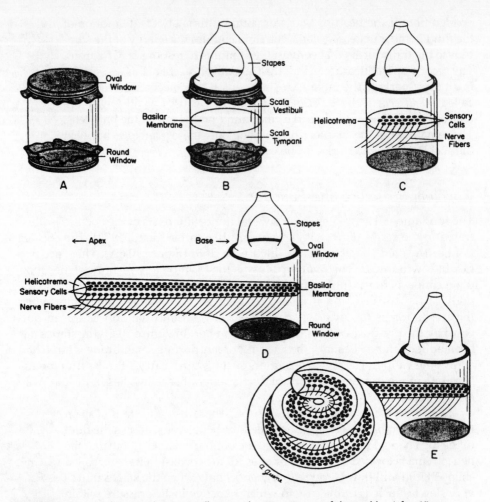

FIGURE 10.6   Schematic drawing to illustrate the components of the cochlea (after Kiang, 1975). As shown in drawings A and B, the cochlea is likened to a hard-walled container with flexible membranes on the top and bottom and another membrane stretched across the middle (C). Drawings D and E elongate the container to better represent the structure of the true cochlea.

In Figure 10.7, we see its components, which include supporting structures, hair cells, and an overlying membrane called the *tectorial membrane* (tectum = roof). This is the view you would have if you unrolled the cochlea as in Figure 10.6D and then sliced it as if you were slicing salami. There are two sets of hair cells—a single row of inner hair cells and three rows of outer hair cells. These cells are so named because they contain hairlike projections called **cilia**. Hair cells are delicate and can be easily damaged through aging, disease, or exposure to certain drugs, or by prolonged exposure to loud noise. Once damaged, the hair cells can regenerate in some species, such as birds, but they do not repair themselves in mammals. Movement of the basilar membrane sets off a shearing motion of the hair cell cilia.

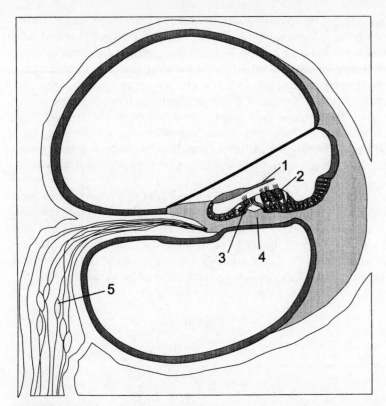

FIGURE 10.7 Cross-section the cochlea and organ of Corti: (1) tectorial membrane, (2) outer hair cells, (3) inner hair cells, (4) basilar membrane, (5) cell body of the auditory nerve.

This motion is translated by the receptor cells into a chemical-electrical signal that is carried to the brain via auditory nerve fibers.

The shape of the basilar membrane influences how sound energy is analyzed by the cochlea. The membrane is relatively narrow at the base, the end near the stapes. It is about ten times wider at the apex. A change in stiffness accompanies the change in width of the basilar membrane so that the base end is about 100 times stiffer than the apex end. The gradation in stiffness is important because it helps to determine how sounds are represented in the cochlea. The stiffness of the basilar membrane near the base of the cochlea creates an efficient response for high-frequency sounds. The more flaccid region near the apex cannot respond to high-frequency energy, so its responses are limited to low frequencies.

The stiffness change from the base to the apex of the cochlea allows the cochlea to analyze the sounds transmitted by the stapes, much like the spectrum analyzer discussed in Chapter 3. The basis of this analysis was described by Georg von Békésy in 1928. He examined the behavior of the cochleas of several species of animals. The bone containing the cochlea was removed from the animal's skull and drilled to expose the membranes in the fluid spaces of the ear. The preparation was placed under a conventional light microscope and then driven mechanically by a sound source. Von Békésy described the motion patterns of the basilar membrane and noted that a *traveling wave* developed along the membrane in response to sound. When high-frequency sounds were employed, the disturbance traveled only a few millimeters from the base of the cochlea. When low frequencies were used, the traveling wave spread from the base to the apex. The place of maximum vibration of the traveling wave was determined by the frequency of the sound. Because each frequency was associated with a specific place of stimulation, the cochlea was said to be *tonotopically organized*.

The illustrations in Figure 10.8 are based on von Békésy's observations (von Békésy, 1960). Three sketches of the basilar membrane are shown. The membrane is "unrolled" as in Figure 10.6D, with the base of the cochlea on the right and the apex on the left. The dashed lines represent the gross patterns of the traveling wave disturbances for 5000, 1000, and 200 Hz, respectively. The numerical scales below the three schematics provide an indication of the distance along the

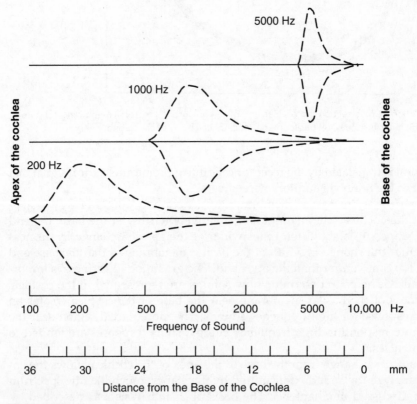

FIGURE 10.8   Traveling waves corresponding to different sound frequencies as described by von Békésy.

basilar membrane in millimeters and the places where individual frequencies would create the maximum disturbances. The traveling waves described by von Békésy appeared to move from base to apex. Frequencies between about 1000 and 20,000 Hz are represented along the 18 mm of the membrane closest to the base of the cochlea. Frequencies between about 100 and 1000 Hz are represented in the "upper" half of the cochlea, between about 18 and 36 mm from the base. Frequencies below about 100 Hz probably result in a wave that sweeps the basilar membrane from end to end without developing a peak in the disturbance pattern.

Von Békésy's work ushered in a new understanding of how the inner ear analyzes sound. His continuing efforts over the next thirty years led to the Nobel Prize in Medicine and Physiology, awarded to him in 1961. Two physicists, Gold and Pumphrey, examined the von Békésy studies and studies of human threshold sensitivity and frequency discrimination and concluded that there had to be some active amplifier process that actually added energy to the signal delivered to the inner ear by the stapes footplate (Gold, 1948, 1989). They reasoned that this amplifier might occasionally become unstable and develop a shrill whistle, like one hears when a public address system produces feedback. They also reasoned that the amplifier elements must be highly tuned. Gold and Pumphrey presented their ideas to scientific experts around 1948, twenty years after von Békésy's report, but they were unable to convince anyone of the merit of their theory and so they pursued other scientific ventures.

About twenty years after Gold and Pumphrey's brief visit to auditory science, evidence for the leakage of energy from the ear back into the air was discovered by David Kemp, who also had a background in physics. Kemp was listening to low-intensity sounds and realized that some unknown source of sound was interacting with the external sound. When he placed a miniature microphone in the ear of a listener, he was he was able to record the "whistle" that reflects the feedback predicted by Gold and Pumphrey (Kemp, 1978). The tones recorded by Dr. Kemp, and from thousands of other subjects since 1978, must reflect an energy source within the inner ear and some disturbance that is transmitted backward through the fluid of the inner ear and middle ear cavity to the eardrum. In this case, the eardrum works like a loudspeaker diaphragm, producing vibrations in the air rather than responding to them! These sounds are called **otoacoustic emissions**. Emissions occur both spontaneously and in response to stimulation and are present in virtually every healthy ear. Kemp found the evidence needed to support the notion that an active amplifier exists inside of the cochlea.

> Did you know that your ears actually emit sound? Most of us "whistle" with our ears!

For a power source, we must look at the details of the organ of Corti. Recall that there are three rows of outer hair cells and only a single row of inner hair cells. Therefore, the outer hair cells outnumber the inner hair cells by about 3:1. There are also a number of other differences between these two types of cells (see Table 10.1). The hair cells differ in shape: The outer hair cells are relatively cylindrical in shape, whereas the inner hair cells are jug-shaped. The position and structural support of the two types of cells also differs. The outer hair cells are in

TABLE 10.1   Differences between Inner and Outer Hair Cells

Outer Hair Cells	Inner Hair Cells
Three rows of cells	One row of cells
Cylindrical in shape	Jug-shaped
Contact with tectorial membrane	No contact with tectorial membrane
Sit on flexible basilar membrane	Sit on bony shelf
Support cells at hair cell base	Support cells surround hair cells
Receive efferent nerve fibers from the brain	Send afferent nerve fibers to the brain

contact with the tectorial membrane, but the cilia of the inner hair cells are free of attachments above their cell bodies. Outer hair cells are situated over the flexible basilar membrane, whereas the inner hair cells sit on a rigid bony shelf. The inner hair cells are firmly encased in supporting structures that surround each inner hair cell, but the outer hair cells are situated on supporting cells at their base. Finally, the inner hair cells receive nearly all of the afferent, or sensory, nerves leading from the ear to the brain. In contrast, the outer hair cells receive nearly all of the efferent or control nerves leading from the brain back to the ear.

These differences point to important functional differences between the outer and inner hair cells. Today, most theories of inner ear function argue that the inner hair cells are the actual sensory transducers. The nerve supply attached to the inner hair cells and measures of their electrical properties during stimulation of the ear are compatible with this notion. The outer hair cells are thought to contribute to the amplification of motion in the inner ear in response to low-intensity sounds. No one has actually "seen" the outer hair cells in operation inside of the ear, but we do know several things about how they work. If outer hair cells are missing, hearing loss occurs in that region. When outer hair cells are compromised or destroyed, the inner hair cells do not function normally. However, if the outer hair cells return to normal function, the inner hair cells do so as well. Likewise, otoacoustic emissions disappear when outer hair cells are compromised, only to reappear if the outer hair cells are restored to normal function.

Outer hair cells have been studied *in vitro*, that is to say, in artificial environments after being removed from an ear. Studied this way, Brownell and his coworkers (1983) discovered a startling fact in the early 1980s: They demonstrated that the outer hair cells changed their lengths in response to chemical stimulation. Other investigations demonstrated that changes in cell length of 5 to 10 percent of the original length can occur in response to electrical, chemical, or mechanical (acoustic) stimulation. When the cell is activated, or depolarized, by a stimulus, *it becomes shorter*! If the cell is returned to its resting electrical (chemical) state, then *its length is restored*! Finally, if the cell is hyperpolarized, the opposite of depolarization, then *its length increases*! As illustrated in Figure 10.9, depolarization of the outer hair cells occurs when the cilia are tilted toward the tallest row. Hyperpolarization would occur if the cilia are forced

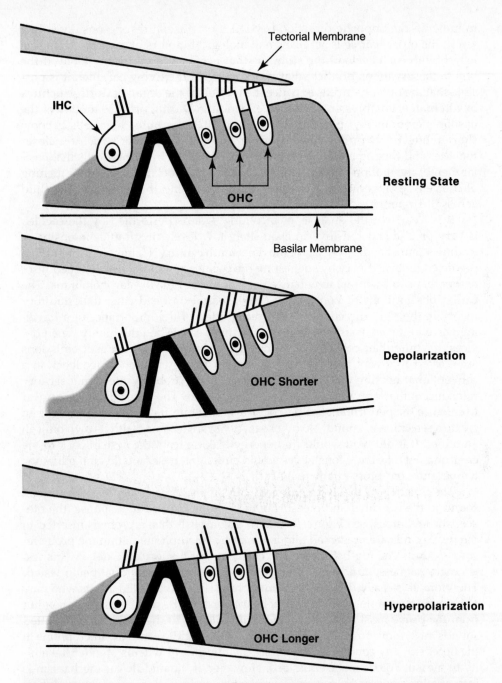

FIGURE 10.9 Action of the outer hair cells (OHC) relative to movement of the basilar membrane. Note the change in length of the outer hair cells and the change in position of the hairs, or cilia, of these cells as the basilar membrane rises or falls. IHC-inner hair cell.

to move in the opposite direction beyond their normal resting positions. In a sense, the outer hair cells act like small biological motors or muscles, changing length with each cycle of the stimulus that is effective in driving them. If the *in vitro* observations predict what is occurring in the living ear, then it is possible that the outer hair cells enhance the motion of the organ of Corti structures by alternately compressing and then expanding. During upward motion of the basilar membrane, as illustrated in Figure 10.9, the outer hair cells become shorter, effectively pulling the tectorial membrane and other structures closer together and forcing endolymph to stream across the inner hair cell cilia. Basilar membrane motion in the opposite direction is associated with a lengthening of the cells, exaggerating the motion and amplifying the motion of the fluid across the inner hair cell cilia.

It is clear that the analysis of incoming sounds performed by the cochlea is very precise and sensitive to exquisitely low levels of stimulus intensity. A leading scientist and physician of the nineteenth century, Helmholtz (1885/1954) predicted today's theory by suggesting the cochlea contained highly tuned resonators that could vibrate to enhance the response of the basilar membrane. The earlier observations of von Békésy (1960), based on dead ears, took auditory theory in the right direction, toward recognition of the importance of a traveling wave in the analysis of sounds by the inner ear. When the highly tuned devices (the outer hair cells) become unstable, spontaneous otoacoustic emissions are created in a way that is probably similar to the creation of feedback in a conventional hearing aid. The inner hair cells are probably the actual sensory transducers that provide information about sound. The outer hair cells appear to enhance the performance of the cochlea so that minute amounts of energy can create a sensation of sound. No other sensory system comes with its own built-in amplifier. If it did, you would find energy leaking from the system back to the environment (like emissions): Eyes would emit light, noses would emit odorants, temperature receptors might emit heat!

The function of the outer hair cells can be tested clinically by presenting a sound in the ear canal and measuring the sounds emitted in response (the otoacoustic emissions, see Figure 10.10). To accomplish this, a probe is inserted in the ear. Sounds are presented and a miniature microphone within the probe records sounds coming back from the cochlea after a short time delay. This test is quick, painless, and requires no response from the individual being tested. Therefore, it is easily done with infants, children, and disabled adults who may not be able to complete other types of hearing exams. Because the sounds coming from the probe must move through the middle ear to the cochlea, and emitted sounds must move from the cochlea through the middle ear to the microphone in the outer ear, any conditions that affect the middle ear will also hinder the ability to measure otoacoustic emissions. However, if the middle ear mechanism is intact, failure to record otoacoustic emissions can signal damage to the outer hair cells within the cochlea. The outer hair cells work very hard to help us to hear, and they are very vulnerable to noise, certain medications, and systemic problems that compromise their energy supply. When outer hair cells are damaged

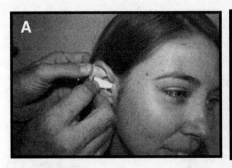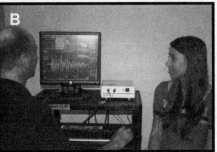

FIGURE 10.10 Otoacoustic emissions testing. (A) A probe is inserted into the ear. (B) Energy generated within the cochlea is displayed on the computer screen.

temporarily by loud noise, we experience a loss of otoacoustic emissions and a temporary loss of hearing. When outer hair cells are destroyed, the loss of emissions and hearing become permanent.

Auditory Connections in the Brain

We hear with our brains, not our ears. Each ear communicates with the central nervous system through afferent (ascending) and efferent (descending) connections. The outer hair cells receive nearly all of the efferent connections from the brain to the ear. The inner hair cells are connected to nearly all of the afferent neurons. The afferent neurons travel from the ear to the central nervous system in the VIIIth cranial nerve, referred to as the auditory nerve. The auditory nerve also contains the neurons from the vestibular system. The neurons from the auditory portion of the VIIIth cranial nerve end when they reach the brainstem. They make connections with neurons in the cochlear nucleus.

As illustrated in Figure 10.11, the neurons that leave the cochlea travel to other places in the central nervous system, where they make connections. The cochlea analyzes sounds into the individual frequencies that are present in a way that is similar to a spectrum analyzer. Individual inner hair cells are responsive to very narrow ranges of frequencies in the spectrum through a process that creates *tonotopic organization* in the cochlea. Neurons carrying information from the inner hair cells to the central nervous system maintain the tonotopic organization. The central nervous system is also organized so that information about individual tones projects to specific places in the brain.

In Figure 10.11, ascending pathways from the right and left ears are shown as solid and dashed lines, respectively. The ascending nerve fibers connect with several groups of neurons (called nuclei) within the brainstem, where auditory information is processed. These nuclei are shown in light gray. There are two sets of nuclei in the brainstem, and some of the ascending auditory information crosses from one side of the

> The messages from the ear to the brain provide information regarding the frequency and intensity of sounds, which you perceive as the pitch and the loudness. So, you actually *hear* with your brain!

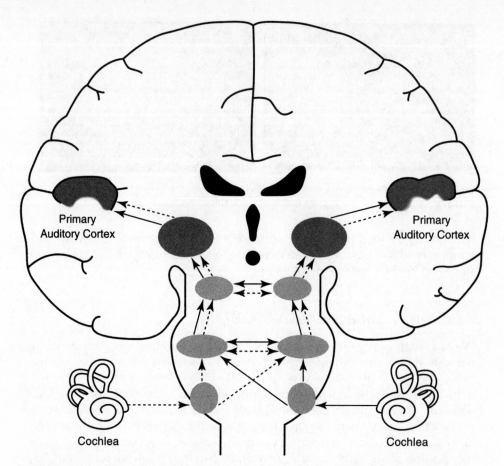

FIGURE 10.11   The central auditory pathways (components not to scale). The nerve fibers (solid and dashed lines) from the cochlea of each ear travel to nuclei in the brainstem (light gray). Nerve fibers from nuclei on each side cross, and information from each ear reaches nuclei on both sides of the cerebrum (areas in dark gray).

brainstem to the other. Neurons in the brainstem send information to the cerebrum, first through subcortical nuclei (dark gray), and from the nerve pathways radiate diffusely to the primary auditory cortex, which is found in the temporal lobe of the brain (see Chapter 2).

It is important to note that the right and left ear inputs are mixed together in the brainstem and that each of the nuclei and fiber tracts above the cochlear nucleus contains neurons that can be traced to both ears. This *binaural* representation helps us to locate sounds in space by comparing the information received from one ear with the information received from the other. The function of each of the major central nervous system structures that contain auditory neurons is not understood completely. However, we know that all of the structures maintain the tonotopic organization that was established in the cochlea. In other words,

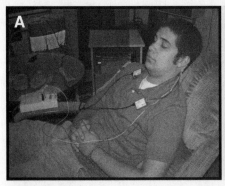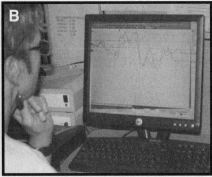

FIGURE 10.12   Electrophysiology is used to test the integrity of the auditory pathways. (A) Electrodes placed on the scalp measure electrical activity generated within the nervous system. (B) The voltage changes associated with the electrical activity are plotted across time on the computer screen. Different peaks in the resulting waveform are generated at different levels of the auditory nervous system.

individual frequencies in simple and complex sounds are represented at specific places within the nervous system from the ear to the cortex.

The conduction of information about sound via nerve impulses along the auditory pathway can be measured. When nerve fibers transmit information, they do so by electrical impulses. These impulses can be detected by metal discs, called electrodes, which are placed on the skin of the head. Changes in electrical voltage are transmitted through wires to a computer that displays this information graphically (see Figure 10.12). The electrical impulses normally move from the auditory nerve through the brainstem in approximately 10 milliseconds. The record of this electrical signal is known as the **auditory brainstem response**, or ABR. The ABR contains a number of peaks and valleys that occur at highly predictable intervals for individuals with normal hearing. However, when hearing is impaired, these peaks can be reduced in amplitude or delayed in time. As we will see in Chapter 12, the ABR can serve as a useful tool for detecting hearing loss that is caused by disruptions to the auditory nervous system.

Information about sound is transmitted through the auditory system to produce an awareness of sound (sensation), but the recognition and interpretation of that information (perception) requires that certain regions of the brain be intact. Much of what we know about the function of individual parts of the auditory nervous system comes from studying humans who have experienced damage to structures due to physical trauma or disease. Mr. Viner provides one such example.

Mr. Viner suffered a small stroke (blockage of blood flow within the brain). This damaged the tissue of the primary auditory cortex on the left side of his brain. However, the surrounding language areas within the left hemisphere were left intact. Because the auditory cortex in his right hemisphere was intact, he could still process sounds and his hearing was normal. Two years later, he suffered a second stroke, this time in the right hemisphere. It was much more extensive, damaging the primary auditory cortex and surrounding cortical regions. Suddenly, Mr. Viner's hearing changed drastically. He could detect when sounds occurred, but he could not "make sense" of them. His wife now had to write notes to communicate, because when she spoke he heard gibberish. In fact, his own speech sounded so abnormal to him, he soon stopped talking as well, resorting to the use of a writing pad to communicate with others.

In Mr. Viner's case, the blood supply to the auditory cortex was interrupted on both sides of the brain. When damage affects only one side, the patient may not experience a hearing loss and may reveal only subtle problems associated with understanding speech in noisy situations. If the auditory cortex is destroyed on both sides, then the patient may have a loss of hearing but will not be deaf. Rather, he or she may have difficulty finding the sources of sounds in space, understanding speech, and making sense of musical sequences. Damage to the auditory nervous system can be visualized using imaging techniques including computed tomography (CT) scans or magnetic resonance imaging (MRI) scans. As Figure 10.13 shows, brain scans can provide images of the auditory nervous system from the cochlea to the brain.

Imaging techniques are also routinely used to detect tumors that put pressure on the acoustic nerve. Damage to the auditory nerve will affect hearing in the ear served by that nerve. The amount of hearing loss due to damage to the nerve is not easy to predict. Persons with auditory nerve damage often have difficulty understanding speech, even more than what is predicted on the basis of their hearing loss for pure tones. In addition, they may not hear intense sounds with appropriate loudness. In contrast, persons who lose outer hair cells reveal a hearing loss and an abnormal growth of loudness when sounds become intense (meaning that sounds may suddenly become uncomfortably loud just a

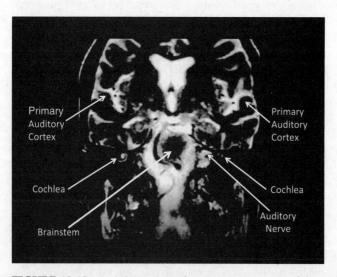

FIGURE 10.13   An MRI scan reveals various components of the auditory system.

few decibels above a level where the sound was comfortable). Reports of subtle symptoms by patients will help a clinician arrive at a clearer picture of the likely underlying causes of the individual's problems.

The auditory system is exquisitely designed to help us become aware of and to use the sounds that occur in our environment. The design enhances our ability to hear by virtue of three important features: (1) resonance properties of the outer ear, (2) transformer action of the middle ear, and (3) active amplification of the energy that arrives at the inner ear. All of the elements of the auditory system operate constantly, because we are never free of auditory stimulation. At a primitive level, the auditory system helps us to ward off danger and to find sources of survival. At a more advanced level, the auditory system connects us with the people in our world through speech, music, and other sounds that we associate with them. In a normally functioning auditory system, all components work together seamlessly. When audiologists screen hearing, they are looking at the integrated functioning of the entire system. Sound must be transmitted through the outer and middle ear, be amplified and transduced properly by the hair cells, and be encoded and transmitted via the auditory nerve. The nerve impulses are then perceived as sound in the central nervous system. When a person performs the simple act of raising a hand to indicate a tone was heard, the entire auditory system must be contributing.

Audiologists document the overall function of the auditory system with a variety of clinical tests. One of the most common is pure tone audiometry. As shown in Figure 10.14, this test involves presentation of sounds, usually through earphones or ear inserts, to one ear at a time and asking the listener to respond when a sound is detected. Almost all of us have experienced this procedure at some time in our lives since this type of test is widely used to screen hearing in schools. In a hearing screening, pure tones are presented at a single low level. To get a more detailed picture of hearing function, audiologists test for hearing thresholds, which are the lowest levels of sound at which a person reliably responds that he or she can hear the tone. These thresholds are then plotted on an audiogram (see Figure 10.14). The audiogram is a graph that plots hearing level (in decibels) against the frequency of the tone presented to the listener. The responses to sounds in the right ear each marked by a circle and an "X" is used to plot responses in the left ear. As shown in Figure 10.15, adults with normal hearing respond to pure tones between 0 and 25 dB HL in each ear. There may be minor variation between ears and to different pure tones, but normal responses fall within this range.

If there is a suspected problem preventing the normal transmission of sound, the audiologist will try to isolate the source of the problem. One approach is to determine whether the problem is occurring at the level of the middle ear or the cochlea. To do this, the audiologist will deliver sounds via a vibrator that rests on the mastoid bone behind the ear (see Figure 10.16). This bone conduction of sound bypasses the outer and middle ear to introduce sound into the cochlea through vibrations of the surrounding bone. When this method of sound presentation is used, additional symbols are used to plot the listener's response to sound (right and left brackets). In Chapters 11 and 12, we will see

A complete hearing test typically includes sounds presented via headphones (air conduction) and sounds presented through a bone vibrator (bone conduction).

Whereas air conduction tests the outer, middle, and inner components all at one time, bone conduction tests only the function of the inner ear.

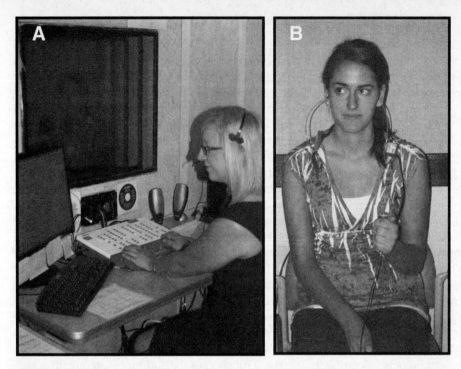

FIGURE 10.14 Pure tone audiometry is used to determine a listener's response to pure tones. (A) An audiologist presents tones to a listener (B) who is wearing ear inserts. The listener pushes a button when a tone is detected.

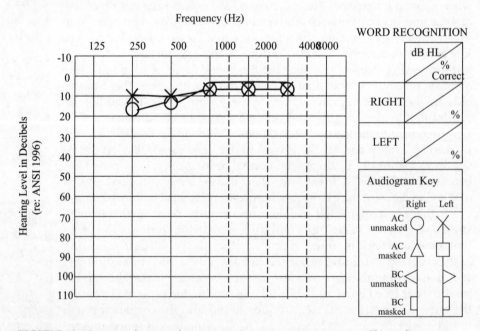

FIGURE 10.15 An audiogram plots a person's responses to pure tones. This audiogram is typical of those with normal hearing.

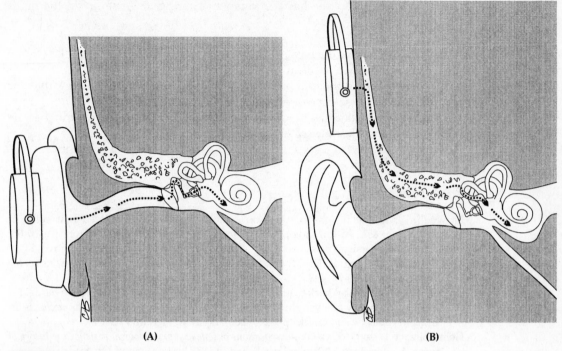

(A)   **(B)**

FIGURE 10.16   Two methods of sound delivery used to test hearing. (A) Sound is delivered from an earphone through the ear canal to the cochlea. (B) A vibrator resting on the mastoid bone delivers sound, which is conducted through the bone to the cochlea.

how pure-tone audiometry and other auditory assessments are instrumental in diagnosing hearing loss in children and adults.

The auditory system is uniquely designed to allow us to be aware of sounds, locate them, and recognize them. For most of us, hearing is the basis for our most important means of connecting with others: language. The auditory system's acoustical, physical, and psychological features are unique, sensitive, and structured to enhance our listening abilities. The most vital parts can be permanently injured by intense stimulation. Once gone, they cannot be repaired. The best hearing aids that we have today cannot restore normal quality to sound, though they provide remarkable assistance to persons with hearing impairments. The best action to take is to avoid situations that are dangerous to your hearing so that you can preserve the unique human link that is associated with the auditory system.

Clinical Problem Solving

Mr. Johnson is 65 years old and has worked for a road construction company for forty years. Although he has been using earplugs to protect his hearing for ten years, he did not think about protecting his hearing when he was much younger. Today, he has a permanent hearing loss, mainly in the high-frequency region.

1. What region of the basilar membrane (base, middle, apex) is likely to be damaged in Mr. Johnson's ears?
2. Which cells in the organ of Corti are likely to be affected by a forty-year history of noise exposure?
3. Give some examples of speech sounds that Mr. Johnson might not be able to recognize because of his hearing loss.

REFERENCES

Brownell, W. E. (1983). Observations on a motile response in isolated hair cells. In W. Webster & L. Aitkin (Eds.), *Mechanisms of hearing* (pp. 5–10). Clayton, Australia: Monash University Press.

Gold, T. (1948). Hearing: II. The physical axis of the action of the cochlea. *Proceedings of the Royal Society, 135,* 492–498.

Gold, T. (1989). Historical background to the proposal 40 years ago of an active model for cochlear frequency analysis. In J. P. Wilson & D. T. Kemp (Eds.), *Cochlear mechanisms: Structure, function and models* (pp. 299–306). London: Plenum Press.

Helmholtz, H. L. von (1954). *On the sensations of tone as a physiological basis for the theory of music.* A. Ellis, Trans. (Original published in 1885 by Longmans, Green).

Kemp, D. T. (1978). Stimulated acoustic emissions from within the human auditory system. *Journal of the Acoustical Society of America, 64,* 1386–1391.

Kiang, N. Y-S. (1975). Stimulus representation in the discharge patterns of auditory neurons. In D. B. Tower (Ed.), *The nervous system: Volume 3: Human communication and its disorders* (pp. 81–96). New York: Raven Press.

von Békésy, G. (1960). *Experiments in hearing.* New York: McGraw Hill.

CHAPTER 11

Disorders of Hearing in Children

James Dean

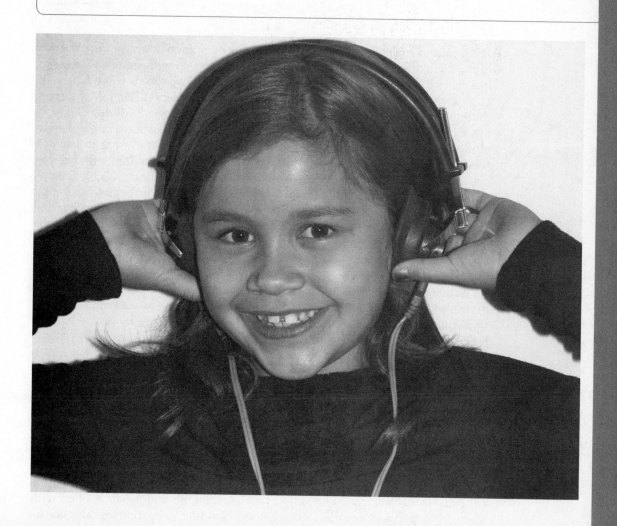

PREVIEW   The birth of a baby is a time of joy and the first wish of the parents is that their newborn child arrives healthy. This is indeed the case for most pregnancies and births, but between one and three of every 1000 newborns will have a permanent hearing loss. Hearing loss can be genetic in origin or caused by other factors like infection or toxins. When hearing loss is suspected, audiologists are called upon to document the type and severity of the loss, and to provide services related to amplification, education, and family support. Audiologists may work with a variety of other professionals to assure that the full range of medical, developmental, and communicative needs of each child are met.

Hearing Loss in Children

The prevalence of childhood hearing loss is more common that most people think. In the United States, approximately 33 babies are born with significant hearing loss every day (White, 1997). Overall, about 2 per 1000 newborns will have a mild or greater hearing loss in at least one ear (Morton & Nance, 2006). Many more children will experience a temporary hearing loss, particularly during the early years of life. In fact, roughly 80 percent of all children will experience some form of middle ear infection before age four. Hearing loss is not always an isolated condition, however; approximately one out of every three children with hearing loss has an additional disability (Gallaudet Research Institute, 2008). Ideally, intervention for hearing loss (known as audiologic habilitation) begins at a young age. In fact, habilitation programs for children born with permanent hearing loss often begin during the first six months of life. Intervention may involve the application of hearing technology such as hearing aids or cochlear implants, but also includes parent counseling, education, and behavioral treatment to support the development of communication skills.

When a hearing loss is first suspected, a pediatric audiologist is one of the first professionals to work with the child and family. Effective assessment and management of hearing loss in children involves knowledge of the biological basis of hearing (as discussed in Chapter 10), as well as knowledge of the types and causes of hearing loss, and what can be done to manage childhood hearing loss.

Types of Hearing Loss

For children, as well as adults, hearing loss arises from a number of different causes. A reduction in hearing acuity may result when sound is prevented from traveling through the ear canal and middle ear to the cochlea. This is referred to as **conductive hearing loss**. A conductive hearing loss can occur when the ear canal is blocked due to impacted wax or when the middle ear is filled with fluid rather than air (see otitis media, below). Conductive hearing loss also occurs when physical abnormalities affect the transduction of sound, as in the case of abnormal fusion of the bones of the middle ear or failed development of the ear canal. As we saw in Chapter 10, the structure of the outer and middle ear provides a boost of about 30–60 decibels to sounds before the signal reaches the inner ear. Without proper function of these structures, the intensity of sounds is reduced. The functional consequences of a conductive hearing loss range from difficulty hearing soft sounds to an inability to hear normal conversations. An example of an audiogram of a child with a conductive hearing loss is presented in Figure 11:1A. As shown, the child is not able to hear sounds presented by air conduction until they are 30–40 decibels or louder. However, the child is able to hear much softer sounds when the ear canal and middle ear are bypassed by presenting sound through bone vibration that directly stimulates the cochlea. In other words, the child's inner ear is working normally, but sound vibrations are not conducted properly through the outer and middle ear. This difference between hearing thresholds for air conduction and bone conduction, is referred to as an air-bone gap. This is the characteristic pattern with conductive hearing loss, where air conduction thresholds are worse than bone conduction.

Hearing loss can also result from damage to the cochlea or the auditory pathways that deliver the information from the cochlea to the brain. This is called **sensorineural hearing loss** because it involves the neural structures of this sensory system (see Chapter 10). The nature of the sensorineural hearing loss depends on the underlying cause (etiology). Losses may occur in one ear only (unilateral), or both ears may be affected (bilateral). Children with sensorineural loss may hear some sound frequencies relatively well and others less well (see Figure 11.1B). They may also have somewhat different levels of hearing loss in each ear. The severity of the sensorineural hearing loss can range from very mild, where there is difficulty hearing soft sounds only, to total deafness.

A child can have both a conductive and a sensorineural hearing loss at the same time. This combination is referred to as **mixed hearing loss**. The audiogram in this case shows that hearing via bone conduction is better than air conduction (an air-bone gap), but the bone conduction thresholds are not within the normal hearing range. In other words, there is both a conductive and sensorineural component to the hearing loss. An example of a mixed hearing loss is displayed in Figure 11.1C.

As with other physical conditions, hearing loss may be present at birth (**congenital**) or it may be develop after birth (**acquired**). More specifically, childhood hearing loss may be the result of something that happened during prenatal development, around the time of birth (perinatal), or acquired after birth (postnatal). Some acquired hearing losses are the result of something that happened during pregnancy or at the time birth but the effects on hearing are delayed, or late in onset.

Childhood hearing loss can be permanent or temporary depending on the cause and the location of the problem within the peripheral or

When testing the hearing of someone with a sensorineural hearing loss, his or her ability to hear pure tones is about the same whether the sounds are presented via earphones or a bone conductor. Why is this true?

Prenatal: the time period before birth (during embryonic and fetal development).
Perinatal: the time shortly before and right after birth (sometimes defined as the interval between the 28th week of pregnancy to a week after delivery).
Postnatal: more than a week after birth.

(A) Conductive Hearing Loss

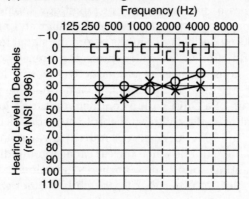
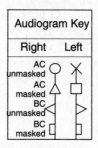

(B) Sensorineural Hearing Loss

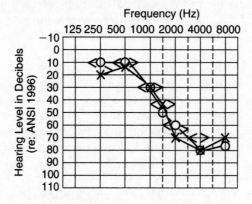
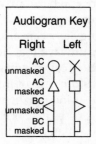

(C) Mixed Hearing Loss

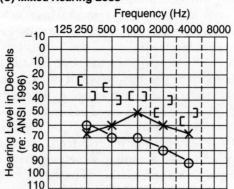
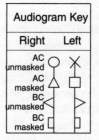

FIGURE 11.1 Examples of audiograms associated with (A) conductive, (B) sensorineural, and (C) mixed hearing loss. Note that in both the conductive and mixed loss types, bone conduction results indicate better hearing than does air conduction. For sensorineural loss, bone conduction results are the same as air conduction results.

central auditory system. Temporary hearing losses occur in children more frequently than permanent hearing loss, and are often associated with transient infections of the middle ear.

Etiology of Hearing Loss

There are a number of genetic and nongenetic factors that can ultimately impact the hearing status of newborns (see Figure 11.2). It is estimated that approximately 50–60 percent of all hearing loss that is congenital, or emerges within the first year, is genetic in origin. In some cases of genetic hearing loss, one or both of the child's parents also have a genetic hearing loss. However, approximately 90 percent of newborns with hearing loss have parents with normal hearing. So, even when a hearing loss is genetic in origin, there may not be other family members with hearing loss. Nongenetic causes of hearing loss make up the remaining 40–50 percent of cases of hearing loss. Some nongenetic hearing losses result from maternal health conditions and infections during pregnancy, and are classified as *environmental,* because the cause is rooted in conditions found in the child's prenatal environment. When the cause of hearing loss is unknown it is called **idiopathic**. We will explore each of these types of hearing loss below.

Genetic Hearing Loss

In most cases of genetic hearing loss, the trait for hearing loss is inherited from the biologic parents. There are also occasions when a spontaneous gene mutation during early pregnancy changes hereditary information encoded by the

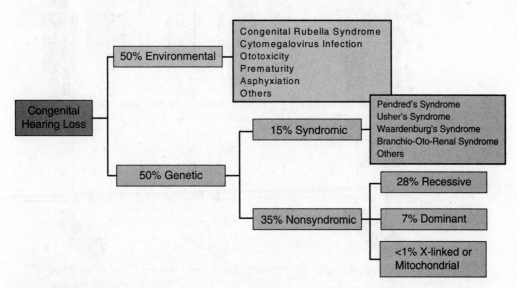

FIGURE 11.2 Environment and genetic contributions to total congenital hearing loss. (prevalence data based on Smith et al., 2005).

developing baby's genes. Chromosome deletions or additions that cause congenital hearing loss can also occur very early in embryonic development. Trisomy 21, which is associated with Down syndrome, is an example of an additional chromosome involving the 21st pair. As we saw in Chapter 2 and 10, trisomy 21, can cause hearing loss along with other congenital anomalies. In most instances, genetically related hearing loss is present at birth, but some types have a delayed onset.

In most cases of inherited hearing loss, both parents have normal hearing, but carry an altered gene that can cause hearing loss. When a child is conceived, each parent passes along one copy of each of their paired **autosomal** chromosomes and one of their two sex chromosomes (the X and Y chromosomes). When each parent carries one altered hearing gene and one normal hearing gene there is a 1 in 4 (25 percent) chance of both parents passing on an altered hearing gene for each pregnancy. When only one parent passes on a gene associated with hearing loss, this one gene is not sufficient to effect hearing. In this case, the offspring will not have a hearing loss, but will be a **carrier** of the hearing loss gene. When both parents pass on the same gene for hearing loss, these two genes acting together result in hearing loss. This type of inheritance pattern is called **autosomal recessive** (see Figure 11.3). Approximately 75–80 percent of all genetic hearing loss is autosomal recessive (Van Camp et al., 1997).

> Many parents are surprised when their child is born with a genetic hearing loss. Why would that be so?

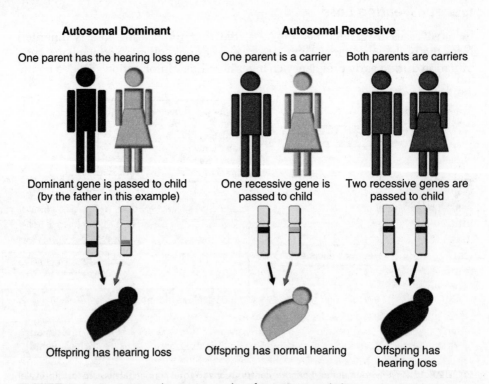

FIGURE 11.3 Dominant and recessive modes of genetic transmission.

Approximately 10–15 percent of all genetic hearing loss is the result of an **autosomal dominant** pattern of inheritance (Van Camp et al., 1997). In this case, only one parent has to pass on an altered gene for hearing to be impaired because it's function is "stronger" than the standard version of the gene, and thus it's action "dominates" in the development of the child. When one parent carries a dominant gene for hearing loss, there is a 1 in 2 (50 percent) chance of each offspring having hearing loss. Other forms of genetic hearing loss include sex-linked (linked to the X or Y chromosome) and mitochondrial (caused by mutation of genes found within the mitochondria of cell bodies), but autosomal dominant and autosomal recessive are the primary genetic forms of hearing loss.

Approximately 30 percent of genetic hearing loss is *syndromic,* meaning that it is one of several signs that occur together. Syndromic hearing loss can be autosomal recessive or autosomal dominant in origin. The syndrome may include additional developmental disabilities that can affect the ability of a child to adapt to or compensate for their hearing loss (Morton & Nance, 2006). Fragile X syndrome is an example of an inherited genetic syndrome that may include hearing loss, along with intellectual and developmental disability that affects speech and language development. Fragile X syndrome is also known to be a genetic cause of autism spectrum disorder. In some types of syndromic hearing loss, the presence of multiple observable physical anomalies and health problems leads to identification of the syndrome at birth. For example, infants with branchio-oto-renal (BOR) syndrome are born with malformations of the neck (brachio), ear (oto) and kidney (renal). When these physical features occur together, the child should be checked for both conductive and sensorineural hearing loss, which is also associated with this syndrome. Syndromic conditions present a challenge to the child and the family as there are interactive and synergistic effects of the multiple disabilities on development. Intervention requires coordination of prolonged, sometimes life-long interdisciplinary assessment and treatment that typically involves an audiologist and speech-language pathologist.

The majority of genetic childhood hearing losses are *non-syndromic* (about 70 percent), meaning there are no additional related anomalies. Non-syndromic hearing losses are typically sensorineural and usually result from autosomal recessive transmission (Van Camp et al., 1997). In cases of non-syndromic hearing loss, the child's appearance may be unremarkable and hearing loss may not be initially suspected. When the hearing loss is missed, delays in speech and language development are likely to occur. Early identification and management of hearing loss is important to help prevent or minimize adverse effects on communication development. Let us consider one case of a child who was born with a congenital hearing loss.

Tilly was born at 40 weeks gestational age. There had been no complications during pregnancy and delivery was noneventful. Tilly was very healthy at birth and there were no obvious physical anomalies. Prior to discharge from the hospital, Tilly had failed two hearing screenings and received a "refer" notation for each ear at both screenings. The parents were advised to have Tilly evaluated by a pediatric audiologist. But after the parents brought her home, Tilly was an active, happy child and they thought she seemed to hear everything going on in the house. There was no history of hearing loss on either side of the parent's family, so the parents concluded that the hearing screening tests had not been accurate.

During a six-month check-up, Tilly's pediatrician reviewed her medical chart and asked the parents if Tilly had seen an audiologist as recommended on discharge from the hospital. The parents explained that they had not, and a referral was made to the community speech and hearing clinic. At the time of the evaluation, a pediatric audiologist did a number of audiologic tests and determined that it was likely that Tilly had a moderate sensorineural hearing loss. The audiologists contacted Tilly's pediatrician and they collaborated to arrange an auditory brainstem response (ABR) test at the regional medical center (see Chapter 10 for explanation of ABR). The ABR test was conducted using a range of sound frequencies, and a moderate sensorineural hearing loss was confirmed bilaterally. Tilly was referred to an ear, nose, and throat specialist who could not find any obvious physical cause for the hearing loss. Genetic testing was done and the etiology of hearing loss was determined to be a genetic, non-syndromic hearing loss called Connexin 26 (CX26). This gene is the most frequent cause of genetic hearing loss (Nance & Kearsey, 2004). Because Connexin 26 is transmitted in an autosomal recessive mode, it is not surprising that Tilly had no other relatives with a hearing loss.

Nongenetic Hearing Loss

Maternal health conditions and prenatal care are key factors influencing the health of a newborn. Medical care during pregnancy enhances *protective factors* and minimizes *risk factors* for congenital birth defects that affect the development of the fetus. Nongenetic, pre-natal risk factors are referred to as environmental or **exogenous** factors because they originate apart from the infant's biological constitution.

Some of the exogenous effects are relatively common conditions experienced by the mother during pregnancy. For example, about 2–4 percent of women experience gestational diabetes mellitus during pregnancy (Braun, Huebschmann, Kim, Lezotte, Shupe, & Dabelea, 2011. In this condition, women develop high blood sugar during their pregnancy, which leads to a number of complications, including a higher risk for delivery complications or illness in the newborn. Many of these conditions can be avoided or treated with good prenatal care. Prompt attention to these conditions can often prevent problems from becoming serious and affecting the developing fetus. Other health conditions can become quite serious for both mother and baby, even with ongoing medical care.

Carla had been pregnant for 25 weeks when she went to her doctor for routine prenatal care. She had been gaining more weight than expected for her time of pregnancy and her hands and feet were a bit swollen. Otherwise, she felt fine. Her doctor, however, was concerned about her blood pressure, which was elevated. This increased her risk for preeclampsia, a condition in which **hypertension** occurs during pregnancy. The doctor scheduled additional visits for Carla, during which the high blood pressure could be monitored. By Carla's next visit, her blood pressure was further elevated and the swelling in her feet and hands had not resolved, indicating preeclampsia. This is a potentially serious condition for both mother and child and can result in premature birth. Carla was also starting to feel ill, with headaches, nausea, and occasional blurry vision. She was put on bed rest and given medication to try to control her high blood pressure. Unfortunately, Carla's preeclampsia continued to worsen, and there was concern for the baby's development. The decision was made to deliver Carla's baby by Cesarean section. Little Theresa Marie was born over six weeks early (at 34 weeks gestation) and weighed 4 pounds, 7 ounces. Among the concerns raised due to her prematurity was the status of her hearing.

Most infants are born at around 40 weeks' gestation. Those born before 37 weeks are considered premature. Prematurity can be caused by a host of factors, some of which can increase the child's risk for health and developmental problems, including hearing loss. Advances in medicine have been associated with improved survival of infants at very young gestational ages and low birth weights. Small and fragile premature babies are inherently at risk because their bodies have not yet developed to a point where they can survive on their own. Birth weight, in particular, is a strong predictor of outcome. For example, a child born at 30 weeks weighing 5 pounds has a better prognosis than one born at 30 weeks weighing 3 pounds. Premature infants are critically ill because they have trouble breathing and swallowing, and they are extremely susceptible to infections. They are typically cared for in a Neonatal Intensive Care Unit (NICU), where they can receive prolonged highly skilled medical care.

> Full-term babies are born after about 40 weeks gestation. Babies born before 37 weeks are considered premature, and are at increased risk for hearing impairment.

Theresa Marie, born at 34 weeks gestational age, was admitted to the Neonatal Intensive Care Unit (NICU) at a medical center because of difficulty with breathing and swallowing. In the NICU she was placed in an incubator bassinet and attached to monitors that measure heartbeat, blood pressure, breathing, and blood oxygen levels. Nurses watched for signs of additional complications, like infection or respiratory distress syndrome. Her bassinet also had overhead warming lights to keep her body temperature stable. There was also an ultraviolet "bilirubin light" to prevent jaundice. Jaundice occurs by a buildup of bilirubin, a yellow chemical that carries oxygen in the blood. Infants with jaundice have a yellow cast to their skin and the whites of their eyes (the sclera). Bilirubin can be toxic, and serious jaundice (hyperbilirubinemia) can lead to hearing loss and other physical complications. Extreme hyperbilirubinemia (kernicterus) can also cause brain damage.

Carla and her husband visited Theresa in the NICU. At first, they were only able to touch her through openings in the incubator, but after two weeks they were able to cuddle and feed her. A week later Theresa was well enough to go home. Just prior to her discharge, a newborn hearing screening was done by a nursing staff member trained to perform the procedure. Theresa received a "pass" on both ears from this screening. The discharge nurse explained the screening results to Theresa's parents. She also advised them to contact Theresa's primary care physician if they had any concerns about her responses to sound at home.

A baby's hearing can also be affected by environmental agents that disturb the development of the embryo or fetus. Such nongenetic factors are referred to as **teratogens**. Examples include toxins, chemicals, radiation, and maternal infections. Teratogenic factors can cause multiple developmental malformations. Therefore, when infants are exposed to teratogens, hearing loss is not the only disability that may arise. The effects of teratogenic exposure will vary with the dose and the time during fetal development when the exposure occurred. Many disabilities caused by teratogens are preventable. For example, Fetal Alcohol Spectrum Disorders (FASD) involve a collection of cognitive and physical signs that can include intellectual disability, poor coordination, dysmorphic facial features, limb and joint abnormalities, and heart defects. The signs of this disorder may be subtle or prominent depending upon the amount and timing of the alcohol exposure and the infant's susceptibility to its toxic effects. Prenatally exposed infants may also experience hearing loss (Cohen-Karem, Bar-Oz, Nulman, Papaioanou, & Koren, 2007). The dysmorphic facial features associated with Fetal Alcohol Syndrome Disorder also increase susceptibility to middle ear infections because of Eustachian tube dysfunction (see Chapter 10). As the name suggests, fetal alcohol exposure is an entirely preventable developmental disorder. Exposure to other ingested or environmental toxins, like heavy metals, solvents, illegal drugs, and tobacco can also affect fetal development, including the development of the auditory system.

Infectious diseases can also function as teratogens. In some cases, the mother may be infected during pregnancy and the infection crosses the placenta to infect the fetus. In other cases, the newborn is exposed to infection during delivery or after birth. A collection of parasitic, bacterial, and viral infections associated with hearing loss are collectively referred to by the acronym TORCH. The TORCH infections include Toxoplasmosis, "Other" (hepatitis B, syphilis, Varicella-Zoster virus, HIV, and parovirus B19), Rubella, Cytomegalovirus, and Herpes simplex. All of these conditions can cause sensorineural hearing loss; however, there is not a simple relationship between the occurrence of TORCH infections and hearing loss. The degree of hearing loss can vary widely among those infected. The onset of hearing loss may be delayed past the time when the infection is present. Cytomegalovirus is an example of an infection that may cause delayed-onset hearing loss. In cases of late-onset hearing loss, a newborn passes a hearing screening prior to their discharge from the hospital and the parents will not suspect that a hearing loss caused by a prenatal or perinatal infection is developing.

Sometimes, hearing loss can be the consequence of the treatment a child needs to survive a serious health condition. These forms of hearing loss are referred to as **iatrogenic**, because they are caused inadvertently through medical care and intervention. Consider the following case:

> *Peyton* was a 7-year-old boy diagnosed with a very adult disease: cancer. Fortunately, his bone cancer was diagnosed relatively early. However, he underwent aggressive chemotherapy to assure that the cancer was eliminated. This left him a bit shorter than the other kids in his class. However, his parents considered this a good trade-off for being cancer-free five years later. Peyton's parents were

surprised when he failed a school hearing screening at age 13. The school audiologist obtained a medical case history from the parents as part of her follow-up procedures for children who fail the screening. She recognized that some forms of chemotherapy could lead to hearing loss in cancer survivors, and suspected this was the case for Peyton. She confirmed a bilateral sensorineural hearing loss that ranged from mild to moderate.

Certain forms of chemotherapy can lead to hearing loss in children years after the treatment has occurred (Gorin & McAuliffe, 2009; Whelan, Stratton, Kawashima, et al., 2011). Drugs administered to treat severe bacterial infections can also lead to hearing loss. For example, a class of drugs known as aminoglycosides is used to treat severe infections. These drugs can be **ototoxic**, leaving the patient with sensorineural hearing loss, and they may also be **vestibulotoxic**, compromising vestibular function and causing balance problems (Guthrie, 2008). Physicians prescribing such drugs collaborate with pharmacists and clinical pathologist to balance the risk of negative side effects like hearing loss against the danger of the infection to the life of the patient. In some cases, like Peyton's, the choice is clear between life and hearing loss.

Middle Ear Infections (Otitis Media)

One of the most common childhood illnesses is a middle ear infection, or otitis media. In fact, otitis media is the most common cause for children visiting a pediatrician (Stool, Berman, Carney, et al., 1994). The term *otitis media* literally refers to the inflammation of the middle ear space, which usually results from an upper respiratory infection. The inflammation causes a fluid buildup behind the eardrum, which restricts eardrum mobility and can cause a conductive hearing loss. Upwards of 80 percent of all children will experience some form of otitis media before age four and rates of otitis media decline after that age (Zielhuis, Rach, & van den Broek, 1989). In many cases, parents may be unaware that their child is having an active bout of otitis media because there may be no clear sign of pain or hearing loss. In other cases of acute otitis media a child's behavior clearly signals that something is wrong, prompting a visit to the pediatrician.

Olivia was normally an active 2-year-old. Over the past day, she seemed more content to sit with her toys than to run around after her 4-year-old brother. When her mother picked her up from daycare, Olivia was crying and the daycare provider reported that she had been cranky all day. Olivia's mother noticed that she was pulling at her right ear. Her mother recognized this as a telltale sign of an ear infection. Olivia had been having recurrent middle ear infections since she was born. At a visit to the pediatrician the following day, an otoscopic exam revealed inflammation of the tympanic membrane and surrounding tissue. Furthermore, the eardrum was red and bulging outwards, indicating that there was a buildup of fluid within the middle ear.

In Olivia's case, the infection was visually obvious with an otoscopic examination. When this is not the case, tympanometry can be a more effective means of diagnosing middle ear pathology, including otitis media (see Chapter 10). Tympanometry measures the mobility of the eardrum and provides evidence of negative pressure or fluid in the middle ear.

Otitis media can occur with or without fluid in the ear. When fluid is present, the condition is referred to as otitis media with effusion. Infants and young children are more prone to developing fluid in the middle ear cavity because the Eustachian tube does not yet effectively drain fluid that builds up in the middle ear cavity. As the child develops, physical changes to the size and angle of the Eustachian tubes will reduce these episodes. Some children are prescribed antibiotics for otitis media. However, Olivia's pediatrician was reluctant to do this because recent research had shown that drugs seem to make little difference in the overall duration of an otitis media episode (Coker, Chan, Newberry, Limbos, Suttorp, Shekelle, & Takata, 2010). If Olivia's bouts increase in frequency, duration, or her level of discomfort increases, the physician may refer her to an otolaryngologist for surgical treatment. This involves inserting a small tube through the tympanic membrane, which allow fluid in the middle ear cavity to drain out through the external ear canal. The tubes also serve to equalize the air pressure between the middle ear and the ear canal, so the tubes are referred to as pressure equalization tubes, or PE tubes.

Otitis media may cause hearing loss that ranges from mild to moderate in severity. The hearing loss is usually temporary, and hearing returns once the infection has cleared. Professionals have been concerned that the presence of fluctuating hearing loss from recurrent otitis media over prolonged periods of time may cause problems for development of auditory, speech, and language skills. However, the scientific studies on the effects of otitis media are largely equivocal regarding its long-term effects on development. Some researchers have found that children's auditory attention may be negatively affected (Asbjørnsen, Obrzut, Boliek, et al., 2005), while other studies show no effect (Arcia & Roberts, 1993). Language development can be affected, but the degree of the effect is quite small and probably not clinically important (Butler, van der Linden, MacMillan, & van der Wouden, 2003; Casby, 2001). Whether a child experiences negative effects from otitis media can be influenced by factors other than the associated hearing loss. For example, attending daycare tends to increase the number of otitis media bouts a child experiences, raising the risk of a negative effect on language development. However, attending a good-quality daycare increases the probability of good language development (Creps & Vernon-Feagans, 2000), which can overcome any detrimental effect of increased bouts of otitis media. Finally, not all otitis media episodes result in significant hearing loss, which is the primary factor thought to be important to speech, language, and academic outcomes. In sum, there is little concern that otitis media itself produces lasting negative effects for children who have no other risk factors for speech, language, or other developmental disorders (Roberts, Hunger, Gravel, et al., 2004).

> For Olivia, the physician's strategy was to wait out this episode of otitis media. She continued with daycare, but her parents began limiting other conditions that raise the likelihood of repeated infections. For example, they limited Olivia's visits to her cousin's house, where both parents smoke. Second-hand smoke raises the risk of

additional infections. The cousins now come to Olivia's house for play dates. Her parents are remaining vigilant and are willing to consider tubes if the frequency of these episodes or their severity increases. Given Olivia's history of recurrent ear infections, the pediatrician recommended that Olivia return for a follow-up visit in four weeks or sooner if she complained of ear pain.

Long-Term Outcomes

The long-term effects of childhood hearing loss vary among individuals and are influenced by a number of factors (see Table 11.1). We will discuss each of these separately, but it is important to appreciate that each factor can influence the effect of others. For example, if time of onset of the hearing loss is at birth, but the child is not identified right away, the impact of the loss will be more significant than if the time of onset was late in childhood (after the child has learned to speak) and the hearing loss was detected right away.

Severity of Hearing Loss

The effect of a hearing loss on speech audibility and clarity varies with the severity of hearing loss. In Figure 11.4, we see categories of hearing loss superimposed on an audiogram. These categories reflect the lowest levels of sound intensity, in decibels, that can be heard. We can also consider the categories relative to what types of sounds can be heard. In Figure 11.5, we see the frequency of occurrence of the different degrees of hearing loss. As Table 11.2 illustrates, individuals with mild loss may be able to hear some speech sounds in normal conversation. However, those with a moderate hearing loss may not be able to make out words when speaking with another person in a normal conversational tone of voice. A child with moderate hearing loss may miss other types of auditory information in the environment as well. For example, the family cat's meow might not be heard. With increasing severity, not only will speech sounds be missed, but many environmental sounds will not be heard. Children with profound losses may not hear the school bell ring or a car horn warning them not to cross the street. Thus, the hearing loss not only affects interpersonal communication, but also the child's ability to interact with the world.

TABLE 11.1   Factors that Affect the Long-term Impact of Childhood Hearing Loss

- Severity of hearing loss
- Time of onset
- Etiology and type of hearing loss
- Age of identification and intervention
- Presence of additional disabilities and general health
- Environmental factors such as:
  - Family nurturing of auditory, speech, language, and learning skills.
  - Access to medical and professional services
  - Availability of appropriate technology

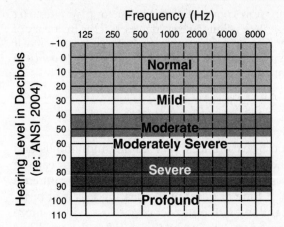

FIGURE 11.4   Classifications of hearing loss by degree as measured by pure tone hearing testing.

TABLE 11.2   The Effects of Hearing Loss

Mild	May hear some speech sounds, but low-intensity sounds are hard to hear.
Moderate	May hear little conversational speech produced at normal loudness levels.
Severe	Will hear essentially no conversational speech, but will hear some loud sounds.
Profound	Will not hear any speech, and only very loud environmental sounds.

Time of Onset

The time of onset is a critical consideration when planning for auditory, speech, and language intervention and educational needs. When a child is born with a significant hearing loss, there may be difficulty developing spoken language in the manner typical of hearing children. Such children benefit from early intervention designed to support the development of communication skills. In contrast, a child who loses hearing after language is well developed can use the already developed skills to mitigate the effects of hearing loss. Therefore, the needs of children with hearing loss present at birth differ considerably from those children who have well-established spoken language.

Etiology and Type of Loss

The etiology of the hearing loss can influence other factors, like the time of onset, and the degree of loss. For example, hearing loss associated with otitis media is conductive and typically results in temporary and relatively mild hearing loss. In contrast, hearing loss associated with the Connexin 26 gene is sensorineural, permanent, and typically more severe than that occurring with

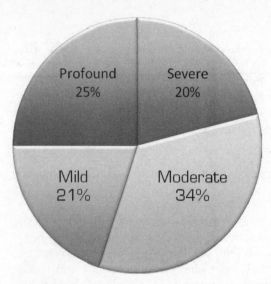

FIGURE 11.5 Distribution of hearing loss by severity.

otitis media. All these factors make a hearing loss linked to Connexin 26 more significant in terms of long-term effects on childhood development.

Age of Identification and Intervention

In 1988, the average age at which children with congenital hearing loss were identified in the United States was 2½ to 3 years of age, and many children were not identified until 5 or 6 years of age (Schow & Nerbonne 2007). With the spread of early hearing detection and intervention (EHDI) programs throughout the United States, the average age at which hearing loss was identified in 2003 had dropped to 2–3 months of age (Harrison, Roush, & Wallace, 2003). The intent of EHDI programs is to identify hearing loss and to facilitate early intervention. The best outcome for children with congenital hearing loss occurs when intervention begins in the first 6 months of life. (Yoshinago-Itano, Sedey, Couler, & Mehl, 1998). We will explore hearing habilitation later in this chapter.

Presence of Additional Disabilities and General Health

Whereas some children experience hearing loss with no other complicating factors, other children have hearing loss as part of a syndrome that may include blindness, physical disability, or intellectual impairment. These children will require more extensive support to maximize their developmental potential, and when the handicapping conditions are severe, they may need lifelong assistance. Overall general health is a factor as well, in that children who experience both hearing loss and ongoing illness may be physically less able to benefit from early intervention programs. Even a child's general health through adolescence can affect long-term outcomes.

Environmental Factors

It is important to note that factors inherent to the child and the nature of the hearing loss are not the only determinants of the long-term effect of hearing loss. We know, for example, that parental engagement is a strong predictor of the success of early intervention programs for children with hearing loss (Moeller, 2000). Furthermore, when a family has access to medical and audiologic services, and a means to pay for these services (through insurance, government assistance, or out-of-pocket), then the child is more likely to have a more positive long-term outcome.

Hearing Assessment

The severity and type of hearing loss is determined through a battery of age-appropriate audiologic tests. An audiogram provides a graphic display of hearing thresholds, and thus indicates the severity of hearing loss. The type of hearing loss is related to the part of the ear that is not functioning normally, and audiologic tests provide information that helps to determine the underlying cause.

Newborn Hearing Screening and Early Hearing Detection and Intervention

In 1993, the United States' National Institutes of Health (NIH) recommended that hearing screening be conducted on all newborn children prior to hospital

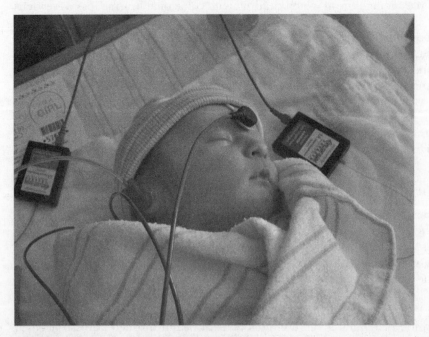

FIGURE 11.6 An infant wears a suction-cup-style earphone during her newborn hearing screening procedure.

discharge (Figure 11.6) Widespread support for this recommendation was prompted by the growing documentation that hearing loss can cause delays in development, and that the identification and intervention for hearing loss in the first six months can reduce language delay (Yoshinago-Itano et al., 1998). Over the ensuing years, the number of newborn hearing screening programs has expanded to include all fifty states and U.S. territories. Recent estimates indicate that approximately 96 percent of all newborns in the United States have a hearing screening before discharge from the hospital. The benefits of newborn screening have become well accepted by the medical and allied health professional communities, as asserted by the U.S. Preventative Services Task Force (2008): "There is good evidence that newborn hearing screening testing is highly accurate and leads to earlier identification and treatment of infants with hearing loss."

Newborn hearing screening programs are part of the National Institutes of Health *Early Hearing Detection and Intervention* program. The goal is to ensure that hearing loss is identified in newborns before discharge from the hospital, and that follow-up medical and audiologic services are provided in a timely manner. The National Institutes of Health has specific goals for early hearing detection and intervention that should occur at one month, three months, and six months, referred to as the 1-3-6 plan.

> A 1-3-6 plan stands for administration of a hearing screening by 1 month of age, confirmation of hearing loss by 3 months of age, and early intervention by 6 months of age.

- Newborn hearing screening using physiologic measures is administered no later than 1 month of age.
- All newborns and infants who do not pass the initial screening are rescreened and should have confirmatory audiologic and medical evaluations no later than 3 months of age.
- All infants with confirmed permanent hearing loss should receive early intervention as soon as possible, no later than 6 months of age.

Federal support for the coordination and funding of statewide newborn hearing screening programs began with congressional passage of the Newborn and Infant Hearing Screening and Intervention Act of 1999. Federal support for statewide early hearing detection and intervention programs is currently provided by P.L. 111-337, *The Early Hearing Detection and Intervention Act (EHDI) of 2010*. Early Hearing Detection and Intervention programs are managed by state agencies that provide annual statistical reports on their programs to the national Centers for Disease Control and Prevention. The mission of this program is to assure that all fifty states and U.S. territories track early hearing detection and intervention programs and ensure that children with hearing loss develop appropriate communication and social skills.

Audiologic Assessment

Infants who do not pass a newborn hearing screening, and those who are known to have risk factors for hearing loss are referred to an audiologist for a comprehensive audiologic evaluation. Children who do not achieve age-appropriate milestones for auditory, speech, and language skills, or show signs of hearing difficulty, are also referred to an audiologist to determine whether hearing loss

TABLE 11.3   Common Signs of Hearing Loss in Children

- No response when called
- Inconsistent response to sound
- Delayed speech and language development
- Unclear speech
- Misunderstanding or not following directions
- Frequent requests for clarification (e.g., saying "huh" and "what")
- Sound turned up on electronic equipment (radio, TV, CD, or mpeg player)

is a significant factor in developmental delay. Some of the common behavioral signs of hearing loss are presented in Table 11.3.

Infants and children suspected of hearing loss may undergo a comprehensive pediatric audiologic assessment. This assessment has multiple goals and may require several visits before a complete diagnosis and plan of intervention can be made. The first goal of a pediatric audiologic assessment is to determine whether a hearing loss is present in one or both ears, and to quantify the degree of hearing loss for each ear. Testing should determine whether the hearing loss is conductive, sensorineural, or mixed in nature. This determination also serves to identify which components of the hearing system are implicated. Periodic reevaluations may be needed to determine whether a hearing loss is stable or is changing over time. The procedures used to meet these goals include the case history, observation of infant/child physical features and behavior, physiologic tests, electrophysiologic tests and behavioral tests.

Case History.   A pediatric case history is typically obtained through a medical chart review and interview of the parent or primary care provider. A good case history should reveal any risks for childhood hearing loss and any signs of hearing loss or developmental delay that the caregivers have observed. Areas covered include medical, neurological, physical, cognitive (intellectual), and sensory functioning. Additional information regarding the daily activities of a child and their daily listening demands should also be obtained. It is important to note that diagnostic audiologic testing should always proceed in the context of a complete case history.

Direct Observation.   Observation of infant and child behavior can be initiated while the family is in the waiting area, with additional observations made throughout the evaluation. With toddlers and children, the observation of "functional behavior" as they play with toys and interact with caregivers provides valuable insight into their auditory, speech, and language skills, as well as information regarding vision and the development of gross and fine motor skills. Such information is important for the selection of developmentally appropriate tests to be used during the formal hearing evaluation.

Observation of physical features is also an important pre-test procedure. Craniofacial and other physical anomalies, such as fused fingers (syndactyly) may be signs of a syndromic hearing loss. An otoscopic inspection of the outer ear, ear canal, and tympanic membrane allows the audiologist to determine factors that may cause a hearing loss. The otoscopic inspection could reveal conditions such as the absence or complete closure of the ear canal (atresia), excess cerumen, red and inflamed tympanic membranes, and tympanic membrane perforations. These conditions require medical treatment and can cause a conductive-type hearing loss.

The Audiologic Test Battery

After completing the case history and observation procedures, the audiologist decides which tests and procedures will be used to evaluate the structure and function of the auditory system from the outer ear to the brain. When selecting tests, the audiologist must consider the child's chronologic age, developmental age, general health, and whether other disabilities are present. An individualized test battery is designed to best meet the diagnostic needs of the child, and may include physiologic and behavioral procedures (see Figure 11.7). The goal is to obtain information regarding different parts of the ear to determine the degree and type of hearing loss and the probable **site of lesion**. It is only through a comparison and "cross check" of test results that site of lesion can be identified. There is no one procedure for testing hearing that is appropriate for all individuals, and the audiologist must be prepared to modify test procedures as necessary. This is particularly true when evaluating children with developmental disabilities.

> The test battery can be thought of as the audiologist's tool kit, used to obtain information about different parts of the ear.

Physiologic Test Procedures. Physiologic tests use sound to trigger a biophysical response that can be measured without active participation by the individual being tested. These procedures are particularly important when evaluating infants, young children, and those with multiple disabilities who are not able to respond behaviorally during testing. The measured responses are compared to normative data. The use of methods that have been shown to produce meaningful and reproducible results in carefully controlled research studies is known as **evidence-based practice**, which is the goal for clinical practice in both audiology and speech-language pathology.

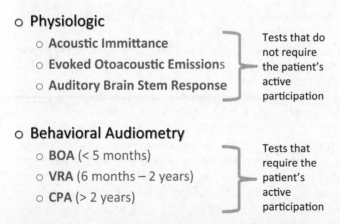

o **Physiologic**
 o **Acoustic Immittance**
 o **Evoked Otoacoustic Emissions**   Tests that do not require the patient's active participation
 o **Auditory Brain Stem Response**

o **Behavioral Audiometry**
 o **BOA** (< 5 months)
 o **VRA** (6 months – 2 years)   Tests that require the patient's active participation
 o **CPA** (> 2 years)

FIGURE 11.7 Classes of diagnostic assessment procedures.

Middle ear function is evaluated using acoustic immittance tests that include **tympanometry** and tests of the **middle ear muscle reflex** as introduced in Chapter 10. Tympanometry is a minimally invasive procedure that helps to identify tympanic membrane abnormalities and to provide information regarding the status of the middle ear. Tympanometry is frequently used to detect such common pediatric conditions such as middle fluid associated with otitis media or the presence of excessive negative air pressure associated with Eustachian tube dysfunction. These conditions and physical anomalies of the middle ear can cause conductive hearing loss.

An assessment of the middle ear muscle reflex is typically performed along with tympanometry. The procedure requires the individual to be quiet and still for a minute or so for each ear. Recall from Chapter 10 that the middle ear muscle reflex arc includes the afferent auditory nerve (cranial nerve VIII) and efferent facial nerves (cranial nerves V and VII). This means that middle ear muscle testing provides information on the function of the auditory neural connections and can be used to detect problems in the neural transmission of information from the inner ear to the brainstem. Abnormal nerve function can cause varying degrees of hearing loss and difficulties in speech perception, even if the middle ear and inner ear are functioning normally.

Evoked otoacoustic emissions (EOAE) tests are another type of physiologic measure that provides information about the status of the inner ear. In Chapter 10, we learned that acoustic emissions are absent if outer hair cells are missing or damaged. We also learned that the inner hair cells (the sensory cells) do not function normally when the outer hair cells are damaged. Therefore, if otoacoustic emissions are absent and the middle ear and outer ear are normal, then there is high probability of a hearing loss of cochlear origin. Otoacoustic emissions test results do not provide information regarding the degree of hearing loss, but they have excellent clinical application when working with infants and children because the absence of emissions alerts the audiologist to the high likelihood of a sensorineural hearing loss. Otoacoustic emissions testing requires the infant or child be calm and quiet, and this may require some creative behavioral management by the audiologist and family to complete the test.

Electrophysiologic tests use sound to trigger a sequence of electrical impulses in the auditory connections that travel from the inner ear toward the brain. These sound-evoked electrical impulses, called the **auditory brainstem response** (ABR), can be detected by electrodes placed on the infant or child's head, and are analyzed by a computer (see Figure 11.8). By controlling the frequency of the sound stimulus and finding the lowest intensity at which the ABR can be detected, the audiologist can estimate hearing thresholds for the speech range frequencies of 500–4000 Hz for each ear. The ABR test can be conducted using air conduction and bone conduction, so the results can be compared to help determine the type of hearing loss. Auditory brainstem response testing requires the infant or child be still, and preferably in a state of natural sleep. In cases when natural sleep recordings are not possible, the child may be tested by an audiologist in an outpatient clinic under anesthesia administered by an anesthesiologist, to ensure optimal recording of the ABR.

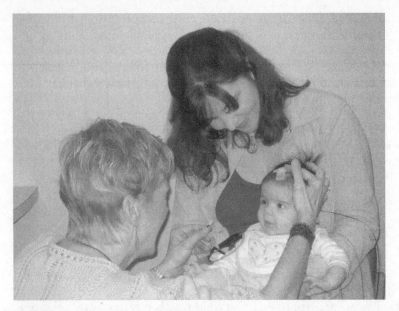

FIGURE 11.8 An audiologist prepares an infant for auditory brainstem response (ABR) testing by placing an electrode on the scalp.

Physiologic test procedures provide a wealth of information that can be used to confirm the presence, severity, and type of hearing loss in very young children who cannot voluntarily participate in the testing.

> *Albert*, age 3 months, was referred for a comprehensive audiologic evaluation because of the concern that he was exposed to cytomegalovirus (CMV) during birth. He passed a newborn screening bilaterally, but the referring physician knew that CMV can cause late-onset hearing loss. The otoscopic inspection and tympanometry were normal for both ears, but otoacoustic emissions were absent in each ear. By comparing and cross checking these test results, the audiologist concluded that there was a high risk of a bilateral sensorineural hearing loss due to a problem with the cochlea. To confirm the presence of the hearing loss and determine its severity, the audiologist performed an auditory brainstem response (ABR) evaluation while Albert slept. Sound was delivered both by air and by bone conduction during the ABR test, and this revealed a mild to moderate sensorineural hearing loss. This finding, considered in the context of the other audiologic findings, confirmed a hearing loss of cochlear origin and early intervention to minimize the adverse effects of hearing loss was initiated.

Behavioral Audiometry

Behavioral audiometry involves a variety of test procedures that rely on the observation of overt changes in behavior in responses to sound. The specific test procedure used depends on the age and ability of the child, but, in general, the purpose is to determine the softest stimulus level at which an infant or child responds to sounds of various frequencies. Behavioral audiometry testing should be conducted in a quiet environment that is free from unwanted auditory and visual distractions. A two-room test suite that prevents extraneous noise from interfering is typically used for testing. In this arrangement, the audiologist is in one room and the child in another. For very young children, a test assistant or parent is present to manage the child during testing.

To establish hearing thresholds, stimuli such as pure tones or warble tones are presented at different frequencies. These frequency-specific test stimuli may be delivered by air conduction or bone conduction to determine whether hearing levels differ for these two methods of testing (see Chapter 10). Bone conduction testing is used specifically to determine whether a hearing loss is conductive or sensorineural in nature (refer back to Figure 11.1). Narrow bands of noise across a range of frequencies may also be used with infants and very young children, because noise stimuli are more acoustically interesting than pure tones, and tend to be better at eliciting a behavioral response in that age group.

Test stimuli are presented to each ear separately using an audiometer that is calibrated to ensure high fidelity sounds are delivered at accurate intensity levels. The sounds are presented to each ear either through soft foam insert earphones or traditional supra-aural earphones. If the child resists wearing earphones or is distracted by them, testing can be done in the sound field with loudspeakers (see Figure 11.9). Testing with loudspeakers does not permit independent assessment of the hearing sensitivity of each ear. Therefore, this method does not allow the audiologist to determine whether there is a significant difference in hearing acuity between ears.

Infants and some young children may not always show clear behavioral responses to sounds during behavioral testing, even when they hear the sounds. Hearing may actually be better than test results indicate for young children. In this

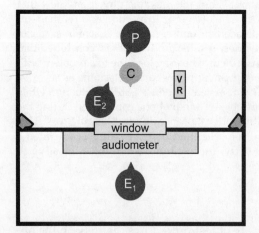

FIGURE 11.9   A typical two-room test suite arrangement for testing children. E_1 = Examiner 1, E_2 = Examiner 2, C = Child, P = Parent, VR = Visual Reinforcer for VRA testing. Speakers for sound field testing are located on the side walls.

case, test results do not reflect true thresholds and are instead called *minimum response levels*. Behavioral testing procedures used for evaluating hearing sensitivity and speech understanding must be appropriate for the age and developmental skills of the child being tested. At approximately 5–6 months of age, an infant can be conditioned to respond voluntarily and repeatedly to auditory stimuli through positive reinforcement. Infants and children with severe intellectual disabilities, for example, cannot always be taught (or "conditioned") to respond to sound voluntarily. In this case, behavioral audiometry test responses are called *non-conditioned*.

Nonconditioned Response Procedures

Behavioral Observation Audiometry (BOA).   BOA is appropriate for infants from the newborn period to 5 months of age and for children with severe intellectual disabilities. It should be used in conjunction with physiologic tests. BOA involves no training of the infant or child. The audiologist watches for changes in the infant's behavior that occur soon after the presentation of the test sounds to observe indications that the infant heard the sound. Infants may have very subtle behavioral responses to soft sounds, so moderately loud auditory stimuli may be used initially to elicit clear, observable responses. The types of behavior changes the examiners look for include cessation of activity, changes in sucking rate, increased movement of extremities or a rudimentary head turn (for infants 3 months of age or older). BOA test results do not reveal true hearing thresholds but rather minimum response levels. They do provide information on a child's awareness of sound, and his or her observed auditory behaviors can be compared to auditory developments milestones.

When possible, a test assistant helps to manage child's behavior during testing, which can improve test reliability. There are certainly times, however, when a child's behavior is misinterpreted. In some instances, an infant may appear to respond to the sound, but the associated behavior is simply by chance, or the infant may have been accidentally cued by the parent's response to the sound. This results in a **false negative** identification. In other words, the result was interpreted as "negative" with regard to the presence of a hearing problem, but that interpretation was wrong. In other circumstances, an infant with normal hearing may not respond to the stimuli for some reason, such as sleepiness, lethargy, or simply lack of interest in the sound presented. In this case, the results are incorrectly interpreted as indicating a hearing loss (a **false positive** identification).

Conditioned Response Procedures

Visual Reinforcement Audiometry (VRA).   Visual reinforcement audiometry is appropriate for use with infants and young children age 5 months to 2 or 2½ years of age. Around age 5–6 months an infant has developed early localization skills and will reflexively look in the direction of the sound source. This localization behavior can be encouraged and developed into a conditioned response by using interesting visual reinforcers as a reward. Visual rewards include animated toys hidden behind dark Plexiglas or video animation screens that light up when the child looks in the correct direction. Figure 11.10 shows a typical two-room test suite arrangement used by audiologists for visual reinforcement audiometry. For this procedure, the child is seated in a high chair or a parent's lap and situated so that the audiologist has a clear view of the child's behavioral changes. An assistant should be present to encourage the child to look in the correct direction when sounds are presented through earphones or loudspeakers, if the child does not do so independently. The assistant can also redirect the child's attention away from visual reinforcer after it is turned off. The assistant may draw the child's attention by using toys, puppets, or video display, in order to prepare the child for the next stimulus trial (see Figure 11.10). Using this procedure, reliable responses for frequency-specific hearing stimuli can be obtained down a level 25 dB HL for children as young as 6 months.

> Test results from bone conduction thresholds are very rarely worse than air conduction, because bone conduction tests only the sensorineural component of the system, whereas air conduction tests the entire hearing mechanism.

Condition Play Audiometry (CPA). Conditioned play audiometry can be used with children 2½–4 years of age and in some cases with children as young as 2 years of age. With this approach, children are taught to put a peg in a pegboard, a block in a bucket, or some other fun activity when they hear a sound, usually a pure tone. Play audiometry is well matched to this developmental age because it is a time when children are inquisitive, social, goal-oriented, and enjoy a fun challenge. It is typically possible to obtain hearing thresholds (the lowest sound that the child can hear) for each ear and for a variety of pure tones. At a minimum, testing should be done for 500–4000 Hz for each ear. The testing begins with earphones (air conduction), and will include bone conduction if significant hearing loss is found.

Speech Audiometry. Tests of speech reception thresholds (SRT) and word recognition can often be done with children who are old enough to repeat spoken words, or to point to pictures of words they hear. The

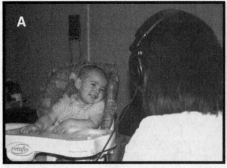
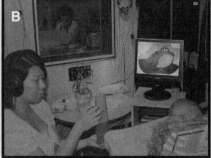

FIGURE 11.10 A baby participates in Visual Reinforcement Audiometry (VRA). (A) An assistant wearing ear muffs to prevent her from hearing test stimuli interacts with the baby. (B) The child hears a sound and turns toward a computer screen that provides a visual reinforcement for that alerting response.

speech reception threshold (SRT) is the lowest intensity level that a child can repeat (or point to pictures of) two-syllable words such as "baseball" and "airplane" 50 percent of the time. The two-syllable words used for this test are those with equal stress on each syllable and are called "spondee" words. Being a "threshold" measure, the SRT is reported in dB HL (Hearing Level). Another test, referred to as the word recognition test, assesses the ability of a child to recognize and repeat common one-syllable words. Testing is done at a conversational speech level for children with normal hearing or at a comfortable loudness level for children with a hearing loss. As with speech reception testing, there are some cases when a child's speech may not be easily understood (see Chapter 4), in which case a set of pictures is provided and the child is instructed to point the word that they hear. Test results are reported as percent correct. A number of word recognition tests are available with vocabulary appropriate for different age groups. Word recognition tests are also available for children whose first language is not English.

Conventional Audiometry.   Starting at age 4–5 years of age, most children will be able to participate in an audiologic evaluation in the same way that adults are tested. That is, they are capable and willing to raise their hand when they hear pure tones and give verbal responses during speech audiometry.

Counseling

Once the audiologic assessment is completed, the test results and their implications are discussed with the family. If parents have just received the news that their child has a hearing loss, they may not be ready to process additional information. Nonetheless, recommendations for intervention and follow-up must be made quickly. An otologic evaluation to determine the etiology of hearing loss is often the next step, and this may involve genetic testing. An ophthalmologic evaluation may also be recommended because of the increased risk for vision disabilities among children with hearing loss. In the case of infants and children under the age 3, information on state and community early intervention programs is provided so that habilitation services can be started early. The essence of the initial counseling session is to educate parents about their child's hearing loss, to let them know that they are not alone, and that community resources are available. A follow-up appointment to answer family questions and inform the family about hearing technology options is also made. Parents want to make informed choices for their children and audiologists are part of a team of individuals who educate and support families.

Interdisciplinary Assessment and Intervention

As we have seen, multiple factors influence the effect of hearing loss on the life of a particular child. Therefore, a holistic approach to assessment and intervention is needed as an individual child is considered. We can see this in the case of Mylar.

Mylar was referred for an audiologic evaluation after being referred from the newborn hearing screening program at the hospital where she was born. Mylar was 6 weeks old at the time of her first visit to the audiologist. Case history information provided by the family revealed no obvious risk factors for hearing loss. The audiologist's observation of her physical characteristics revealed a small baby (birth weight 4 lbs. 13 ounces) with a very small head size (microcephaly). Her ears were set low on the head and her neck was short and it seemed like her shoulders were in a permanent "shrug." Her muscle tone was very low (hypotonia) and she made frequent random eye movements that seemed like they were not under her control.

> Low birth weight is a risk factor for hearing impairment. Average newborn birth weight is 7 pounds, with a range of 5.5 to 10 pounds.

When an audiologist notes multiple physical anomalies, there is usually concern that there might be an underlying **syndrome** that includes hearing loss. As mentioned earlier, children with syndromic hearing loss are at risk for multiple developmental delays. When this is the case, the audiologist will contribute to an interdisciplinary team that assesses the overall functioning of the child and manages his or her needs. In Mylar's case, the audiologic assessment included a tympanometry, otoacoustic emissions, electrophysiology, and auditory behavioral response testing.

The audiologist confirmed the presence of a bilateral, moderate-to-severe sensorineural hearing loss. These results were forwarded to Mylar's pediatrician. The audiologist also facilitated a follow-up physician appointment and initiated an interdisciplinary referral process through a state agency serving infants with developmental disabilities.

Interdisciplinary assessment may be coordinated through the child's pediatrician, "medical home." A medical home is not a specific place, but identifies an interdisciplinary practice for family-centered health-care service delivery. When an infant has a syndrome or multiple disabilities, other professionals will participate in the assessment. In Mylar's case, additional assessment included an ophthalmologic examination to assess vision. Referral to an otolaryngologist was needed to evaluate the physical anomalies involving the ears and facial features. A pediatric neurology evaluation was scheduled because the low muscle tone suggested a problem involving the peripheral nervous system (see Chapter 2). A speech-language pathologist completed a swallowing evaluation (see Chapter 6) because the infant's low weight suggested feeding problems. Subsequently, a nutritionist became involved to address Mylar's low weight. In cases like this, when multiple professionals are involved in the assessment of a child, a service plan coordinator is assigned to manage the many appointments and to facilitate smooth communication between the various professionals on the team (see Figure 11.11).

Following completion of the team assessment it was determined that Mylar had a severe, bilateral sensorineural hearing loss, congenital cataracts, neurodevelopmental delays, swallowing difficulty (dysphagia), and failure to thrive. A subsequent

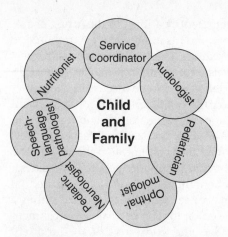

FIGURE 11.11 Mylar's interdisciplinary team. Multiple professionals interact with Mylar and her family to assess all of the areas of concern and arrive at a diagnosis for the child.

comprehensive medical and developmental assessment at a children's hospital yielded a diagnosis of Cerebro-Oculo-Facial-Skeletal (COFS) syndrome. This is a degenerative disorder of the brain and spinal cord that begins before birth and is genetic in origin.

Once a diagnosis is determined, specific recommendations for audiologic follow up can be made and written into a service plan that addresses the full spectrum of the child's needs. Audiologic recommendations for infants frequently include periodic audiologic assessment to determine whether the hearing loss is stable or progressive, to monitor the use and benefit from amplification methods, and to initiate family-centered audiologic habilitation services. Each of these components is covered in other sections of this chapter.

Following the diagnosis of bilateral sensorineural hearing loss, Mylar was fitted with binaural hearing aids at age 3 months and comprehensive interdisciplinary intervention services were in place by age 6 months. These achievements met the best practice benchmarks of the Early Hearing Detection and Intervention 1-3-6 plan. Follow-up audiologic evaluations revealed that her hearing loss was stable. Periodic functional assessments of her auditory function when wearing hearing aids revealed evidence of positive changes in Mylar's auditory skill development. She had gone from being nonresponsive to most environmental sounds before being fitted with hearing aids to showing increased awareness of speech and environmental sounds and beginning to develop sound localization skills. "My favorite part of the day is when I put Mylar's hearing aids in every morning," Mylar's mother reported. "When I turn them on, she stops and listens and I know she can hear me."

Amplification

Most infants and children with bilateral hearing loss, and many with unilateral hearing loss, benefit from some form of personal amplification device. Medical clearance for hearing aid use should be obtained after an otologic evaluation is completed. Ideally, the time between identification and the fitting of amplification will be minimal, however, parents are not always prepared to make quick decisions about amplification. The audiologist must respect a family's need to take time for decision making, but the benefits of fitting amplification with minimum delay need to be discussed openly.

It is generally accepted that hearing loss of 25 dB HL or greater impedes a child's ability to perceive speech adequately for optimal development of speech and language. Although no hard and fast rules exist regarding the degree of hearing loss for which amplification should be used, the American Academy of Audiology (2003) provides general guidelines.

The primary goals of hearing aid selection and fitting are to (a) ensure that conversational-level speech is audible, (b) to keep amplified speech within a comfortable listening range, and (c) to ensure that loud speech and environmental sounds do not reach unsafe listening levels. Other concerns that are important for children include selecting hearing aids that are durable and flexible in terms of their ability to be fine-tuned. Specifically, it is critical that modifications can be made easily as the listening demands change, and as more is learned about the child's hearing sensitivity.

There are many styles of hearing aids, but digital programmable behind-the-ear hearing aids, coupled to the child's ear with a soft earmold are the most common type used by pediatric audiologists. These hearing aids meet the requirement of durability and flexibility and are typically compatible with hearing assistance technology. Hearing aids have microphones that pick up sound waves, which are converted to a digital code. Once sound has been digitized, it is amplified and filtered before being converted back to sound waves that are delivered to the ear canal though an earmold. Figure 11.12 shows a schematic of a behind-the-ear style hearing aid.

> The primary goal of hearing aid use is to ensure that speech is audible at a variety of loudness levels.

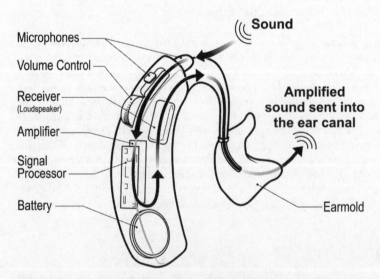

FIGURE 11.12 Schematic of a behind-the-ear hearing aid. Sound is received by a microphone in the hearing aid body and transmitted through the internal components (dashed line) to the ear.

Decisions regarding the selection and programming of hearing aids for infants and children are based on the results of a comprehensive audiologic testing battery. A computer is used to program hearing aids using information about the child's age, as well as the degree, type and slope of hearing loss. When hearing aids are fitted, it is important to verify that sound is amplified appropriately for the child's needs, and not to unsafe levels. This is done by measuring the sound amplified by the hearing aid in the ear canal with a probe microphone system. During this test, a soft tube attached a microphone is placed in the ear canal, and the hearing aid earmold is then put in the ear and the hearing aid is turned on. Sounds from a small loudspeaker are picked up by the hearing aid microphone, and the amplified signal from the hearing aid is measured in the ear canal. Figure 11.13 shows the probe microphone arrangement.

Implantable Auditory Prostheses

In some instances, a sensorineural hearing loss is too severe to benefit from traditional hearing aids that introduce sound through the ear canal. Permanent damage or malformation of the outer or middle ear can also prevent the use of a traditional hearing aid. Instead, implantable auditory devices (prosthetics) may be used to introduce sound through alternative routes.

Bone-Anchored Hearing Aids

A bone-anchored hearing aid transmits sound through bone conduction, so that sound travels through the skull directly to the cochlea. It can be useful for

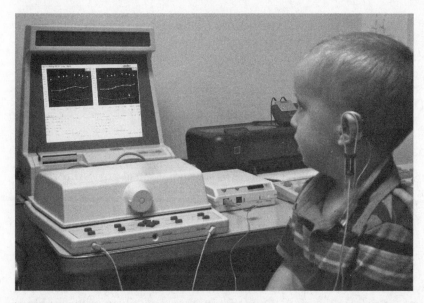

FIGURE 11.13 A probe microphone is used to measure the sound delivered by a hearing aid into the ear canal.

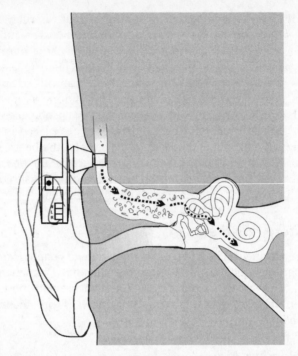

FIGURE 11.14 A schematic of a bone-anchored hearing aid. The aid is anchored to the bone just behind the ear using a titanium post. Sound is conducted through the bone to the inner ear.

individuals with a conductive hearing loss resulting from atresia (absence of external ear canal) or those with permanent middle ear problems, because bone conduction bypasses the outer and middle ear structures. A bone-anchored aid is small device (about the size of your thumb from the tip to the knuckle) that is connected to a titanium post surgically implanted in the skull as shown in Figure 11.14.

Cochlear Implants

Cochlear implants are not hearing aids. They are digital signal processing devices that provide the experience of sound by delivering electrical stimulation within the cochlea. They can be useful for children who have profound sensorineural hearing loss. A cochlear implant has external and internal components, as illustrated in Figure 11.15. The external components include a microphone, digital sound processer, and transmitter that delivers sound to the internal components, which are surgically implanted. The internal components include a receiver connected with wire to a series of electrodes placed within the coils of the cochlea. The electrodes deliver electrical stimulation to the nerve fibers of the auditory nerve (cranial nerve VIII).

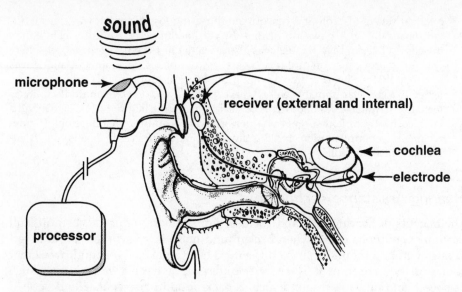

FIGURE 11.15 A schematic of a cochlear implant.

The general guidelines for cochlear implantation with children were first published by the U.S. Food and Drug Administration (FDA) in 2002. They were revised in 2011, as summarized in Table 11.4.

> *Camden*, a healthy newborn, was born at full term to a young couple. He passed a newborn hearing screening bilaterally before being discharged with his mother 48 hours after birth. During the first five months, he showed clear signs of responding to sounds around the home and started to turn his head toward his parents when they spoke. At age 6 months he was rushed to the hospital because of high fever and vomiting. He was diagnosed with bacterial meningitis, admitted to the hospital, and successfully treated. After coming home, Camden no longer responded to his parent's voices or sounds around the home.

> Camden was referred to an audiologist by his pediatrician because of concern regarding his lack of response to sounds. The diagnostic hearing evaluation, including an auditory brainstem response test (ABR; see Chapter 10), confirmed a

Meningitis is an inflammation of the membranes that cover the brain and spinal cord. It is usually caused by a viral or bacterial infection.

TABLE 11.4 Guidelines for Appropriate Candidates for Cochlear Implantation in Children

- Newborn to 2 years of age with bilateral profound sensorineural hearing loss.
- Older than 2 years with bilateral severe to profound sensorineural hearing loss.
- Shows little or no benefit in audition or speech development from hearing aids.
- Has no medical or anatomical contraindication for surgery.
- Has access to appropriate education and rehabilitation follow-up.
- Has access to an environment that supports successful learning and habilitation with an implant.

bilateral severe-to-profound sensorineural hearing loss. Camden was quickly fitted binaurally with powerful behind-the-ear hearing aids. Auditory habilitation (discussed later in this chapter) was also started. Over the next four months there was no improvement in auditory awareness or speech development and it was apparent that the hearing aids did not provide significant benefit. Camden was referred to a cochlear implant center, where he was evaluated by a multidisciplinary team to determine candidacy for a cochlear implant (see Figure 11.16). Two months later, cochlear implant surgery was performed. His auditory habilitation program resumed after implantation, and this time he showed progress in developing listening and speaking skills.

Hearing Assistance Technology

The benefits of hearing aids and cochlear implants are reduced when difficult listening conditions exist. When background noise is present, or sound reverberates within a room, it can be difficult to hear a particular sound over other sounds in the environment. The relative difference between a wanted sound such as speech and unwanted sound such as background noise is usually described as the **signal-to-noise ratio** (sometimes referred to as SNR). When the signal, such as a speaker's voice, is high relative to the background noise, listening is relatively easy. However, when the signal is low, or the background noise is high, listening can be very difficult. Difficult acoustic conditions often exist in classrooms. The conflict that poor room acoustics can create between a signal and the background noise can negatively affects communication and learning.

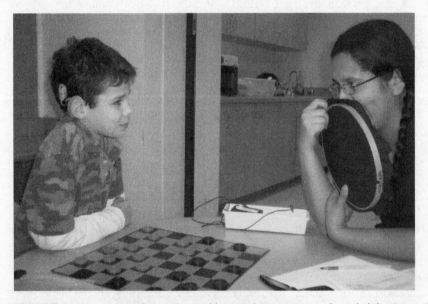

FIGURE 11.16 A young boy with a cochlear implant receives auditory habilitation training. The child's view of the clinician's mouth is blocked to prevent lipreading.

For this reason, students with hearing loss may benefit from hearing assistance technology that serves to improve listening conditions.

The term **hearing assistance technology** refers to devices that enhance communication or media access for deaf and hard of hearing persons. A personal FM system is one type of hearing assistance technology that enhances communication by reducing the adverse effects of poor room acoustics. An example of an FM system can be seen in Figure 11.17. These systems transmit acoustic information via radio waves using the same technology as an FM radio in a car, but a personal FM system transmits over a relatively short distance (e.g., within

A signal-to-noise ratio of 0 dB means that speech and noise are equal in intensity.

A signal-to-noise ratio of 10 dB means that the speech signal is 10 dB more intense than the competing noise.

A signal-to-noise ratio of –10 means that speech is 10 dB weaker than the competing noise.

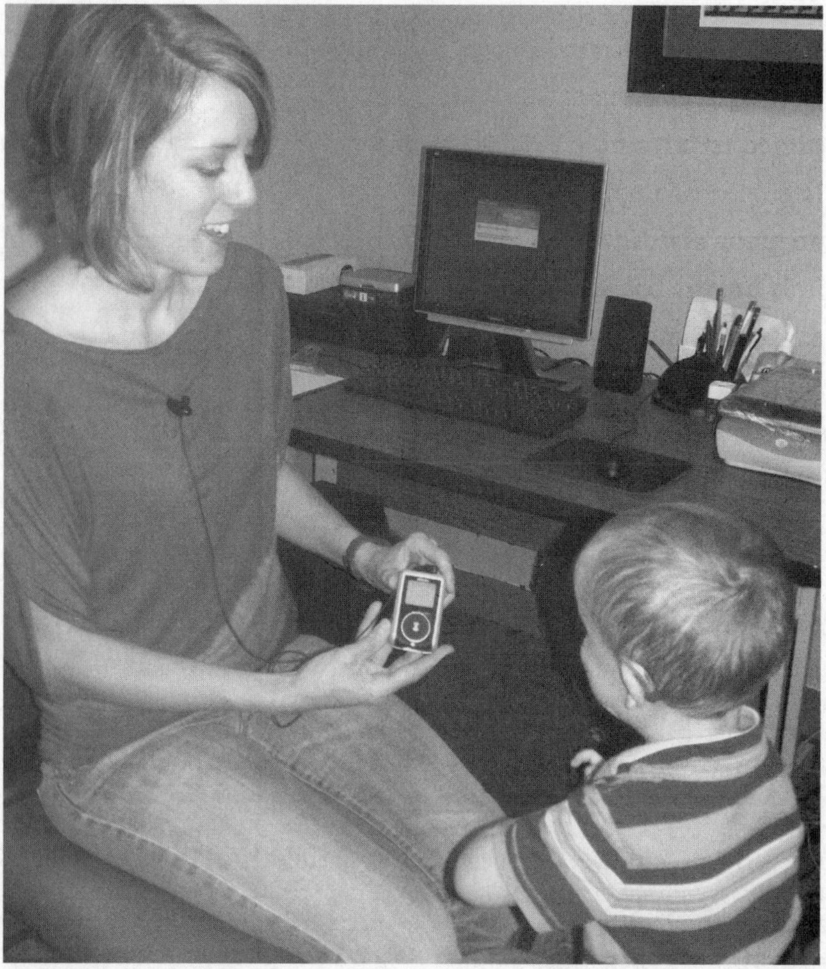

FIGURE 11.17 An audiologist demonstrates an FM (frequency modulated) system to a child. The microphone clipped to the audiologist's shirt picks up her voice, which is then transmitted to the child's hearing aid.

a classroom or theater). An FM system includes several components that serve to transmit the signal from a speaker directly to a listener. These include (1) a microphone worn by the talker (e.g., the teacher), (2) an FM radio frequency transmitter that sends the teacher's speech across a room to the listener, and (3) small receivers connected to the hearing aids or implantable device worn by the listener. The microphone serves to isolate the speaker's voice so that it is heard clearly over any background noise. The radio frequency transmission sends the signal from the microphone directly to the receiver attached to the hearing aid worn by the child, ensuring that the speech signal is easier to hear over classroom noise. Proper use of hearing assistive technology in classrooms serves to improve speech audibility (Thibodeau, 2010), as well as the attention, communication, and academic performance of the wearers (Langlan, Sockalingam, Caissie, & Kreisman, 2009).

When an FM system is fitted in a school setting, an educational audiologist ensures that the FM receivers work with the student's hearing aids properly, and makes adjustments to the hearing aid and FM system in accordance with the child's hearing loss. The educational audiologist also works with classroom teachers to confirm that the FM system is consistently providing good benefit to the students. Children who have a unilateral hearing loss, and even some who do not have a hearing loss but have difficulty processing spoken language, may also benefit from the use of hearing assistance technology. For example, some children who have normal hearing but poor ability to attend to, or process, auditory information may have improved understanding of speech when using an FM system. Another useful amplification system involves the use of loud speakers attached to an FM receiver and amplifier that are placed strategically within a classroom.

Hearing Habilitation and Communication

The goal of hearing screening, both for newborns in hospitals and for school children, is to detect hearing loss as soon as possible after onset. However, detection is not of much benefit if effective services to support children with hearing loss are not also provided early. Fitting a hearing aid or turning on a cochlear implant does not always assure that normal communication skills will follow. **Habilitation** services provide the link between the hearing levels that the child will achieve (with or without assistive technology) and the their ability to maximize the benefit from that hearing.

When a hearing loss is detected, parents need information concerning the nature and degree of the hearing loss, what this is likely to mean for their child's development, and the options for managing the consequences of the hearing loss. An audiologist is often the primary source of this information and serves a vital role in the initial counseling of parents. We have discussed in this chapter various forms of technological assistance available to children with significant hearing loss or deafness. Parents need to make decisions concerning whether to use these types of devices, or whether to rear their child as a member of the Deaf community. This is a highly personal decision, which is influenced by many factors. For example, some Deaf parents of Deaf children may not see a need for hearing technology because their family communicates solely with American Sign Language, is fully integrated into the Deaf community, and education provided solely in sign language is readily available at a local school for the Deaf. Other Deaf parents may welcome the option of hearing aids or cochlear implants. Hearing parents likewise weigh many factors in decision making regarding their children. Parents need and want realistic information about the potential benefits and limitations of various approaches to hearing loss management (Sjoblad, Harrison, Roush, & McWilliam, 2001). The audiologist's job is to fairly represent the range of options available to parents, the benefits and limitations of these options, and to help parents access the community resources available to their child.

> Wendy's mother, Erica, recounted her feelings at the time her daughter's hearing loss was diagnosed. "I was shocked when I learned that Wendy had a hearing loss. This had never happened in my family." Wendy's father, Dan, was equally caught off guard. "When Wendy arrived, I counted her fingers (10) and toes (10). Perfect! She was just beautiful. And two days later, it seemed like she was no longer our perfect baby." "The staff audiologist was really helpful in terms of reassuring us that Wendy could still have a great life," recounted Erica. "During follow-up visits we learned about hearing aids, cochlear implants, and early intervention. Hearing aids were the right option for Wendy, but I really worried how our family would react to her with hearing aids. It would have really hurt if our relatives had treated her differently, but it turned out we shouldn't have worried at all. We've since heard the same from other parents like us." "The big thing for me," related Dan, "was that we completely underestimated hearing aid care and maintenance. I just figured they put the aids on Wendy and that would be that. Boy, did I learn fast. Batteries wear out. The earmolds need cleaning. There was just more maintenance than I expected."

Children with hearing loss are eligible for a variety of habilitative services. The best communication outcomes for young children with hearing loss are achieved when services are initiated within the first year of life (Moeller, 2000; Yoshinaga-Itano, Sedey, Coulter, & Mehl, 1998). Habilitation services for children this age are available through a variety of sources, including university clinics and private practice clinics. Most commonly, these children are served through government agencies, such as the Department of Developmental Disabilities and local schools. Federal law (**IDEA**, see also Chapter 8) supports services for infants and preschool children that is family-centered and typically delivered in the home. Parents and professionals, including audiologists, speech-language pathologists, deaf educators, and other developmental specialists, work together to develop an *Individualized Family Service Plan* to identify the services the child will receive and who will be involved. As the name of the service plan implies, services are tailored to the individual needs of the child and the family. For a child with moderate hearing loss without other handicapping conditions, this might mean training parents in the care and maintenance of a hearing aid, and speech-language therapy to develop oral language and social communication skills. A child who is not only deaf, but also has cerebral palsy that limits the ability to physically interact with the world, might receive services to reduce the physical handicap as well. Parents are central to the process of planning and implementing treatment, as parental involvement in early intervention is a strong predictor of communicative outcome for children with hearing loss (Moeller, 2000).

> Erica and Dan enrolled their daughter in a home-based hearing habilitation program. Either Erica or Dan is present for each session with Wendy so that they can help facilitate her speech and language development. "The services have been great for Wendy," said Erica. "But if I had one thing to tell other parents, it would be to 'have patience.' You are not going to see results immediately. But they will come. Each milestone was like a little victory. Wendy is 3 now and is doing great."

Some children who have received high-quality early intervention may have no further need for support services other than periodic checks of hearing status. However, many children with hearing loss require support throughout the school years. When they transition from home-based services under the Individualized Family Service Plan to school-based services, the school personnel and the parents develop an Individualized Educational Plan. As with the Individualized Family Service Plan, the *Individualized Educational Plan* is tailored to the specific needs of each child, and is intended to maximize the child's ability to participate in and benefit from the educational environment. The plan considers the modality of the child's communication (e.g., sign language, spoken language, or use of an augmentative device [see Chapter 4]). It also takes into account the full range of handicapping conditions that may impact the child's ability to function in school.

Many states have residential or day schools for the deaf (or for the deaf and blind). These schools provide those enrolled with a community of students who have hearing loss. Parents may prefer these schools as an educational option because the educators have particular expertise regarding the needs of students with hearing loss and classes often have low student-to-teacher ratios. Decades ago, the majority of children considered to have educationally significant hearing loss attended these schools. Currently, most school-age children with hearing loss attend their neighborhood school. Local school districts may employ a number of professionals with expertise in the education of children with hearing loss. This may include educational audiologists, speech-language pathologists with training in hearing habilitation, and special education teachers who have expertise in deaf education, and reading specialists. Additional professionals, including occupational therapists and physical therapists, may become involved in educational programs for children who have hearing loss in the presence of a broader syndrome. Local schools also provide the advantage of learning and interaction with the typically developing children who also attend the neighborhood school.

There is a broad range of school-based services to accommodate the needs of the individual student. A child with a mild hearing loss, for example, may function well if the teacher simply seats him or her in a space that minimizes distractions and the teacher manages the class in a way that reduces the overall ambient noise. Teachers may consult with an educational audiologist concerning how they can improve the overall hearing environment within their classroom. This might include simple modifications like the use of visual aids during teaching, or pacing discussions so that children are not talking over each other (Brackett, 1997). In other cases, technological solutions, like classroom amplification, may be necessary. Children with moderate-to-severe hearing loss may benefit from the services of a speech-language pathologist to improve their speech production. Some children with hearing loss struggle with literacy skills, particularly if their oral language skills are behind those of their peers. Supporting the development of reading and writing may require services from the speech-language pathologist (see Chapter 8) or class time spent with a reading specialist.

The overall goal for children with hearing loss during the school years is to help them develop the social, communication, and academic skills needed for success in life. This is necessarily a multidisciplinary effort, with audiologists, speech-language pathologists, medical professionals, and educators each playing a role to address all the needs of the child and family. As we have seen in this chapter, supporting children with hearing loss is most successful when hearing loss is identified as early as possible after onset and effective means of treatment (both technological and behavioral) begin as soon as possible after the nature and severity of the loss is determined.

Clinical Problem Solving

Annalisa failed her newborn hearing screening two days after birth. She subsequently failed a second screening. She was scheduled for a full audiometric evaluation within the next week.

1. What types of tests might the audiologist use to determine if she has a hearing loss?
2. If she turns out to have a severe sensorineural hearing loss, what forms of technology might be appropriate for her at her age?
3. What other means of supporting her overall development might her parents want to pursue?
4. To assure the best outcome, what timeline might the audiologist adhere to for diagnosing her hearing loss and beginning a management plan?

REFERENCES

American Academy of Audiology (2003). *Pediatric Amplification Protocol*. Washington, DC: Author.

Asbjørnsen, A. E., Obrzut, J. E., Boliek, C. A., Myking, E., Holmefjord, A., Reisæter, S., & . . . Møller, P. (2005). Impaired auditory attention skills following middle-ear infections. *Child Neuropsychology, 11*, 121–133.

Arcia, E., & Roberts, J. E. (1993). Otitis media in early childhood and its association with sustained attention in structured situations. *Journal of Developmental and Behavioral Pediatrics, 14*, 181–183.

Brackett, D. (1997). Intervention for children with hearing loss in general educational settings. *Language, Speech, & Hearing Services in Schools, 28*, 355–361.

Braun, P. A., Huebschmann, A. G., Kim, C. A., Lezotte, D. C., Shupe, A., & Dabelea, D. (2011). Effect of maternal birthplace on gestational diabetes prevalence in Colorado Hispanics. *Journal of Immigrant Minority Health, 13*, 426-433.

Butler, C. C., van der Linden, M. K., MacMillan, H. L., & van der Wouden, J. C. (2003). Should children be screened to undergo early treatment for otitis media with effusion? A systematic review of randomized trials. *Child: Care, Health and Development, 29*, 425–432.

Casby, M. W. (2001). Otitis media and language development: A meta-analysis. *American Journal of Speech-Language Pathology, 10*(1), 65–80.

Coker, T. R., Chan, L. S., Newberry, S. J., Limbos, M. A., Suttorp, M. J., Shekelle, P. G., & Takata, G. S. (2010). Diagnosis, microbial epidemiology, and antibiotic treatment of acute otitis media in children: a systematic review. *JAMA, 304*, 2161–2169.

Creps, C. L., & Vernon-Feagans, L. (2000). Infant daycare and otitis media: Multiple influences on children's later development. *Journal of Applied Developmental Psychology, 21*(4), 357–378.

Cohen-Karem, R., Bar-Oz, B., Nulman, I., Papaioanou, V. A., & Koren, G. (2007). Hearing in children with fetal alcohol spectrum disorder (FASD). *Canadian Journal of Clinical Pharmacology, 14*, e307-e312.

Gallaudet Research Institute. (2003). Regional and National Summary Report of Data from the 2002–2003. Annual Survey of Deaf and Hard of Hearing Children and Youth. Washington, DC: GRI, Gallaudet University.

Gorin, S. S., & McAuliffe, P. (2009). Implications of childhood cancer survivors in the classroom and the school. *Health Education, 109*, 25–48.

Guthrie, O. W. (2008). Aminoglycoside induced ototoxicity. *Toxicology, 249*, 91–96.

Harrison, M., Roush, J., & Wallace, J. (2003). Trends in age of identification and intervention in infants with hearing loss. *Ear and Hearing, 24*, 89–95.

Langlan, L. A., Sockalingam, R., Caissie, R., & Kreisman, B. M. (2009). The benefit of sound-field amplification in First Nations elementary school children in Nova Scotia, Canada. *Australian and New Zealand Journal of Audiology, 31*(2), 55–71.

Moeller, M. P. (2000). Early intervention and language development in children who are deaf and hard of hearing. *Pediatrics, 106*, 1–9.

Morton , C. C., & Nance, W. E. (2006). Newborn screening—a silent revolution. *New England Journal of Medicine, 354*(20), 2151–2164.

Nance, W. E., & Kearsey, M. J. (2004). Relevance of connexin deafness in (DFNB1) human evolution. *American Journal of Human Genetics, 74*, 1081–1087.

Roberts, J., Hunter, L., Gravel, J., Rosenfeld, R., Berman, S., Haggard, M., & . . . Wallace, I. (2004). Otitis media, hearing loss, and language learning: Controversies and current research. *Journal of Developmental and Behavioral Pediatrics, 25*, 110–122.

Schow, R. L., & Nerbonne, M. A. (2007). *Introduction to audiologic rehabilitation.* Boston: Pearson Education.

Sjoblad, S., Harrison, M., Roush, J., & McWilliam, R. A. (2001). Parents reactions and recommendations after diagnosis and hearing aid fitting. *American Journal of Audiology, 10,* 24–31.

Smith, R. J., Bale Jr., J. F., & White, K. R. (2005). Sensorineural hearing loss in children. The *Lancet, 365,* 879–890.

Stool, S. E., Berg, A. O., Berman, S., Carney, C. J., Cooley, J. R., Culpepper, L., Eavey, R. D., Feagans, L. V., Finitzo,T., Friedman, E. M., Goertz, J. A., Goldstein, A. J., Grundfast, K. M., Long, D. G., Macconi, L. L., Melton, L., Roberts, J. E., Sharrod, J. L., & Sisk, J. E. (1994). *Otitis media with effusion in young children. Clinical practice guideline, Number 12.* Agency for Health Care Policy and Research (AHCPR) Publication Number 94-0622. Rockville, MD: U.S. Department of Health and Human Services, Public Health Service.

Thibodeau, L. (2010). Benefits of adaptive FM systems on speech recognition in noise for listeners who use hearing aids. *American Journal of Audiology, 19*(1), 36–45.

U.S. Preventative Services Task Force. (2008). Universal screening for hearing loss in newborns: U.S. Preventative Service Task Force recommendation statement. *Pediatrics, 122,* 143–148.

Van Camp G., Willems, P. J., & Smith, R. J. (1997). Nonsyndromic hearing loss: Unparalleled heterogeneity. *American Journal of Human Genetics, 60,* 758–764.

Whelan, K., Stratton, K., Kawashima, T., Leisenring, W., Hayashi, S., Waterbor, J., Blatt, J., Sklar, C. A., Packer, R., Mitby, P., Robinson, L. L., & Mertens, A. C. (2011). Auditory complications in childhood cancer survivors: A report from the childhood cancer survivor study. *Pediatric Blood Cancer, 57,* 126–134.

White, K. R. (1997, October). *The scientific basis for newborn hearing screening: Issues and evidence.* Invited keynote address to the Early Hearing Detection and Intervention (EHDI) Workshop sponsored by the Centers for Disease Control and Prevention, Atlanta, Georgia.

Yoshinaga-Itano, C., Sedey, A. L., Coulter, B. A., & Mehl, A. L. (1998). Language of early- and late-identified children with hearing loss. *Pediatrics, 102,* 1168–1171.

Zielhuis, G., Rach, G., & van den Broek, P. (1989). Screening for otitis media with effusion in preschool children. *Lancet, 11,* 311–313.

READINGS FROM THE POPULAR LITERATURE

Bowers, T. (1999). *Alandra's lilacs.* Washington, DC: Gallaudet University Press. (hearing parents, deaf child)

Cohen, L. H. (1994). *Train go sorry: Inside a deaf world.* New York: Vintage Books. (deafness)

Greenburg, J. (1971). *In this sign.* New York: Henry Holt. (novel about a deaf family)

Keller, H. (1961). *The story of my life: The autobiography of Helen Keller.* New York: Dell. (deaf-blind)

Kisor, H. (1990). *What's that pig outdoors: A memoir of deafness.* New York: Hill and Wang. (deafness)

Sidransky, R. (1990). *In silence: Growing up hearing in a deaf world.* New York: St. Martin's Press. (hearing child, deaf parents)

Walker, l. A. (1986). *A loss for words: The story of deafness in a family.* New York: Harper & Row. (hearing child, deaf parents)

Disorders of Hearing in Adults

Linda Norrix
Frances P. Harris

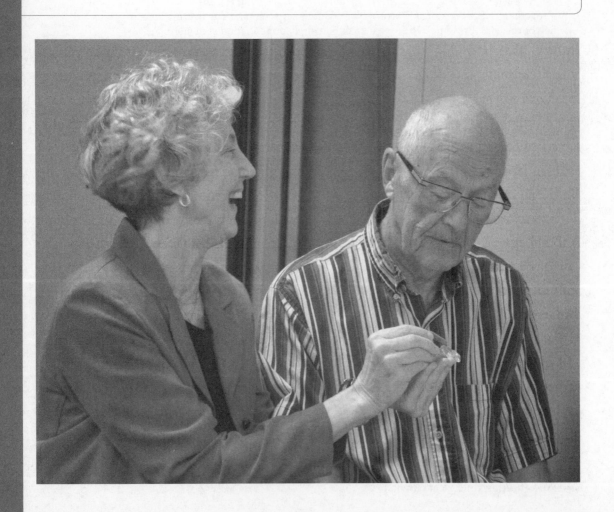

Acquired hearing loss is one of the most common age-related changes experienced by adults. The cause may be associated with prolonged exposure to noise, specific medical conditions, or simply the effects of aging. Regardless of the underlying etiology, hearing loss can have a significant negative effect on communication, and in turn disrupt family relationships, social interactions, work performance, and overall well-being. The audiologist plays a central role in documenting the degree and type of hearing loss and evaluating its impact on the individual's life. In addition, the audiologist can offer a variety of means to improve hearing performance, including amplification, assistive and alerting devices, as well as strategies to maximize communication.

PREVIEW

More than 34 million Americans report difficulty hearing (Kochkin, 2009). The majority of these individuals developed their hearing impairment in adulthood, but, of course, childhood hearing impairments also persist in this population. As reviewed in the preceding chapter, hearing *impairment* is defined as a loss or abnormality in the structure or function of the auditory system. The impairment may result in reduced sensitivity for detection of sound, poor understanding of speech, or both. The degree of impairment can be measured using standardized techniques to quantify the hearing loss, and the audiologist plays a major role in determining, implementing, and interpreting the appropriate tests (Martin & Clark, 2011). As with any communication impairment, however, personal and environmental factors influence the extent to which a hearing impairment affects the person's life. For example, an individual with a high-frequency hearing impairment who is socially active, is likely to report more difficulties understanding speech in noisy environments compared to someone with the same impairment who has few social contacts. Audiologists working with adults aim to understand not only the degree of hearing impairment, but also the extent of the disability. They appreciate that hearing loss may limit an individual's involvement in social activities and may lead to reduced life participation due to social isolation, reduced economic resources, and difficulty maintaining independence. In clinical practice, the audiologist's goal is to optimize the client's ability to live a full life in both the workplace and society. By considering the hearing impaired individual's abilities, restrictions, and limitations in the context of his or her personal situation, an appropriate rehabilitation plan may be developed.

Conductive Hearing Loss

A conductive hearing loss occurs when the sound cannot reach the inner ear efficiently, so that the sensory receptors in the inner ear are not adequately stimulated (see Chapter 10). The audiogram for a conductive loss will show elevated thresholds by air conduction and normal thresholds by bone conduction, so that an air-bone gap will be present (see Chapter 11). In other words, sound vibrations are not properly transmitted through the outer or middle ear, thus reducing hearing by air conduction, but the neural mechanism of the inner ear is not affected, so hearing is fine when the inner ear is stimulated directly. The person with a conductive hearing loss can typically recognize words without difficulty, provided that speech is loud enough to be heard.

Whereas conductive hearing loss is relatively frequent in childhood, it is not as common in adults. Causes of conductive impairments include excess *cerumen*, or ear wax, blocking the ear canal, fluid behind the eardrum within the middle ear space (see Chapter 11 for a discussion of middle ear fluid in children), a perforated eardrum, or damage to the ossicles within the middle ear. **Otosclerosis** is an example of a disorder that occurs in adulthood and causes a progressive conductive hearing impairment. In otosclerosis, bony tissue is replaced by spongy or fibrous bone growth. The most common place for this abnormal bone growth to occur is in the area of the oval window, resulting in reduced motion of the stapes so the mechanical vibrations are not properly transmitted from the middle ear to the inner ear. Otosclerosis typically develops in both ears, rather than in just one. It is more common in women than in men, and in Caucasians than in Asian or African Americans. Genetics seem to play a role, and a family history is often reported (Balloh, 1998).

> Conductive hearing loss often may be restored by medical or surgical intervention.

> *Ms. Garrett*, age 35 years, reported that over the last several years she has had difficulties understanding speech in background noise, localizing sounds, hearing people talk when they were on her left, and using the telephone with her left ear. Figure 12.1 illustrates Ms. Garrett's audiogram and word recognition ability. Notice

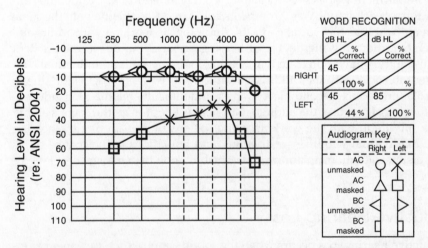

FIGURE 12.1 Audiogram illustrating a conductive hearing loss in the left ear due to otosclerosis. Note that it was necessary to use masking at levels of 50 dB and above to prevent crossover of sounds to the opposite ear. Masked thresholds are represented by squares on the audiogram. AC-air conduction; BC-bone conduction.

that when tested in the left ear at a normal conversational level (45 dB HL), she repeated only 44 percent of the single-syllable words correctly. This was because the speech signal was not entirely audible to her. A medical evaluation confirmed that Ms. Garrett has otosclerosis, and although the condition may eventually affect both ears, only her left ear was affected at that time.

Ms. Garrett's audiogram provides an indication of the frequencies where her hearing is reduced, but to appreciate the effect of hearing loss on her ability to understand speech, it is helpful to examine the relative contribution of the different frequency and intensity combinations for speech audibility. Such a graph is shown in Figure 12.2, which contains one hundred dots concentrated in the frequency range for speech: the denser the distribution of dots, the greater the amount of speech energy that falls within that frequency band. An **articulation** or **audibility index** is calculated by assigning 0.01 (one percent) to each dot that is within a person's audibility range. Ms. Garrett's left ear air conduction thresholds are superimposed on the graph.

You can count 36 dots that fall above Ms. Garrett's audiometric curve (between her thresholds and 110 dB HL), which indicates an audibility index of 0.36. This value indicates that she is hearing only about 36 percent of the sound necessary to understand speech. The audibility index can then be used in a formula to estimate how well she will be able understand syllables, words, or sentences in typical conversation (Mueller & Killion, 1990). Those measures of intelligibility can be compared with how well Ms. Garrett performed when her hearing for speech was tested directly. As expected, she only understood about half of the speech stimuli presented at typical loudness levels. However, when words were presented at a higher intensity level (85 dB HL), Ms. Garrett's word recognition ability was excellent (100 percent correct).

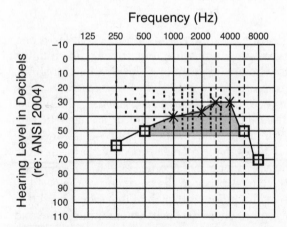
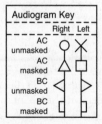

FIGURE 12.2 The left ear thresholds of an individual with unilateral otosclerosis superimposed on the Count-the-Dot audiogram for calculation of the articulation index. The shaded portion of the graph indicates the frequency range and hearing levels that are audible when speech is presented at a normal conversational level. Based on Mueller & Killion (1990).

What is an air-bone gap? What does it indicate with regard to the ear?

Ms. Garrett's profile indicates that she is an excellent candidate for a hearing aid because her hearing loss is conductive, which results in little or no sound distortion. With appropriate amplification, the individual with a conductive hearing impairment will have few if any limitations or restrictions in daily life. Depending on the cause of the hearing loss, surgery or medical treatment may improve or even restore hearing.

Ms. Garrett had surgery to eliminate the conductive hearing loss due to otosclerosis. The surgery, performed by an ear, nose, and throat (ENT) specialist, is known as a **stapedectomy** and often reduces or nearly eliminates the conductive component of a hearing impairment. During her surgery, the footplate of the stapes was removed and replaced with a wire prosthesis. Ultimately, there was nearly complete elimination of the conductive hearing impairment, so that Ms. Garrett had a return of normal bilateral hearing.

Sensorineural Hearing Loss

The majority of hearing impairments in adulthood are sensorineural, where there is damage to the inner ear or cochlea, the nerve leading to the brainstem, or both (see Chapter 10). The audiogram for such hearing impairments shows relatively equivalent hearing thresholds for air conduction and bone conduction because in either case, the neural impulses are not properly transmitted to the brain stem. In other words, the audiogram does not show an air-bone gap as observed in a conductive hearing loss (Northern & Downs, 2002). Four common conditions associated with sensorineural hearing impairments in adulthood are aging, noise exposure, Ménière's disease, and ototoxicity.

Aging Process

The proportion of people with hearing loss increases with age. While 18 percent of American adults 45–64 years have a hearing impairment, this number increases to 47 percent for adults who are 75 years or older (National Institute on Deafness and Other Communication Disorders, 2010). A decrease in hearing acuity associated with the aging process is known as **presbycusis**. A lifetime of environmental noise exposure, disease processes, drug effects, and genetic predisposition to hearing impairment influence the function of the cochlea and contribute to presbycusis. Although changes to the cochlea probably begin earlier in life, it is generally not until middle age or later that people begin to have difficulties understanding speech. Initial changes occur in the basal end of the cochlea, that is, the region that is near the oval window rather than the apex. Recall that the basal end of the cochlea is the region where the basilar membrane is thin and responds best to high-frequency sounds (see Chapter 10).

Because low-frequency hearing is relatively normal, individuals with early presbycusis typically report that they can hear people talk, but that they cannot understand what is being said. This is because they hear the lower-frequency vowel sounds, but the consonants, which are composed of high frequency, low-intensity energy, may be inaudible. This causes a problem because the consonant sounds are the most important for understanding spoken words. Figure 12.3 depicts the general frequency and intensity characteristics of five different classes of speech sounds: voiced consonants, nasals, vowels, voiceless stops, and voiceless fricatives (Olsen, Hawkings, & Van Tasell, 1987). Notice that voiceless stops and fricatives are high in frequency compared to nasals and vowels. Voiceless stops and fricatives, therefore, are easily missed by the person with a high-frequency hearing loss. Perceiving the place of articulation (e.g., distinguishing /b/ from /d/ from /g/) is also dependent on high-frequency cues. Without using speechreading or contextual cues, a person with a high-frequency hearing loss might report hearing "ben" for "den" or "gay" for "day" or "bay." Another common complaint of individuals with high-frequency hearing loss is the inability to understand speech in the presence of background noise, because the noise will obscure, or "mask" the weaker components of the speech signal (e.g., the high-frequency consonants and place-of-articulation cues). Rooms with reverberation (echoes) are also difficult listening environments for those with hearing impairment.

> Presbycusis typically affects the understanding of consonants more than vowels. Why is that so?

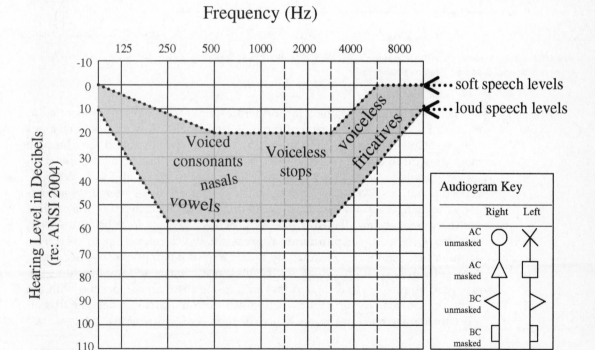

FIGURE 12.3 The frequency and decibel levels of various classes of speech sounds. Based on Olsen, Hawkins, & Van Tasell (1987).

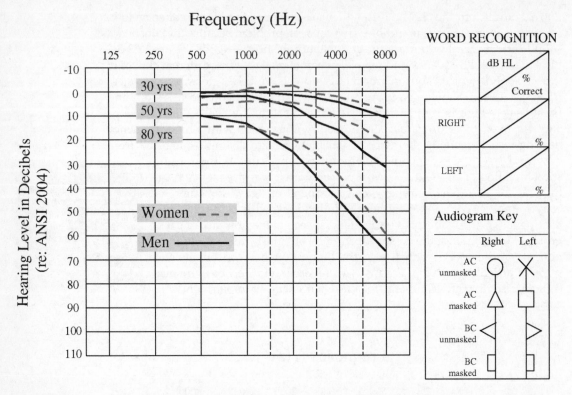

FIGURE 12.4   Hearing thresholds at three ages. Note that thresholds at the higher frequencies show the most change with age. Based on Pearson et al. (1995).

Typical hearing thresholds for individuals of various ages are illustrated in Figure 12.4. Notice that hearing of the high frequencies shows marked changes with age. However, in the oldest individuals, low-frequency sounds also become more difficult to detect. It is also the case that hearing thresholds decline at an earlier age and more quickly in men than women (Pearson et al., 1995). With advanced presbycusis, a loss of neurons in the central nervous system may accompany the changes within the cochlea, resulting in central presbycusis or a **central auditory processing disorder** (see retrocochlear hearing loss, below). A sign of central presbycusis is **phonemic regression**, which refers to poor word recognition that cannot be explained by the degree of hearing loss for pure tones. A common report of individuals with central presbycusis is "I can hear fine, but everyone mumbles." Central auditory processing disorders associated with the aging process may be difficult to distinguish from the cochlear damage that almost always accompanies aging, hence the term sensorineural hearing loss.

> *Mr. Robinson*, age 70 years, came to the clinic to have his hearing evaluated. He was accompanied by his two daughters, who reported that their father was answering questions inappropriately and constantly saying "huh." Although Mr. Robinson

admitted that he had some difficulty hearing, he commented that his hearing "was not all that bad" and that he would be able to hear better if people "would speak more clearly." Figure 12.5 illustrates Mr. Robinson's audiogram. He has central presbycusis. He shows signs of a central auditory processing disorder along with cochlear impairment. This is evident because his ability to understand words is poorer than expected based on his pure-tone audiogram. His word recognition ability was 28 percent in his left ear and 32 percent in his right ear when words were presented at a sound level well above his thresholds.

It is estimated that more than 50 percent of individuals over 65 years of age will have a central auditory processing disorder in addition to cochlear hearing loss (Stach, Spretnjak, & Jerger, 1990). This population has greater difficulty extracting speech from noise, understanding speech when reverberation is present, and benefitting from amplification devices than those with hearing impairment who do not have central auditory processing disorders.

The increased prevalence of central auditory processing disorders with advanced age is important to consider when working with people over age 65 years. As the baby boomer generation ages, there will be more older people living in retirement and nursing home facilities. It is estimated that by the year 2030, the nursing home population will reach 3 million residents (Sahyoun, Pratt, Lentzner, Dey, & Robinson, 2001). Of these, nearly half will have a hearing impairment that interferes with communication (Schow & Nerbonne, 1980) and all are likely to be interacting and socializing in challenging listening conditions. For example, communication often occurs in meeting rooms, dining areas, and recreational rooms that are likely to be noisy. Hearing-related communication impairments may adversely affect patient-staff relationships, and hearing-impaired residents may be inappropriately perceived as being withdrawn, uncommunicative, or confused.

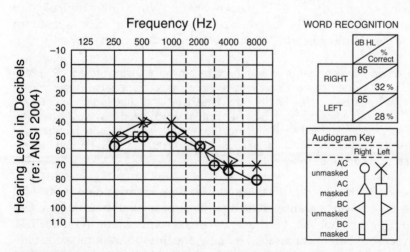

FIGURE 12.5 Audiogram illustrating a sensorineural hearing loss. The poor word recognition scores suggest a central auditory processing disorder in addition to cochlear damage.

Hearing impairment can also be associated with poor performance on cognitive tests, especially when administered verbally. In fact, if cognitive testing is implemented without adequate amplification, then a significant proportion of those tested are likely to appear demented (or more demented) than they actually are (Weinstein & Amsel, 1986). This is important to keep in mind, because even when nursing home residents have their own personal hearing aids, many of them are likely to be malfunctioning (Erber & Heine, 1996; Thibodeau & Schmitt, 1988). In addition, few health care providers have received formal training in the management of patients with communication disorders. Because of the high prevalence of hearing loss in the older population, an audiologist might be employed to provide audiologic evaluation, fit hearing aids, and train staff members on how to use strategies to enhance communication as well as how to troubleshoot hearing aids. These services are important to prevent social isolation due to hearing loss, which can dramatically decrease quality of life for those in nursing home facilities.

> Noise exposure can result in hearing loss in the high frequencies.

Many factors contribute to hearing impairment among older adults. Each person's hearing capabilities and communication contexts are unique, and treatments must be tailored to individual needs. Although challenging, hearing rehabilitation with older adults can be particularly rewarding work for the audiologist.

Noise Exposure

The National Institute on Deafness and Other Communication Disorders (2011) estimates that 26 million Americans are exposed to dangerously high sound levels on a regular basis. These potentially hazardous noise levels occur in the workplace, at home, and during recreational activities. It is well documented that noise exposure can cause a "threshold shift" initially observed around 4000 Hz. That is, hearing a tone in the 4000 Hz frequency region will be more difficult after noise exposure than before. The long-term effects of noise exposure account for 16 percent of the disabling hearing impairments in adults worldwide.

> *Mr. McGee*, age 52 years, has been employed in a manufacturing plant for 25 years. He also enjoys carpentry work and snowmobiling as recreational activities. He reported that he hears ringing in his ears (**tinnitus**) and that speech sounds are muffled. The audiologist employed by his company evaluated his hearing (see Figure 12.6) and compared the results to previous evaluations. She noted a threshold shift—that is, his hearing for the frequencies 3000, 4000, and 6000 Hz had become poorer since his previous tests.

A reduction in threshold at 4000 Hz (4k Hz) with improvement at 8000 Hz is known as a "4k notch" because of the dip that appears on the audiogram (see Figure 12.6). This threshold shift is due to damaged sensory cells in the cochlea, resulting in sensorineural hearing loss. Initially, the threshold shift may be temporary. After removing oneself from the high noise levels, thresholds may return to normal. This is known as a *temporary threshold shift*. However, it is likely that

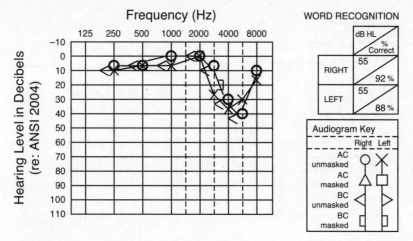

FIGURE 12.6 Audiogram illustrating a sensorineural hearing loss centered around the 4000 Hz region as a result of excessive noise exposure.

some damage to the sensory cells occurs with each exposure. After repeated exposure for a longer period of time, or with personal susceptibility to noise damage, recovery may not be complete. The result can be a *permanent threshold shift*. Similar to persons with presbycusis, individuals with noise-induced hearing loss have difficulty understanding speech in noisy environments and in rooms with high levels of reverberation.

> Mr. McGee received a complete audiometric evaluation and was counseled about the harm that noise exposure causes, as well as the effects of his high-frequency hearing loss on communication ability. He was shown how to wear earplugs appropriately and instructed to limit his exposure to noise and wear hearing protectors at work as well as during recreational activities that involve high noise levels.

> Noise-induced hearing loss is preventable. What steps can you take to reduce your risk?

Ménière's Disease

> *Mrs. Hill*, age 55 years, experiences episodic attacks of vertigo, nausea, tinnitus, and a sensorineural hearing loss in the right ear that is more severe in the low frequencies than in the high frequencies. A feeling of pressure in her right ear often precedes the attacks. The most distressing symptom for her is the vertigo that comes on suddenly with little warning. Because of the unpredictability of these attacks and the embarrassment she feels, Mrs. Hill is no longer employed and has stopped socializing with friends. She was diagnosed with **Ménière's disease** ten years ago. The hearing loss has become slightly worse over the last five years. Figure 12.7 displays her audiogram.

Approximately 615,000 people in the United States suffer from Ménière's disease (National Institute on Deafness and Other Communication Disorders, 2010).

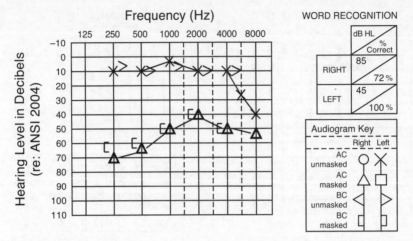

FIGURE 12.7 Audiogram illustrating a right sensorineural hearing loss due to Ménière's disease.

Although the exact cause of Ménière's disease is unknown, it is thought to be due to an excess buildup of inner ear fluid called *endolymph*. Ménière's disease is coincident with fluctuating hearing thresholds and is often unilateral. One-third of those with the disease will develop it in both ears. It is common for the first episode to occur during early to mid-adulthood. As the disease progresses, the low-frequency hearing loss becomes more severe and permanent. The role of the audiologist with this population is to provide information about the disease and the available audiologic rehabilitation methods. Amplification may be necessary depending on the nature and degree of hearing impairment. In some cases, individuals with Ménière's disease get some relief from the effects of tinnitus by wearing a small device akin to a hearing aid that makes noise and serves to mask the ringing in their ears.

Ototoxicity

Ototoxicity results when certain drugs damage the inner ear, resulting in sensorineural hearing loss. The damage is usually in the high frequencies and can be reversible or permanent. Ototoxic drugs are often used for treatment of life-threatening medical conditions. The audiologist's role is to obtain periodic audiograms prior to, during, and after drug therapy. For those individuals who develop hearing loss, the audiologist provides rehabilitation services that may consist of selecting and fitting appropriate amplification, support, and encouragement. Education about hearing conservation is also important, because individuals on drug therapies may be more susceptible to noise damage than those not receiving such therapies.

Retrocochlear Hearing Loss

When the pathology is beyond the cochlea, so that it involves the eighth nerve or is within the central auditory system, the hearing impairment is known as **retrocochlear**. Individuals with retrocochlear pathology may retain the ability to perceive pure tones but have extreme difficulty understanding speech, especially in difficult listening environments.

Vestibular Schwannoma

> *Ms. Parker*, age 56 years, came to the ENT clinic because she was having pain on the left side of her face, tinnitus in the left ear, and dizziness. Her audiogram revealed a sloping, mild-to-moderate sensorineural hearing loss in the left ear and mild high-frequency sensorineural hearing loss in the right ear (Figure 12.8). Her word recognition performance was excellent in the right ear when words were presented at normal and loud conversational levels (50 and 90 dB HL, respectively). The left ear results revealed good word recognition at 70 dB HL, but poor recognition when words were presented at 90 dB HL.

This dramatic decrease in word recognition as the presentation level of the words is increased is known as **rollover** and is often associated with pathology in the auditory nervous system.

> The audiologist evaluated Ms. Parker using the auditory brainstem response (ABR) test (see Chapter 11). Electrodes were placed on the surface of her scalp, and clicking sounds were presented to each ear. The electrodes detected the brain's electrical

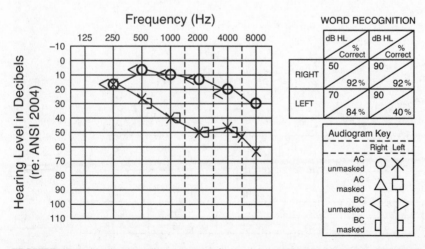

FIGURE 12.8 Audiogram illustrating a left sensorineural hearing loss associated with a vestibular schwannoma. Note that the word recognition score for the left ear (seen at upper right) decreased when words were presented at 90 dB HL compared to 70 dB HL (rollover).

activity that occurred in response to the clicks. Samples of the electrical activity that occurred after each click were recorded and processed with a computer.

An ABR typically includes several positive peaks of electrical activity that occur within milliseconds following each click. Delayed electrical peaks, in the absence of a conductive hearing loss, or delayed intervals between the peaks are strong indicators that pathology is located in the neural pathways of the auditory nerve or brainstem (see Chapter 10).

In addition to the sensory hearing impairment documented by the elevated pure tone air and bone conduction thresholds, there was evidence of retrocochlear pathology on the left side. Ms. Parker's ABR (auditory brainstem response) results are shown in Figure 12.9. The peaks for waves III and V for the left ear were at 4.36 ms and 6.64 ms, respectively, which was much longer than the latencies for the comparable brainwaves from the right ear (3.84 ms and 5.92 ms, respectively). Ms. Parker subsequently had an MRI of the internal auditory canal (the bony canal through which the auditory nerve passes when it leaves the cochlea). The MRI image confirmed that a tumor had developed on the VIIIth cranial nerve, which transmits auditory and vestibular information. The tumor was surgically removed, and confirmed to be a **vestibular schwannoma** (also referred to as an **acoustic neuroma**). Unfortunately, the surgery left Ms. Parker with no measurable hearing in her left ear. Being active in her vocation and community, she found that the unilateral hearing loss restricted her participation in everyday activities. As is common with unilateral hearing loss, she had difficulty localizing sounds, understanding speakers positioned on the side of the poorer ear, and understanding speech in noise. The audiologist fit her with a hearing aid that placed a microphone at the unusable left ear and a receiver on the good right ear. This arrangement allows the microphone to pick up the signal reaching the impaired ear and send it to the good ear to facilitate sound detection.

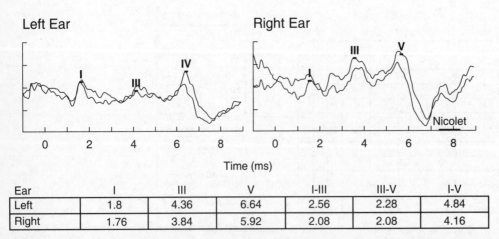

Ear	I	III	V	I-III	III-V	I-V
Left	1.8	4.36	6.64	2.56	2.28	4.84
Right	1.76	3.84	5.92	2.08	2.08	4.16

FIGURE 12.9   The auditory brainstem response of a patient with a left vestibular schwannoma. When clicks were presented to the left ear, waves III and V were abnormally delayed compared to the waves associated with right ear click stimulation.

A hearing aid arrangement in which a microphone placed on an unaidable ear sends the signal to the good ear is known as *contralateral routing of signals*, or a CROS hearing aid. Wearing a CROS hearing aid makes it easier for the individual with a unilateral hearing impairment to hear sounds directed to the impaired ear. It also restores a sense of sound balance and an improvement in the **signal-to-noise ratio** when the signal is on the side of the poorer ear. A recent medical device called the Bone-Anchored Hearing Aid (BAHA) is also available for single-sided deafness. With this device, an abutment is surgically implanted into the skull. A processor, worn on the head, changes sound into vibrations that are sent via the skull to the good cochlea. Although this device does not provide hearing for the "deaf" ear, sounds that originate on the side of the deaf ear are more accurately perceived in the good ear and provide a sensation of hearing on both sides.

Although vestibular schwannomas affect only 1 out of 100,000 people, if undetected this condition can result in death due to pressure on brainstem structures from tumor growth. If detected early and surgically removed, hearing may be preserved. Therefore, patients experiencing unilateral hearing loss or unilateral tinnitus should be tested to determine whether a vestibular schwannoma is the cause of their symptoms.

Diseases of the Central Auditory System

Audiologists may also evaluate and participate in the rehabilitation of patients who have lesions to the brain or brainstem that affect hearing (see Chapter 10 for a discussion of the central auditory pathways). Such disorders include multiple sclerosis, strokes, and cortical or brainstem tumors. A lesion of the brain can disturb the blood supply to the cochlea, resulting in damage to the hair cells and a reduced ability to perceive sound. However, most often a central auditory disorder will cause difficulties with speech processing without affecting pure-tone hearing sensitivity. Individuals with central auditory lesions report difficulties listening in background noise, with reverberation, when visual cues are not available, and when speech is spoken at a rapid rate. An older person with a central auditory lesion will likely also have some difficulty hearing pure tones due to the effects of aging on the cochlea.

Mixed Hearing Loss

Finally, a hearing loss that has both conductive and sensorineural components is known as a *mixed hearing loss*.

> *Mrs. Leon*, age 84 years, reported a sudden decrease in her hearing. Her family, who accompanied her to the evaluation, reported that for many years she had some difficulties understanding speech and had to turn the television to higher-than-normal loudness levels in order to hear most programs. Recently, her neighbors

had complained about the loud noise coming from her apartment. Mrs. Leon reported a sudden hearing loss coincident with a cold that she developed approximately two months prior. She expressed much concern about her deteriorating hearing ability, as it was a sign of "getting old" and "one more thing going wrong."

Mrs. Leon's audiometric results are displayed in Figure 12.10. The audiogram shows that she has a mixed hearing loss. Notice that there is a 30 to 40 dB air-bone gap, which reflects the conductive part of the hearing loss, and a mild-to-moderate 30 to 50 dB sensorineural hearing loss (thresholds for bone conduction range from 30 to 50 dB HL). The conductive component of her hearing impairment was due to bilateral middle ear infection (otitis media, see Chapter 11). The sensorineural component was diagnosed as presbycusis. Pressure equalization tubes were placed in her ears by an ENT specialist. After medical intervention, the audiologist recommended hearing aids and assisted her in the rehabilitation process. Mrs. Leon adapted quite well to her new hearing aids and showed a renewed interest in communicating with her family and friends. Comforted by the knowledge that she was not rapidly going deaf, and assisted with amplification, she was better able to participate in community functions and religious services.

Conductive, sensorineural, and retrocochlear pathologies can co-exist. Through comprehensive testing and careful case history taking, the audiologist determines the degree of hearing impairment, site of pathology, and functional difficulties the client exhibits so that appropriate referrals and remediation plans can be developed and implemented.

Psychosocial Impact of Hearing Loss

It is obvious that hearing serves some very basic functions in life, including the ability to recognize sounds that serve to signal or warn us about things in the

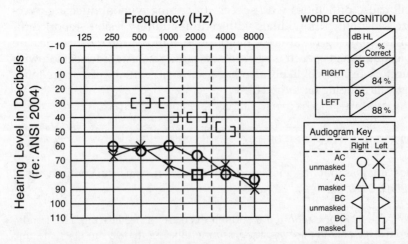

FIGURE 12.10 Audiogram illustrating a mixed hearing loss due to otitis media (which caused the conductive component) and presbycusis (which caused the sensorineural component).

environment. For individuals who grew up in a world of sound, the ability to hear and communicate in the spoken modality is a fundamental aspect of their psychological and social life experience. Even a mild acquired hearing loss can have a significant impact on interpersonal relations, and more severe hearing impairment can have dramatic consequences on psychological and emotional well-being. Hearing connects us to the world of sound, and adults who acquire their hearing loss experience psychosocial effects to different degrees. This is not always dependent on the severity of the hearing loss, rather, the person's reaction and adjustment to it.

> *Mr. Cohen*, a 42-year-old salesman, experienced a sudden, severe, bilateral sensorineural hearing loss. Mr. Cohen had provided the sole financial support for his family, which included three children. Because of the severity of the loss and the communication demands of his job, he made the decision to quit working. His wife became employed, and Mr. Cohen became more responsible for daily activities in the home. He often declined social invitations because he tired easily when trying to participate in the conversations. He relied on his wife to interpret for him and often pretended to understand what people were saying.

A hearing impairment often impacts the entire family and significant others. In fact, the initial visit to the hearing clinic often comes at the urging of a spouse or partner. Family members may become frustrated at continually repeating and interpreting for the individual with a hearing loss. The extra effort required to include the hearing-impaired individual in conversations and spectator activities such as plays, movies, and lectures can put stress on family relationships and result in exclusion of the hearing-impaired person. It is not uncommon to hear an older person with hearing loss say, "If I don't do something about my hearing, my spouse will leave me." Even said in jest, this statement reflects the seriousness of communication breakdown and its impact on relationships. Likewise, hearing impairment can interfere with activities of daily living. Communicating on the telephone and asking a passerby for directions are just two examples of the many activities that may become quite difficult with hearing impairment.

The audiologist must be knowledgeable and competent to assess the effects of hearing loss on functional communication, including how it influences the psychosocial, educational, and occupational wellbeing of the individual (ASHA, 2002). Training the hearing-impaired individual and significant others to use effective communication strategies and offering counseling for those adjusting to hearing loss are two very important services that an audiologist provides.

Audiological Evaluation

Hearing Screenings

The audiologist may screen for hearing loss or may oversee the hearing screening program. The purpose of screening is to identify individuals who have a high probability of hearing loss, so that they can be referred for appropriate diagnostic testing. ASHA recommends that adults be screened at least every ten years through age 50 and then at three-year intervals (ASHA, 1995). Common settings for screenings include health fairs and medical facilities. It is particularly important to identify hearing loss in nursing home residents because of the high prevalence of hearing impairments in the older population.

Hearing screenings are conducted by presenting pure tones at predetermined levels. The American Speech-Language-Hearing Association (1997) has recommended that if an adult responds to pure-tone air conducted stimuli at 25 dB HL at 1000, 2000, and 4000 Hz in both ears, then he or she passes the screening (see Figure 12.11). If no response is obtained at one or more frequencies in *either* ear, then the individual fails the screening. The 25 dB HL level was recommended because even mild hearing loss can negatively influence a person's health and well-being.

In addition to pure-tone screening, a hearing disability index should be used to identify individuals who perceive themselves as having a disability (ASHA, 1997). Self-assessment measures gauge the clients' perceptions by asking them to rate the degree to which their hearing loss interferes with daily activities or social

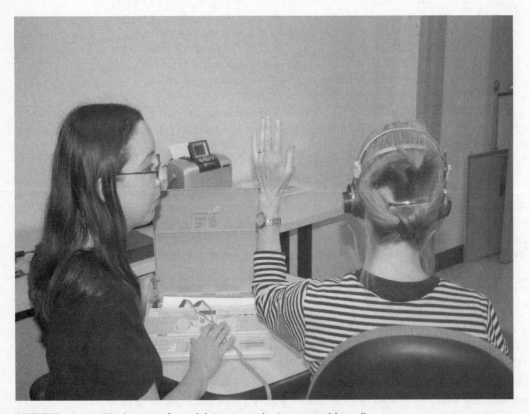

FIGURE 12.11   The hearing of an adult is assessed using a portable audiometer.

interactions. Such measures help identify those individuals who believe that they have a disability, and who are likely candidates for rehabilitation. Individuals who fail the pure-tone screening and report problems with hearing in their daily lives should be counseled regarding hearing impairment and the need for a referral for a complete hearing assessment.

Hearing Assessment

A second task of the audiologist is to assess a client's hearing status. A complete audiologic evaluation will determine the need for medical referral, additional audiologic follow-up, or both. The test results will assist a physician in diagnosing and treating the patient. A complete evaluation also provides the basis for a rehabilitation plan.

An audiologist looks in the ear canal with an otoscope before beginning to test hearing. Ask an audiologist what kinds of "surprise findings" she has encountered.

The audiologic evaluation begins with a case history. The audiologist obtains information about the hearing difficulties that the person is experiencing, family history of hearing loss, medical history, and previous experience with hearing aids. Next, the audiologist examines the patient's external ears with a handheld **otoscope** or **video otoscopy**. With video otoscopy, enlarged images of the tympanic membrane and ear canal can be projected on a video monitor (see Figure 12.12). A photo print of these structures can be made to document pathology and medical treatment outcomes. If excess *cerumen* (wax) is observed in the ear canal, then it must be removed prior to audiologic testing. Cerumen removal can

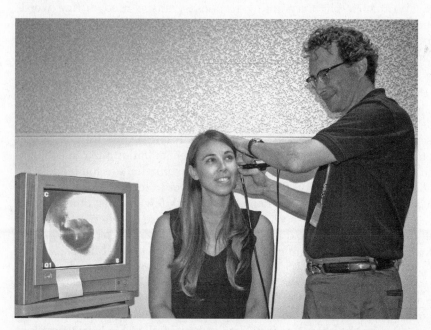

FIGURE 12.12 An audiologist uses video otoscopy to examine the ear canal and tympanic membrane. These structures can be seen on the computer monitor to the left.

be performed by an audiologist with specialized training or by appropriate medical personnel. Audiologic testing is performed to determine if a hearing impairment exists, the type of impairment (conductive, sensorineural, or mixed), and the severity of the impairment for various frequencies and for speech. We can examine the stages of the audiologic evaluation by following the case of Mr. Peterson.

> *Mr. Peterson* came to the clinic because he was having difficulties hearing his co-workers. He reported more difficulty hearing from his right ear than his left. After a case history was obtained and an otoscopic examination revealed the ear canals to be free of cerumen, immittance measures were obtained (see Chapter 11 for a discussion of immittance). Next, Mr. Peterson was seated inside a sound-treated booth, and miniature earphones were inserted in his ear canals. The audiologist tested the hearing of each ear individually using an audiometer. The test began with the audiologist playing prerecorded, two-syllable words (such as "cowboy" and "armchair") to Mr. Peterson. The lowest level at which he was able to repeat the two-syllable words 50 percent of the time was recorded for each ear. These were his speech recognition (reception) thresholds (SRTs). Next, the pure-tone air conduction and bone conduction thresholds were obtained. Finally, word-recognition ability was assessed. Single-syllable words were presented at normal and loud conversational levels, and the audiologist recorded the percentage of words that Mr. Peterson repeated correctly.

Audiologists also test adults who are not able to respond verbally to the test stimuli, such as adults with developmental disabilities, severe head injury, or stroke. Written or picture-pointing responses can be used during word-recognition testing. *Otoacoustic emissions* (see Chapter 10) also can be used to screen for hearing loss in difficult-to-test adults, because such tests do not require a volitional response. If a person fails the screening, then an auditory brainstem response threshold search can be implemented.

Assessing Participation Restrictions

For those hearing impairments that are not medically correctable, the audiologist has the task of developing and implementing a rehabilitation plan in conjunction with the patient. Results from the audiologic evaluation are combined with information about the individual's daily life in order to formulate an appropriate plan. Some individuals may be homebound, with few visitors; others are involved actively with work or social activities. There are a variety of potential communication needs, and the difficulties each person perceives may be greater or less than what the audiogram might suggest (Matthews, Lee, Mills, & Schum, 1990; Weinstein & Ventry, 1983). For that reason, self-assessment tools have been used to gauge functional communication.

The audiologist must understand the individual's hearing abilities as they relate to communication demands. An understanding of each patient's hearing and his or her communication needs will assist the audiologist in jointly developing rehabilitation goals with the patient and the patient's family.

Management Strategies

According to ASHA (2002), "Audiologic/aural rehabilitation (AR) is an ecological, interactive process that facilitates one's ability to minimize or prevent the limitations and restrictions that auditory dysfunctions can impose on well-being and communication, including interpersonal, psychosocial, educational, and vocational functioning" (p. 90). The audiologist achieves these goals with a variety of methods. One of the most important goals of rehabilitation is to facilitate accurate understanding of speech. This may involve the use of hearing aids.

Hearing Aids

Hearing aids are electronic devices that amplify sound. To provide maximum benefit to an individual client, they must be selected and fit appropriately. The hearing aid selection and fitting process includes *assessment*, *selection and fitting*, *verification*, *orientation*, and *validation* (ASHA, 1998). By completing each of these stages carefully, the audiologist increases the likelihood that clients will not only receive amplification that is appropriate for them but also that they will use it successfully. Hearing aids come in various styles (Figure 12.13). Most hearing aids are ear-level devices and include the behind-the-ear, open-fit, in-the-ear, in-the-canal, and completely-in-the-canal styles. Special fittings, such as the CROS aid described earlier for Ms. Parker, are also available.

All hearing aids, no matter the style, have the same basic components: a microphone for sound input and conversion to an electrical signal, an amplifier to increase the level of sound, a receiver to convert the electrical signal to an

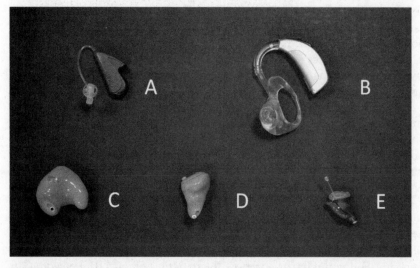

FIGURE 12.13   Common types of hearing aids. From left to right, top to bottom: open-fit (A), behind-the-ear (B), in-the-ear (C), in-the-canal (D), and completely-in-the-canal (E).

acoustic signal, and a battery to power the device. The circuitry of a hearing aid, and how it processes the electrical signal, may vary across instruments. Most hearing aids in today's market are digital rather than analog. This means that the hearing aid uses a computer chip and mathematical algorithms to manipulate the incoming signal after it is converted to a series of digits. The digital signal is tailored to the individual's audiometric configuration. For example, if a client has a hearing loss in the high frequencies only, then the hearing aid would produce more amplification in the high-frequency range and little if any amplification in the lower frequencies.

Decisions concerning the circuitry of the hearing aid are determined primarily by *assessment* of the degree of the hearing loss. Hearing aid *selection* depends on both the nature of the hearing impairment and the client's preferences and lifestyle. For example, the largest size behind-the-ear hearing aid may have the most flexibility for fitting any magnitude of hearing loss but may not be accepted by a client as readily as a smaller style. However, smaller hearing aids cannot always compensate for more severe hearing losses and may be more difficult for many older adults to insert and remove. For clients with binaural hearing loss, the use of two hearing aids (binaural amplification) is generally recommended because of the advantages for localizing sound and for understanding speech in background noise. Guidance and counseling are important to help each client to understand the advantages and disadvantages of each style so that an appropriate selection may be made. The advanced technology now available in hearing aids makes them more flexible; however, many of the limitations of using amplification for an individual with a sensorineural hearing loss remain. Two of these limitations include distortion of the signal and intolerance for loud sounds. Having realistic expectations improves satisfaction with a hearing aid.

Hearing aids are custom-fitted to the client's ear. After *fitting* the hearing aid, the audiologist must *verify* the fitting to assure that it is correct and appropriate for the client. One verification method involves the insertion of a small probe microphone in the ear canal, near the tympanic membrane. The microphone measures the characteristics of sounds near the plane of the eardrum. These recordings are referred to as *real-ear* or *probe-microphone measurements*. Sounds of various frequencies or recorded speech are presented through a loudspeaker while the probe microphone measures the sound pressure level with the hearing aid in the ear and turned on (aided condition) and without the hearing aid in the ear (unaided condition). The difference in sound pressure level between the aided and unaided conditions tells the audiologist how much gain in sound level the hearing aid provides at different frequencies. Because probe microphone measurements require no response from the patient, they are reliable and can be used to verify hearing aid fittings even with a difficult-to-test patient. Although this is the preferred verification method, other means of verification are available if real-ear measurements cannot be made.

During the *orientation* stage, the patient is instructed in the use and care of the hearing aids. Following the orientation, the patient is given a trial period with the devices during which time any problems with the fitting may be resolved.

Let us examine this aspect of the rehabilitation process by following Mrs. Leon, the woman who received pressure equalization tubes to correct the conductive component of a mixed hearing impairment (see Figure 12.10 for a review of Mrs. Leon's audiogram).

> Written and oral instructions were provided to Mrs. Leon and her family regarding her hearing aids. A gradual listening program was recommended. Mrs. Leon was instructed to wear the hearing aids initially in quiet environments such as when watching television or having a conversation with one or two people. After she became comfortable using the hearing aids in quiet, she was instructed to wear them in noisier environments. Listening activities were also recommended. Mrs. Leon was instructed to make a list of common, everyday background sounds in her environment (e.g., water running, the refrigerator humming) and to listen to these sounds while wearing the hearing aids. She was informed that these exercises would assist her in relearning how to tune out or ignore the background noises that she may not have heard for quite some time due to her hearing loss.

> A needs assessment tool was administered to her both before and after a trial use period with her hearing aids. She indicated that she wanted to hear the minister in her church during the Sunday sermon. The needs assessment revealed that the hearing aids had achieved this goal for her, thus validating one aspect of the fitting.

Although hearing aids are the most common form of treatment for sensorineural hearing impairment, only one in four individuals with hearing impairments use them (Kochkin, 2009). The low percentage of hearing aid users is likely due to denial, embarrassment, or a belief that a hearing aid will not help. The statistics are unfortunate given the research that shows hearing aid use to be associated with improvements in social, emotional, psychological, and physical well-being (National Council on the Aging, 1999). These improvements in quality of life are found not only for those with severe hearing loss, but for those with mild loss as well.

Technological advances as well as skillful counseling are likely to increase the number of adults who become successful hearing aid users. Two of the strongest predictors of hearing aid success are a patient's motivation and his or her perception of handicap. An individual who purchases a hearing aid because he or she is missing out on conversation during social interactions is much more likely to make a successful adjustment than is a person who has stopped socializing and purchases a hearing aid because of family pressure. Presbycusic listeners with severe central auditory processing disorders are also less likely to benefit from wearing hearing aids.

Assistive Listening and Alerting Devices

An **assistive listening device** is any device, excluding hearing aids, designed to improve a hearing-impaired individual's ability to communicate and therefore function more independently than without the device. Closed captioning of television broadcasts is one example of an assistive device that can be used in the home. A **closed caption decoder** displays the television dialogue in written form at the bottom of the television screen. Many public venues, such as theaters and meeting halls, are equipped with frequency-modulated or **FM systems**, infrared systems or teleloop systems. These systems use special forms of energy conversion (such as light, radio frequency, or electromagnetic) to send signals such as a speaker's voice or a movie sound track to a listener equipped with a receiver and earphones or a hearing aid with an appropriate connection. Because these systems are wireless, the hearing-impaired individual and the talker are able to move around freely within the listening environment. Other types of assistive listening devices are designed for one-on-one communication. For example, a simple amplified handset is often sufficient to allow the hearing-impaired individual to communicate over the telephone. For more profound hearing losses, the telephone message can be typed by a relay operator and transmitted to a special **telecommunication device for the deaf (TDD)** for the hearing-impaired individual to read. Special captioned telephones and Internet services can also convert speech to a written message to be displayed to the listener.

In addition to assistive listening devices, **alerting devices** are also available. These include devices that provide a visual signal for common environmental sounds (e.g., the ringing of a phone or a doorbell), vibrotactile devices, such as an alarm clock that vibrates the pillow, or special smoke alarms. Finally, hearing-ear dogs are also trained to help alert their owners to auditory signals.

Not all hearing-impaired persons come to the audiologist's office with the intent to purchase hearing aids or assistive listening and alerting devices. Mrs. Lough is an example of a client who continued to deny that she had a hearing problem and had no intention of trying amplification.

> *Mrs. Lough* came in for testing urged by her husband, who was having difficulty communicating with her. He reported that when she does not hear him (which is most of the time), he raises his voice, and then Mrs. Lough gets angry because she feels like he is yelling at her. Mrs. Lough's first comment to the audiologist was "I hope you're not going to fit me with hearing aids because I don't want them." She had tried hearing aids twice previously at other clinics and was very dissatisfied with them. The hearing evaluation was performed, and as Figure 12.14 indicates, Mrs. Lough had a moderate sensorineural hearing loss in both ears. Her word recognition ability was fair at a high presentation level. Once the testing was completed, the audiologist used a handheld amplifier to describe the hearing impairment and its implications for understanding speech. Oral and written information was provided to Mrs. Lough and her husband about hearing aids (what hearing aids could and could not do) and strategies that could facilitate the communication process. Assistive listening devices were also discussed as an alternative to hearing aids. Mrs. Lough was resistant to purchasing any type of amplification, including assistive listening devices.

Unfortunately, sometimes counseling cannot undo the negative impact of prior bad experiences with amplification or poor motivation to communicate

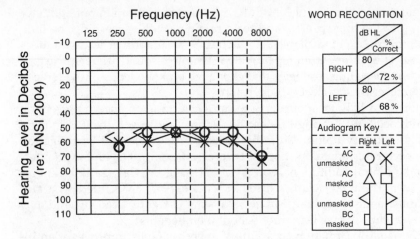

FIGURE 12.14 Audiogram of a moderate sensorineural hearing loss with fair word recognition ability. Although amplification would make more speech sounds audible to this client, she refused to try it.

more effectively. To benefit from amplification, a patient must accept the hearing loss and be ready to work with the audiologist to improve his or her communication abilities.

Cochlear Implants

For those with severe to profound hearing loss who do not benefit substantially from amplification, cochlear implants might be recommended. When implanted in adulthood, the cochlear implant has been more successful in adults with acquired hearing loss than with adults who have been deaf since childhood. As we saw in Chapter 11, the implant consists of multiple electrodes surgically placed within the cochlea. The electrodes conduct electrical current that directly stimulates auditory nerve fibers to produce hearing sensations. Audiologists play an important role in education and counseling of potential candidates for cochlear implants. Although inserted into the cochlea by a surgeon, the audiologist activates and maps the implant approximately four weeks after surgery. Mapping involves determining the appropriate levels of electrical stimulation for each electrode. The audiologist also participates in the follow-up and long-term rehabilitation plan that involves teaching the client to use available auditory cues in conjunction with speechreading.

Auditory Training and Speechreading

Historically, **auditory training** and speechreading were used to teach children who were deafened before or shortly after birth to understand speech. However,

> Wireless technologies provide a means to amplifiy the sound of a movie or television program, without increasing other sounds in the environment.

> When an adult with an acquired sensorineural hearing loss gets a cochlear implant, the brain relearns how to interpret the neural signals from the ear.

these techniques may be useful for adults who use amplification but still have difficulty understanding speech. Auditory training involves teaching the individual to optimize use of available sound cues. Several approaches to auditory training exist. These range from repetitively listening to sound sequences (e.g., /ba/ vs. /da/) to teaching strategies that capitalize on knowledge of the topic of conversation to assist speech comprehension.

The short- and long-term effects of auditory training on speech perception in those with acquired hearing loss are not known. However, there is indirect evidence that auditory training in individuals learning a second language can facilitate speech discrimination (Logan, Lively, & Pisoni, 1991) and even effect changes in the central auditory nervous system (Kraus, McGee, Carrell, King, & Tremblay, 1995; Tremblay, Kraus, Carrell, & McGee, 1997). Structured programs to assist adults to improve their listening skills are currently available and may prove to be beneficial as we learn more about their benefits.

Adding visual information to auditory speech signals improves identification relative to auditory input alone (Hardison, 1998). **Speechreading** is a technique that capitalizes on this improvement. In face-to-face communication, listeners can improve their ability to understand speech considerably by watching the speaker's mouth as words are formed (Sumby & Pollack, 1954). Attending to the speaker's face provides information about the place of articulation (see Chapter 3). This provides a significant benefit because these acoustic cues are most severely affected by background noise and high-frequency hearing loss.

> For those who wear glasses, do you ever feel like you can't *hear* without your glasses on? Why is that?

The ability to speechread varies widely across individuals. However, there are some factors that can increase the likelihood of success (see also Montgomery, 1993, for suggestions to maximize speechreading in combination with amplification). Training in speechreading might include strategies such as making sure that a speaker's face is visible and well lit so that mouth movements and position of the articulators can be seen. A client also learns to focus on understanding phrases and ideas, rather than phonemes and words.

Counseling and Communication Strategies

The audiologist provides critical information to the client and significant others. Individuals must understand the nature of their hearing impairment and its implications for day-to-day life. Furthermore, it is important for hearing-impaired individuals and their significant others to understand the limits of available technologies and rehabilitative methods. For example, the client should understand that hearing aids will not restore normal hearing. Strategies to improve the communication process are also discussed with the patient and family members. Kaplan (1988) listed several strategies that can be used by both the hearing-impaired person and the person speaking. For example, the client with a hearing loss may be advised to ask a speaker to repeat or rephrase a statement that was not understood. Hearing-impaired individuals are also counseled to read reviews prior to seeing a movie to better follow the plot. Significant others might be advised to face the client when speaking and to talk more slowly.

In addition to informational counseling, the audiologist must be sensitive to how an individual reacts to his or her hearing impairment and to any psychosocial adjustment problems related to the impairment. Tanner (1980) provided an excellent article about loss related to communication disorders and Kübler-Ross's (1969) five stages of the grieving process (i.e., denial, anger, bargaining, depression, acceptance). It is important to keep in mind that an individual may not only be grieving the loss of hearing but also the loss of independence, vocation, or self-identity. Support groups for persons with hearing loss offer an excellent opportunity to share experiences and feelings with others experiencing similar problems.

Support Groups

Members of national and local support groups work together to improve communication and teach self-management skills. Information about hearing impairment is often provided at support group meetings, as are discussions about communication problems and solutions. The meetings provide an opportunity for the hearing-impaired individual to practice assertive communication strategies in a nonthreatening environment. The groups also offer opportunities for members to be proactive in political issues related to the civil rights of those with a hearing loss. For example, members of Self-Help for the Hard of Hearing (SHHH, now the Hearing Loss Association of America, HLAA) were actively involved in developing regulations for section 255 of the Telecommunications Act of 1996. This section requires telecommunication products and services to be accessible to people with disabilities. The group was also instrumental in developing regulations for the Americans with Disabilities Act (ADA) of 1990. The ADA was designed to ensure that those with disabilities (including hearing loss) are not discriminated against in employment, public accommodations, transportation, state and local government services, and telecommunications.

Clinical Problem Solving

Mr. Westrich, age 76, reported that he has difficulty understanding his wife and grandchildren when they talk. He also has difficulty understanding speakers on television. He suggested that "all newscasters must go to the same school of mumbling." At family gatherings, he relies on his wife to repeat what people have said and often gets left out of conversations. He was a pilot in the military for thirty years and enjoyed hunting before he retired. Figure 12.15 displays his audiogram and word-recognition ability.

1. What type of hearing loss does Mr. Westrich have?
2. What factors are likely to have contributed to Mr. Westrich's hearing loss?

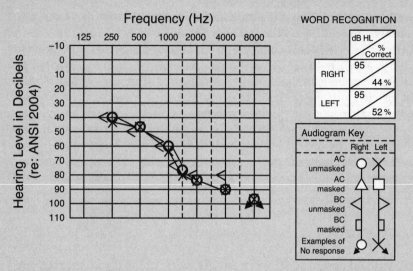

FIGURE 12.15 Audiogram of a client who came to the clinic because of difficulties communicating with his family.

3. What types of speech sounds will be the most difficult for Mr. Westrich to understand?
4. Is Mr. Westrich a candidate for amplification? Why or why not?
5. What types of communication strategies might Mr. Westrich use when communicating? What might the speaker do to facilitate Mr. Westrich's speech understanding?

REFERENCES

American Speech-Language-Hearing Association (ASHA). (1995, February). Report on audiological screening. *American Journal of Audiology, 4,* 24–40.

American Speech-Language-Hearing Association (ASHA). (1997). *Guidelines for audiologic screening* (pp. 49–59). Rockville, MD: Author.

American Speech-Language-Hearing Association (ASHA). (1998). Guidelines for hearing aid fitting for adults. *American Journal of Audiology, 7,* 5–13.

American Speech-Language-Hearing Association (ASHA). (2002). *Knowledge and skills required for the practice of audiologic/aural rehabilitation.* Rockville, MD: Author.

Americans With Disabilities Act of 1990, Pub. L. No. 101–336, §2, 104 Stat. 328 (1991).

Balloh, R. W. (1998). *Dizziness, hearing loss, and tinnitus.* Philadelphia: F.A. Davis.

Erber, N. P., & Heine, C. (1996). Screening receptive communication of older adults in residential care. *American Journal of Audiology, 5,* 38–46.

Hardison, D. M. (1998). Acquisition of second-language speech: Effects of visual cues, context and talker variability (Doctoral dissertation, Indiana University, 1998). *Dissertation Abstracts International, 59*(5-A), Z5053.

Kaplan, H. (1988). Communication problems of the hearing-impaired elderly: What can be done? *Pride Institute Journal of Long Term Home Health Care, 7,* 10–22.

Kochkin S. (2009). MarkeTrak VIII: 25-year trends in the hearing health market. *Hearing Review, 16,* 12–31.

Kraus, N., McGee, T., Carrell, T. D., King, C., & Tremblay, K. (1995). Central auditory system plasticity associated with speech discrimination training. *Journal of Cognitive Neuroscience, 7,* 25–32.

Kübler-Ross, E. (1969). *On death and dying.* New York: Macmillan.

Logan, J. S., Lively, S. E., & Pisoni, D. B. (1991). Training Japanese listeners to identify /r/ and /l/: A first report. *Journal of the Acoustical Society of America, 89,* 874–886.

Martin, F. N., & Clark, J. G. (2011). *Introduction to audiology* (11th ed.). Boston: Pearson/ Allyn & Bacon.

Matthews, L. J., Lee, F., Mills, J. H., & Schum, D. J. (1990). Audiometric and subjective assessment of hearing handicap. *Archives of Otolaryngology—Head and Neck Surgery, 116,* 1325–1330.

Montgomery, A. A. (1993). Management of the hearing-impaired adult. In J. Alpiner & P. McCarthy (Eds.), *Rehabilitative audiology: Children and adults* (pp. 311–330). Baltimore: Williams & Wilkins.

Mueller, H., & Killion, M. (1990). An easy method for calculating the articulation index. *Hearing Journal, 3,* 14–17.

National Institute on Deafness and Other Communication Disorders. (2011, February). Noise-induced hearing loss. Retrieved September 7, 2011, from www.nidcd.nih.gov/ health/hearing/noise.html#who

National Institute on Deafness and Other Communication Disorders. (2010, June). Quick statistics. Retrieved August 16, 2011, from www.nidcd.nih.gov/health/statistics/ quick.htm

National Council on the Aging. (1999). *The consequences of untreated hearing loss in older persons.* Conducted by the Seniors Research Group. Retrieved March 23, 2007, from www.ncoa.org/ news/hearing/01_intro.htm

National Institute on Deafness and Other Communication Disorders. (2010, September). *Ménière's disease.* Retrieved August 16, 2011, from www.nidcd.nih.gov/health/balance/meniere.html.

Northern, J. L., & Downs, M. P. (2002). *Hearing in children* (5th ed.). Baltimore: Lippincott Williams & Wilkins.

Olsen, W., Hawkins, D., & Van Tasell, D. (1987). Representations of the long-term spectra of speech. *Ear and Hearing, 8*(5), 1003–1085.

Pearson, J. D., Morrell, C. H., Gordon-Salant, S., Brant, L. J., Metter, E. J., Klein, L. L., & Fozard, J. L. (1995). Gender differences in a longitudinal study of age-associated hearing loss. *Journal of the Acoustical Society of America, 97,* 1196–1205.

Sahyoun, N. R., Pratt, L. A., Lentzner, H., Dey, A., & Robinson, K. N. (2001). *The changing profile of nursing home residents: 1985–1997.* Aging Trends, No. 4. Hyattsville, MD: National Center for Health Statistics. Retrieved March 23, 2007, from www.cdc.gov/ nchs/data/agingtrends/04nursin.pdf

Schow, R., & Nerbonne, M. (1980). Hearing level in nursing home residents. *Journal of Speech and Hearing Disorders, 45,* 124–132.

Stach, B. A., Spretnjak, M. L., & Jerger, J. (1990). The prevalence of central presbycusis in a clinical population. *Journal of the American Academy of Audiology, 1,* 109–115.

Sumby, W. G., & Pollack, I. (1954). Visual contributions to speech intelligibility in noise. *Journal of the Acoustical Society of America, 26,* 212–215.

Tanner, D. (1980). Loss and grief: Implications for the speech-language pathologist and audiologist. *Asha, 22,* 916–928.

Thibodeau, L. M., & Schmitt, J. (1988). A report on condition of hearing aids in nursing homes and retirement centers. *Journal of the American Academy of Audiology, 21,* 99–112.

Tremblay, K., Kraus, N., Carrell, T. D., & McGee, T. (1997). Central auditory system plasticity: Generalization to novel stimuli following listening training. *Journal of the Acoustical Society of America, 102,* 3762–3773.

Weinstein, B. E., & Amsel, L. (1986). Hearing loss and senile dementia in the institutionalized elderly. *Clinical Gerontology, 4,* 3–15.

Weinstein, B. E., & Ventry, I. M. (1983). Audiometric correlates of hearing handicapped inventory for the elderly. *Journal of Speech and Hearing Disorders, 48,* 379–384.

READINGS FROM THE POPULAR LITERATURE

Biderman, B. (1998). *Wired for sound: A journey into hearing.* Toronto: Trifolium Books. (cochlear implant to restore hearing)

Chorost, M. (2006). *Rebuilt: My journey back to the hearing world.* New York: Mariner Books. (cochlear implant in adult years)

Harvey, M. (2004). *Odyssey of hearing loss: Tales of triumph.* San Diego, CA: DawnSign Press. (10 individual accounts of deafness)

LaCrosse, B. (2003). *Silent ears, silent hearts: A deaf man's journey through two worlds.* Roseville, MI: Deaf Understanding. (Deaf culture)

Lane, H. (2000). *The mask of benevolence: Disabling the Deaf community.* San Diego: Dawn Sign Press. (deafness)

Lane, H., Bahan, B., & Hoffmeister, R. (1996). *A journey into the Deaf world.* San Diego: Dawn Sign Press. (Deaf culture)

Merker, H. (1999). *Listening.* Dallas: Southern Methodist University Press. (sudden adult-onset hearing loss)

Nieminen, R. (1990). *Voyage to the island.* Washington, DC: Gallaudet University Press. (deaf woman, teaching deaf children)

Niesser, A. (1990). *The other side of silence.* Washington, DC: Gallaudet Press. (deafness)

Padden, C., & Humphries, T. (1990). *Deaf in America: Voices from a culture.* Cambridge, MA: Harvard University Press. (Deaf culture)

Romoff, A. (1999). *Hear again: Back to life with a cochlear implant.* New York: League for the Hard of Hearing Publications. (adult restoration of hearing via implant)

Sacks, O. (1989). *Seeing voices: A journey into the world of the deaf.* New York: Harper Perennial. (deafness and Deaf culture)

Schaller, S. (1995). *A man without words.* Berkeley: University of California Press. (adult learning to talk)

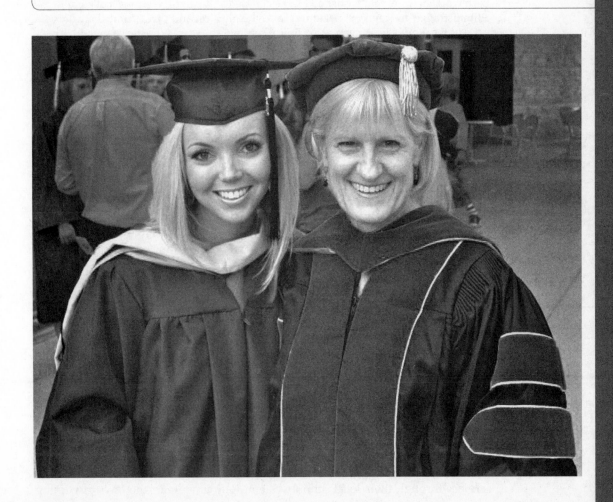

CHAPTER 13

Professional Issues

PREVIEW

In this book, we have reviewed normal communication processes and disorders of communication that require the professional services of speech-language pathologists and audiologists. Along the way, we have introduced various aspects of clinical practice. In this final chapter, we will provide an overview of professional work settings, discuss interdisciplinary interactions, and address some professional issues such as standards, ethics, and certification requirements. Future advances in the understanding of communication processes and disorders will influence approaches to evaluation and treatment. In addition, professional practice patterns are likely to undergo change in response to social, political, and economic influences. In this final chapter, we will provide personal insights from colleagues regarding the actual practice of the professions, and will touch on some foreseeable future trends.

Speech-language pathologists and audiologists work in a variety of settings. Each work environment is shaped by the clinical caseload, professional colleagues, administrative and support personnel, and the physical and procedural characteristics of the work site. A change in clinical setting can mean a drastic change in the characteristics of one's employment. Some professionals enjoy the opportunity to shift the nature of their work by changing clinical environments over the course of their career. Even those who remain in one type of setting are likely to experience considerable variety in their professional activities from day to day and year to year.

Clinical Settings

School Settings

Public and private schools employ 54 percent of all speech-language pathologists and 9 percent of all audiologists, making them the most common work settings for ASHA members (ASHA, 2010b). The start of school-based speech and hearing programs dates back to 1910 in the Chicago public school system (Paden, 1970). Programs developed because educators recognized that speech and hearing problems affected performance in the classroom, and they deemed it appropriate to provide services onsite. The scope of public school services has expanded over the years to include any child who has a communication disorder that negatively affects his or her education. Services for "educationally handicapped children" became nationwide in 1975 with the passage of Public Law 94-142, the Education for All Handicapped Children Act. Subsequent public laws were passed that govern services for children within the schools. Public Law 95-561 expanded remedial services by providing federal support to improve children's basic educational skills, including listening and speaking. With the passage of Public Law 99-457 in 1986, preschool children who appear to have a speech, language, or hearing problem became eligible for assessment and remediation services through their local school system. Refinements in the laws governing

> Approximately half of all speech-language pathologists are employed in school settings.

service delivery to infants, preschoolers, and school-age children continue with the most recent legislation, the No Child Left Behind Act of 2001 and the Individuals with Disabilities Education Improvement Act (IDEA) of 2004. The public schools also conduct periodic hearing screening programs that may involve the direct or indirect participation of the audiologist.

Speech-language pathologists in the public schools may work with children individually, in small groups, or in an entire classroom. The caseload can vary from multiply handicapped children to those with specific speech or language difficulties. Some professionals serve children in only one school, whereas others are itinerant, traveling to several schools. Audiologists provide a range of services to public school children, including screening, diagnostic, and aural habilitation programs. They also assist students with the wide variety of personal and classroom amplification systems. One notable feature of work in the public school setting is the nine- to ten-month academic calendar, with a long summer break or extended breaks throughout the year. This schedule holds appeal for some professionals, particularly if their own children are of school age.

> Nearly three-quarters of all audiologists are employed in medical settings.

Medical Settings

Medical settings are the second most common employment sites for speech, language, and hearing professionals. In 2010, 72 percent of audiologists and 38 percent of speech-language pathologists worked in medical settings (ASHA, 2010b). These work sites include a broad spectrum of health care delivery environments, including hospital-based acute care and rehabilitation units, inpatient and outpatient rehabilitation facilities, residential health care facilities, private practice offices, and medical clinics. Even within one hospital, speech-language pathologists and audiologists may work in a variety of settings. In the 1970s and 1980s, it was common for audiology and speech-language pathology to comprise a single unified department, but that is no longer standard practice. In most hospitals, speech-language pathologists and audiologists are members of various medical teams or departments within the hospital. For example, audiologists may be associated with otolaryngology or physical medicine and rehabilitation. Speech-language pathologists are often members of multidisciplinary teams that focus on different stages of the rehabilitation process, from acute to subacute to outpatient rehabilitation. Similarly, some teams focus on specific disorders, such as dysphagia or cognitive assessment and rehabilitation. It is most common for speech-language pathologists to work within a rehabilitation department, but in some hospitals they may be allied with other medical specialties, such as neurology, neurosurgery, pediatrics, surgery, or physical and rehabilitation medicine. The particular demands of medical settings have been addressed in several excellent resources, including a practitioner's guide (Johnson & Jacobson, 2007) and the *Journal of Medical Speech-Language Pathology.*

Just as clinical practice in the public schools has been influenced by public laws, service delivery in medical settings is greatly influenced by forces such as health care legislation, managed care, and health insurance policies. Hospital stays have shortened considerably in recent years, and there has been an increase in service delivery in the home, provided through home health care agencies. Patients tend to receive therapy for shorter durations than in the past, and clinicians must clearly justify their patients' need for therapy and the benefits of their services. These changes have been accompanied by an emphasis on the functional outcomes of treatment, so that clinicians focus on very practical aspects of the patients' needs and how treatment will make a difference in their everyday lives.

Academic and Clinical Training Programs

Clinical training in the evaluation and treatment of communication disorders is conducted in many colleges and universities. The departments that provide coursework and professional preparation in speech-language pathology and audiology have various names, such as Speech, Language, and Hearing Sciences, Audiology and Speech-Language Pathology, and Communication Disorders. Clinical training involves academic course work at the undergraduate and graduate levels and supervised clinical training. Most university programs include an on-campus clinic for student training opportunities and off-campus practicum training with cooperating clinical placement sites in the community. University clinics typically serve both children and adults who have hearing, language, articulation, voice, and fluency problems. The clinics may offer students the opportunity to observe evaluation and treatment procedures in communication disorders prior to beginning direct clinical work. They also provide supervised clinical training for graduate students. Many training programs confer bachelor's, master's, and doctoral degrees.

University programs also contribute to the knowledge base of the professions through the conduct of basic and applied research. The research endeavors within a particular department reflect the areas of interest of faculty members. Students may become involved in research in a variety of informal and formal ways through work-study programs, volunteering, independent study, and thesis options. Research doctoral degree programs (e.g., PhD, ScD) are research oriented and require completion of original research in the form of a dissertation. There are also doctoral programs that focus on the clinical aspects of the professions, such as the AuD, doctorate of audiology, which is the entry level degree for clinical practice in audiology. A small number of institutions offer a clinical doctorate in speech-language pathology.

Community Speech and Hearing Centers

Many of the first speech and hearing service programs in the United States were provided in community speech and hearing centers. Such clinics are often housed in freestanding buildings rather than within an educational or medical facility. Community clinics are not as common as they once were, but those that still exist often derive some of their financial support from supplemental sources.

For example, they may be funded by agencies such as the United Way or county public health programs, philanthropic groups such as Scottish Rite, or national organizations such as the Easter Seal Society. The clientele may be specific to certain disorders, such as children with cerebral palsy, or may include a wide variety of disorders that affect individuals of all ages.

Private Practice

Some audiologists and speech-language pathologists provide clinical services in private practice settings. In 2010, 19 percent of certified audiologists were in full-time private practice, and another 8 percent worked in part-time private practice. In speech-language pathology, about 6 percent of certified professionals were in full-time private practice, and another 11 percent worked part-time in private practice (ASHA, 2010b). These individuals may provide services in their own office, at patients' homes, or through contractual arrangements with other care providers (e.g., hospitals, schools, nursing facilities). Practitioners who work part-time in a private practice may spend the rest of the day in another clinical setting (such as a public school or hospital). Private practitioners treat a wide variety of disorders. Adults may seek a private practice speech-language pathologist to continue treatment for a chronic condition, such as aphasia or a motor speech disorder. Parents may contract a private practitioner to supplement the services their child receives through the schools or to treat conditions not otherwise covered in school-based programs (e.g., tongue thrust). Schools, hospitals, and other agencies may contract with private practitioners in order to relieve personnel shortages. In such cases, the private practitioner operates as an independent contractor to these businesses and organizations rather than as one of their employees. This autonomy often appeals to clinicians who choose to maintain a private practice.

Interdisciplinary Interactions

Almost all speech-language pathologists and audiologists work in conjunction with other professionals to some degree. Some of the cases presented earlier in this text provide examples of interdisciplinary interactions in the treatment of communication disorders. We can find out more about the nature of these interactions by reading about the experiences of clinicians who work on interdisciplinary teams. We will also consider the professionals who comprise these teams and work with speech-language pathologists and audiologists in a variety of settings.

Team Approach in Public Schools

We begin with professionals who work with children in a public school setting. These individuals are jointly involved at all levels of case management, from the initial referral through the day-to-day implementation of therapy goals.

Patty is a speech-language pathologist with ten years' experience in the public school setting. She currently works with Cheryl, an occupational therapist (OT), and Jean, a physical therapist (PT), along with psychologists and several preschool and special education teachers. "An obvious motor impairment or speech-language problem is usually the cause for referral at our center. But often, with years of experience, you can just watch a child and know that this child needs to be seen by other professionals," Cheryl reported. The initial screening team in this school consisted of the classroom teacher, speech-language pathologist, and psychologist, with additional professionals brought in as needed.

All team members participate in joint evaluation of the child. However, their participation fluctuates according to the relevance of each assessment task to their area of expertise. For example, Patty may do the formal language testing of a child, but she may also observe during the PT's assessment of gross motor activities, because she knows that children are likely to use the most spontaneous language during that time. Cheryl reported that the group has come to work smoothly because each has gotten to know what the others do. "Initially, it was intimidating, not knowing when it was my turn to do something. Then [over time] it just kind of smoothed out." "We pretty much follow the child's lead," added Patty. "When I'm preparing my next set of materials, Cheryl is already in there doing her next activity. The nice thing is it really speeds up the evaluation, so the child doesn't get bored."

The group pointed out several factors that made their work as an evaluation team effective. "First, it really helped that we all had experience with this population. Then, it was a matter of picking up on each other's pace," reported Jean. Patty added, "It's also a matter of knowing which activities are most likely to provide me with language information. Or when I'm presenting information, Cheryl might say, 'You want to hold that at an angle because you can tell he's got low vision,' which helps me get optimal performance." The group agreed that teams work well when there is a respect for other professions and some knowledge of what each can contribute. The members must understand that the domains represented by each profession really do affect one another. As Cheryl put it, "I think that if you go in thinking that your own profession is the only one that is going to make a difference for the child, you're missing out on an integrated picture of the whole child."

This group offered many examples of ways in which the goals of different therapists interrelate for a particular child. For example, the positioning guidelines from the physical therapist may also be used by the occupational therapist and speech-language pathologist to provide the stability the child needs for learning to occur. To maximize their efforts, the therapists often develop methods that address multiple goals at the same time.

Patty related, "If I am working to increase requests by a child, I can have the child ask for materials during an art project. When the request is made, I hand the crayon or straw to the child. I can do that in a way that reinforces the reaching or grasping behaviors I know Cheryl is working on as well." Often, motor activities can serve as the reinforcement for training speech goals. One popular activity is an obstacle course that primarily serves OT and PT goals. Children are "allowed" to run the course after producing three correct articulation targets. Jean remarked that she often watches Patty to see the level at which she presents language to the child: "It doesn't do me any good if a child can't perform a movement because he didn't understand my directions." In return, Patty has "borrowed" techniques from both Cheryl and Jean because she has noticed their effectiveness in helping children maintain their attention during various activities.

In the example above, we have seen how some professionals may work together in public schools. Let us now take a closer look at the professional interactions of a speech-language pathologist in a pediatric clinic.

Team Approach in a Pediatric Clinic

Lora is a speech-language pathologist who serves as the coordinator of her hospital's cleft palate team (see Chapter 4 for a discussion of this condition). This team consists of an audiologist, geneticist, nurse, otolaryngologist (ENT), pediatrician, plastic surgeon, dentist, orthodontist, prosthodontist, and social worker, all of whom interact as a full team or as individuals with the parents and child.

"We get notified [that a child has been born with a cleft palate] from the birthing clinic. If it's feasible, we try to do a hospital visit within that first 24 to 48 hours," Lora reports. This visit usually involves a speech-language pathologist, a social worker, and a nurse. These individuals provide the parents with initial information concerning their child's condition, what can be done, and what to expect as the child develops. Lora also provides important information about feeding the child. Lora commented, "We feel that this early visit provides a valuable service."

Soon after, the audiologist will see the child to evaluate hearing status and to counsel the parents about possible concerns with hearing health as their child develops. Other early appointments will be with the geneticist, ear-nose-throat doctor, and the plastic surgeon. "As the child grows," related Lora, "he or she will be seeing the ENT, plastic surgeon, and some of the other team members on a regular basis. Then our program requires that the child visit the entire team, which meets once a month, for certain procedures to be approved. They want [the treatment] to be a team consensus to be sure that it is the appropriate treatment for the child." Procedures that routinely involve team discussion include pharyngeal flap, bone grafts, and lip and nose revisions. The team may brainstorm ideas about the timing and course of treatment, taking into consideration the various aspects of the child's condition.

The team meeting starts with a preconference. "I type a summary of what surgeries have already been done, the diagnosis, presenting concerns, and [histories of all other services] ahead of time," reported Lora. "One of the physicians will act as the presenting or attending physician, who will say what the main concerns are. If any questions come up right then, we will discuss them." Then the parents come into the meeting, and the team members have an opportunity to examine the child. This is also an opportunity for the parents to provide all the professionals with input on treatment decisions and to ask questions about possible future intervention. "We really try to encourage the parents to consider themselves a member of the team," said Lora, "and I know that it can sometimes be a bit intimidating for some of them."

The team meeting is an opportunity for the parents and professionals to see how all the components of intervention come together for the child. Through these meetings, Lora has learned from the other professionals about state-of-the-art techniques for the management of cleft palate. In addition, she has provided the team with valued contributions. She provides this example: "I've had to sell the team on the usefulness of videoendoscopy (see Chapter 6), and they've pretty much bought into it now. We've had a couple of cases where we discovered that the child didn't need surgery [based on the videoendoscopy results]. I feel really good about how that has developed." Lora concludes with this thought, "I know that I have grown tremendously in this role professionally. I used to be so intimidated. I would dread the conference and I would know inside 'Oh, it's three days away,' and now I've been doing it for six years. I've grown much more confident. Over time, I've earned the other team members' respect. And I had to earn it."

Team Approach in a Medical Setting

Tom is a speech-language pathologist with twelve years of professional experience. Most of his work has been in medical settings with adults with acquired communication disorders, typically related to stroke or head injury. Tom currently works in a hospital-based skilled nursing unit that provides subacute care. The patients in the program are medically stable, but in need of rehabilitation and nursing care. Many of them were transferred to the unit after a stay in the acute care unit of the hospital, where they were admitted following a medically significant event, such as a stroke. Other patients were admitted directly to the subacute unit for a period of diagnostic and rehabilitative care to improve their independent living skills. Although the facility where Tom works is in a hospital setting, many skilled nursing facilities are not located on a hospital campus.

Tom is part of a multidisciplinary rehabilitation team that includes a physical therapist, occupational therapist, dietician, nurse, and medical doctor. His workspace is part of a common rehabilitation area where the physical therapist and occupational therapist also work with patients. Interdisciplinary interaction is completely natural and occurs in both planned and spontaneous ways. For example, Tom had a patient who fatigued easily and had a limited amount of time when he was awake, alert, and able to participate in therapy. In order to maximize the patient's optimal treatment time, Tom conducted speech and language therapy at the same time that the PT was working with the patient on balance. The simultaneous attention to two tasks, balance and speech, offered an additional challenge to the patient that was more representative of real life than treating each in isolation. In other cases, therapy goals may be common across several disciplines and may be referred to as *conjoint treatment goals*. Tom told of a patient with a hip fracture who could not remember the precautions he was given by the physical therapist to protect his healing hip; therefore, part of the cognitive training that Tom implemented with this patient included strategies to assist him in learning the hip precautions. In this case, all of the therapies had common treatment goals that related to safety and achieving independent living.

Team interaction is a big part of what Tom enjoys about his current job. In fact, he selected his current work site because the team approach appealed to him. He said, "it is important to go beyond what you have been taught" to be successful in a given setting. Working side by side with other professionals is one way to continually expand and integrate professional knowledge.

The Professional Association: The American Speech-Language-Hearing Association

History and Purpose

The professions of speech-language pathology and audiology emerged and grew over the course of the twentieth century. In the early 1900s the focus was on speech disorders, particularly articulation and stuttering. In 1925, a group of professionals devoted to the treatment of communication disorders started an association called the American Academy for Speech Correction (Paden, 1970). The profession of audiology developed after World War II, owing to the needs of many soldiers who returned home with acquired hearing loss (Cherry & Giolas, 1997). As the audiology profession was established, audiologists were included among the ranks of professionals dealing with communication disorders. In 1948, the professional organization became the American Speech and Hearing Association (ASHA; asha.org). As clinical attention to language impairments increased, the profession changed the name again in 1978 to the American Speech-Language-Hearing Association, although the ASHA acronym was retained. Currently, about 145,000 speech-language pathologists, audiologists, and speech, language, and hearing scientists hold ASHA membership (ASHA, 2010b). Another relevant organization is the American Academy of Audiology, which has a membership of more than 10,000 audiologists who are "dedicated to providing quality hearing care services through professional development, education, research, and increased public awareness of hearing and balance disorders" (American Academy of Audiology, 2011).

Although there are other related professional organizations to which audiologists and speech-language pathologists belong, ASHA is the primary professional organization for speech, language, and hearing professionals. The mission of ASHA is to promote the interests of the professions and to advocate for people with communication disabilities. The purposes are reflected in the Association bylaws (ASHA, 2008), which are paraphrased here:

1. To encourage basic scientific study of the processes of individual human communication with special reference to speech, language, hearing, and related disorders.
2. To promote high standards and ethics for the academic and clinical preparation of individuals entering the discipline of human communication sciences and disorders.
3. To promote the acquisition of new knowledge and skills for those within the discipline.
4. To promote investigation, prevention, and the diagnosis and treatment of disorders of human communication and related disorders.
5. To foster improvement of clinical services and intervention procedures concerning such disorders.
6. To stimulate exchange of information among persons and organizations, and to disseminate such information.
7. To inform the public about communication sciences and disorders, related disorders, and the professionals who provide services.
8. To advocate on behalf of persons with communication and related disorders, such as dysphagia.
9. To promote the individual and collective professional interests of the members of the Association.

ASHA is an organization that is intended to serve the interests of the membership. There are two bodies that govern and establish the policies of the Association: the Legislative Council and the Executive Board. The Legislative Council establishes the policies of the organization and is composed of elected representatives from every state; the Executive Board consists of officers elected by the ASHA membership, as well as the Executive Director of the Association. Many of the ASHA policies, such as defining the scope of practice of the professions, have significant impact on speech-language pathologists and audiologists, and therefore are of great interest to members of the Association. The executive board also manages the affairs of the Association, and board members often serve as official representatives of the Association. The committees, task forces, and boards that operate within the ASHA structure provide opportunities for the membership to significantly contribute to the professions.

Certification and Accreditation

Most practitioners in speech-language pathology and audiology in the United States are members of ASHA and have received the Certificate of Clinical Competence (CCC) in audiology, speech-language pathology, or both, from ASHA. To be eligible to obtain the CCC, ASHA requires the completion of graduate course work and graduate clinical practicum from a program certified by ASHA (ASHA, 2005, 2009). Academic preparation includes basic sciences and professional coursework that meets the ASHA standards. Clinical observation and supervised practicum must be completed across a range of ages and disorders as specified by ASHA (2005). Following the completion of the graduate degree, the CCC applicant must spend a Clinical Fellowship Year (CFY) working in an approved clinical setting under the direct supervision of a clinically certified clinician. The applicant also must pass a certification examination. ASHA membership is not required for certification by the organization, but the number of nonmembers holding certification is small. Most states require a license to practice, although those requirements are often consistent with the standards set forth by ASHA for the CCC. Evidence of continuing education also may be required for periodic state licensure renewal.

Continuing Education

ASHA is devoted to continuing education and advancement of scientific clinical knowledge in the professions. The Association publishes several scholarly journals that are available to members and are carried in many libraries: *American Journal of Audiology; American Journal of Speech-Language Pathology; Journal of Speech, Language, and Hearing Research;* and *Language, Speech, and Hearing Services in Schools.* These journals contain research articles that have been reviewed by experts in the professions (a process called peer review) and have been deemed worthy of publication. A monthly newspaper called *ASHA Leader* helps keep members abreast of current events of interest to the profession. Another continuing education opportunity is provided by the annual ASHA Convention. This convention often draws more than 10,000 participants, who have the opportunity to listen to professional presentations, view new books and clinical materials, and meet for a variety of formal and informal gatherings. Although the ASHA Convention is the largest educational event each year, there are many other learning activities available throughout the year that are sponsored by ASHA, state and local organizations, academic programs, and private groups. The opportunities include workshops, telephone seminars, videoconferences, and electronic learning activities, such as web-based workshops.

Ethical Conduct

A primary concern of ASHA is for certified speech-language pathologists and audiologists to practice their professions ethically. Consequently, all certified audiologists or speech-language pathologists (regardless of ASHA membership) must adhere to the Association's Code of Ethics (ASHA, 2010a). The Code of Ethics provides guidelines for professional practice and is a helpful resource when ethical questions arise (Figure 13.1). A timely example of the value of the Code of Ethics pertains to the discussion of clinical cases via electronic mail and listserv

Code of Ethics

Preamble

The preservation of the highest standards of integrity and ethical principles is vital to the responsible discharge of obligations by speech-language pathologists, audiologists, and speech, language, and hearing scientists. This Code of Ethics sets forth the fundamental principles and rules considered essential to this purpose.

Every individual who is (a) a member of the American Speech-Language-Hearing Association, whether certified or not, (b) a nonmember holding the Certificate of Clinical Competence from the Association, (c) an applicant for membership or certification, or (d) a Clinical Fellow seeking to fulfill standards for certification shall abide by this Code of Ethics.

Any violation of the spirit and purpose of this Code shall be considered unethical. Failure to specify any particular responsibility or practice in this Code of Ethics shall not be construed as denial of the existence of such responsibilities or practices.

The fundamentals of ethical conduct are described by Principles of Ethics and by Rules of Ethics as they relate to the responsibility to persons served, the public, speech-language pathologists, audiologists, and speech, language, and hearing scientists, and to the conduct of research and scholarly activities.

Principles of Ethics, aspirational and inspirational in nature, form the underlying moral basis for the Code of Ethics. Individuals shall observe these principles as affirmative obligations under all conditions of professional activity.

Rules of Ethics are specific statements of minimally acceptable professional conduct or of prohibitions and are applicable to all individuals.

Principle of Ethics I

Individuals shall honor their responsibility to hold paramount the welfare of persons they serve professionally or who are participants in research and scholarly activities, and they shall treat animals involved in research in a humane manner.

Rules of Ethics

A. Individuals shall provide all services competently.
B. Individuals shall use every resource, including referral when appropriate, to ensure that high-quality service is provided.
C. Individuals shall not discriminate in the delivery of professional services or the conduct of research and scholarly activities on the basis of race or ethnicity, gender, gender identity/gender expression, age, religion, national origin, sexual orientation, or disability.
D. Individuals shall not misrepresent the credentials of assistants, technicians, support personnel, students, Clinical Fellows, or any others under their supervision, and they shall inform those they serve professionally of the name and professional credentials of persons providing services.
E. Individuals who hold the Certificate of Clinical Competence shall not delegate tasks that require the unique skills, knowledge, and judgment that are within the scope of their profession to assistants, technicians, support personnel, or any nonprofessionals over whom they have supervisory responsibility.
F. Individuals who hold the Certificate of Clinical Competence may delegate tasks related to provision of clinical services to assistants, technicians, support personnel, or any other persons only if those services are appropriately supervised, realizing that the responsibility for client welfare remains with the certified individual.
G. Individuals who hold the Certificate of Clinical Competence may delegate tasks related to provision of clinical services that require the unique skills, knowledge, and judgment that are within the scope of practice of their profession to students only if those services are appropriately supervised. The responsibility for client welfare remains with the certified individual.
H. Individuals shall fully inform the persons they serve of the nature and possible effects of services rendered and products dispensed, and they shall inform participants in research about the possible effects of their participation in research conducted.
I. Individuals shall evaluate the effectiveness of services rendered and of products dispensed, and they shall provide services or dispense products only when benefit can reasonably be expected.
J. Individuals shall not guarantee the results of any treatment or procedure, directly or by implication; however, they may make a reasonable statement of prognosis.
K. Individuals shall not provide clinical services solely by correspondence.
L. Individuals may practice by telecommunication (e.g., telehealth/e-health), where not prohibited by law.

FIGURE 13.1   ASHA Code of Ethics
Used with permission of the American Speech-Language-Hearing Association.

M. Individuals shall adequately maintain and appropriately secure records of professional services rendered, research and scholarly activities conducted, and products dispensed, and they shall allow access to these records only when authorized or when required by law.

N. Individuals shall not reveal, without authorization, any professional or personal information about identified persons served professionally or identified participants involved in research and scholarly activities unless doing so is necessary to protect the welfare of the person or of the community or is otherwise required by law.

O. Individuals shall not charge for services not rendered, nor shall they misrepresent services rendered, products dispensed, or research and scholarly activities conducted.

P. Individuals shall enroll and include persons as participants in research or teaching demonstrations only if their participation is voluntary, without coercion, and with their informed consent.

Q. Individuals whose professional services are adversely affected by substance abuse or other health-related conditions shall seek professional assistance and, where appropriate, withdraw from the affected areas of practice.

R. Individuals shall not discontinue service to those they are serving without providing reasonable notice.

Principle of Ethics II

Individuals shall honor their responsibility to achieve and maintain the highest level of professional competence and performance.

Rules of Ethics

A. Individuals shall engage in the provision of clinical services only when they hold the appropriate Certificate of Clinical Competence or when they are in the certification process and are supervised by an individual who holds the appropriate Certificate of Clinical Competence.

B. Individuals shall engage in only those aspects of the professions that are within the scope of their professional practice and competence, considering their level of education, training, and experience.

C. Individuals shall engage in lifelong learning to maintain and enhance professional competence and performance.

D. Individuals shall not require or permit their professional staff to provide services or conduct research activities that exceed the staff member's competence, level of education, training, and experience.

E. Individuals shall ensure that all equipment used to provide services or to conduct research and scholarly activities is in proper working order and is properly calibrated.

Principle of Ethics III

Individuals shall honor their responsibility to the public by promoting public understanding of the professions, by supporting the development of services designed to fulfill the unmet needs of the public, and by providing accurate information in all communications involving any aspect of the professions, including the dissemination of research findings and scholarly activities, and the promotion, marketing, and advertising of products and services.

Rules of Ethics

A. Individuals shall not misrepresent their credentials, competence, education, training, experience, or scholarly or research contributions.

B. Individuals shall not participate in professional activities that constitute a conflict of interest.

C. Individuals shall refer those served professionally solely on the basis of the interest of those being referred and not on any personal interest, financial or otherwise.

D. Individuals shall not misrepresent research, diagnostic information, services rendered, results of services rendered, products dispensed, or the effects of products dispensed.

E. Individuals shall not defraud or engage in any scheme to defraud in connection with obtaining payment, reimbursement, or grants for services rendered, research conducted, or products dispensed.

F. Individuals' statements to the public shall provide accurate information about the nature and management of communication disorders, about the professions, about professional services, about products for sale, and about research and scholarly activities.

G. Individuals' statements to the public when advertising, announcing, and marketing their professional services; reporting research results; and promoting products shall adhere to professional standards and shall not contain misrepresentations.

Principle of Ethics IV

Individuals shall honor their responsibilities to the professions and their relationships with colleagues, students, and members of other professions and disciplines.

Rules of Ethics

A. Individuals shall uphold the dignity and autonomy of the professions, maintain harmonious interprofessional and intraprofessional relationships, and accept the professions' self-imposed standards.

B. Individuals shall prohibit anyone under their supervision from engaging in any practice that violates the Code of Ethics.

C. Individuals shall not engage in dishonesty, fraud, deceit, or misrepresentation.

D. Individuals shall not engage in any form of unlawful harassment, including sexual harassment or power abuse.

E. Individuals shall not engage in any other form of conduct that adversely reflects on the professions or on the individual's fitness to serve persons professionally.

F. Individuals shall not engage in sexual activities with clients, students, or research participants over whom they exercise professional authority or power.

G. Individuals shall assign credit only to those who have contributed to a publication, presentation, or product. Credit shall be assigned in proportion to the contribution and only with the contributor's consent.

H. Individuals shall reference the source when using other persons' ideas, research, presentations, or products in written, oral, or any other media presentation or summary.

I. Individuals' statements to colleagues about professional services, research results, and products shall adhere to

FIGURE 13.1 (continued)

prevailing professional standards and shall contain no misrepresentations.

J. Individuals shall not provide professional services without exercising independent professional judgment, regardless of referral source or prescription.

K. Individuals shall not discriminate in their relationships with colleagues, students, and members of other professions and disciplines on the basis of race or ethnicity, gender, gender identity/gender expression, age, religion, national origin, sexual orientation, or disability.

L. Individuals shall not file or encourage others to file complaints that disregard or ignore facts that would disprove the allegation, nor should the Code of Ethics be used for personal reprisal, as a means of addressing personal animosity, or as a vehicle for retaliation.

M. Individuals who have reason to believe that the Code of Ethics has been violated shall inform the Board of Ethics.

N. Individuals shall comply fully with the policies of the Board of Ethics in its consideration and adjudication of complaints of violations of the Code of Ethics.

FIGURE 13.1   (continued)

discussion groups. There are many opportunities for clinicians to solicit the opinions and advice of other professionals regarding the diagnosis or treatment of a particularly difficult or unusual case by Internet and email interactions. When seeking information, common sense would suggest that it would be inappropriate for a clinician to reveal the name or other identifying information about a specific patient in the context of a listserv discussion (Principle I). However, it might not be so obvious that it is unethical to conduct evaluation or treatment solely by correspondence, as indicated by Principle I-I (see Figure 13.1). That principle should caution clinicians who seek and offer advice about practice via email, because there are potential problems when diagnostic treatment suggestions are given by someone who has not seen the actual patient. Therefore, advice proffered by mail (electronic or otherwise) should be taken as suggestions rather than prescriptions for treatment. The Code of Ethics can help clarify these issues for the clinician.

Student Membership

There is a student organization, the National Student Speech Language Hearing Association (NSSLHA), that undergraduate and graduate students may join as they pursue preprofessional education in speech-language pathology, audiology, and the associated sciences. Many colleges and universities have NSSLHA chapters. NSSLHA membership offers students the opportunity to receive professional journals, participate in educational activities, and even become involved in association governance activities. NSSLHA also has its own journal: *Contemporary Issues in Communication Science and Disorders*.

Special Interest Groups

Although members of ASHA are generally trained to manage a broad array of communication disorders, many members have special interests in particular disorders or aspects of the profession. In 1988, special interest divisions were established to allow ASHA members with common interests to identify themselves and affiliate with one another. The groups have different objectives,

TABLE 13.1 Special Interest Groups of the American Speech-Language-Hearing Association

Division 1:	Language Learning and Education
Division 2:	Neurophysiology and Neurogenic Speech and Language Disorders
Division 3:	Voice and Voice Disorders
Division 4:	Fluency and Fluency Disorders
Division 5:	Speech Science and Orofacial Disorders
Division 6:	Hearing and Hearing Disorders: Research and Diagnostics
Division 7:	Aural Rehabilitation and Its Instrumentation
Division 8:	Public Health Issues Related to Hearing and Balance
Division 9:	Hearing and Hearing Disorders in Childhood
Division 10:	Issues in Higher Education
Division 11:	Administration and Supervision
Division 12:	Augmentative and Alternative Communication
Division 13:	Swallowing and Swallowing Disorders (Dysphagia)
Division 14:	Communication Disorders and Sciences in Culturally and Linguistically Diverse Populations
Division 15:	Gerontology
Division 16:	School-Based Issues
Division 17:	Global Issues in Communication Sciences and Related Disorders
Division 18:	Telepractice

but their common purposes are to advance the education of their affiliates and represent their special interests within ASHA. There are eighteen special interest groups, which are listed in Table 13.1. In addition to ASHA members and international affiliates, members of NSSLHA may choose to affiliate with one or more of the divisions, which may provide them with insight into current issues in prospective areas of interest. Affiliation with special interest groups is optional; affiliate dues may be paid at the same time that ASHA or NSSLHA dues are paid.

Trends In the Profession

Specialty Recognition

Professional preparation in speech-language pathology and audiology is relatively broad based, and there are many clinical populations and settings from which to choose. However, many professionals find over time that they tend to specialize in a particular area (or areas) of clinical practice. In 1994, the Legislative Council of ASHA approved a program for specialty recognition within the professions of speech-language pathology and audiology. This voluntary program allows practitioners within a given specialty to petition for the establishment of specialty recognition in their area of expertise. Clinical Specialty Boards established by ASHA oversee the application process, but the initiative to establish specialty recognition comes from a group of professionals in a given practice area. So, in effect, speech-language pathologists and audiologists who have become specialists in a particular area take the responsibility to establish the criteria for such specialization. In some cases, a Special Interest Group may choose to petition for specialty recognition, in other cases, the petitioner may be a related professional organization. The specialty recognition process is in its infancy. Students and new professionals in speech, language, and hearing may be interested in researching the status of specialty recognition as they prepare to enter their profession.

Use of Support Personnel

The use of support personnel is an emerging trend within the professions. There are different levels of support personnel, including speech-language pathology assistants, or aides, audiometric technicians, or audiology assistants. These individuals work in a variety of settings under the supervision of an ASHA-certified speech-language pathologist or audiologist. In a recent national survey, 37 percent of speech-language pathologists and 43 percent of audiologists reported the use of support personnel in their work place (ASHA, 2009). Unlike the requirements for clinical certification of speech-language pathologists and audiologists, there is no widely accepted training standard for support personnel. However, ASHA has provided guidelines for the training, credentialing, use, and supervision of these individuals in clinical and educational settings (ASHA, 2004). In addition, the ASHA Code of Ethics provides principles related to work performed by support personnel. The use of support personnel is intended to occur as an adjunct to and under the supervision of clinically certified personnel. When managed properly, a program that includes both certified personnel and support personnel can be effective. Let's take a look at one such team.

> *Kendall,* an ASHA-certified speech-language pathologist, "inherited" a speech aide when she took a part-time job at a state residential facility for adults with severe developmental disorders. Her aide, Julie, had been working at this center for twenty years, the last six as a speech aide. Julie has a high school education and received on-the-job training for her current position. Kendall and Julie have been working together for three years.

> Kendall is responsible for initial assessments of the center's residents. She interviews the center staff concerning the residents' level of functioning and develops programs designed to increase their functional communication. She discusses a new program with Julie to get her insights on how it might be integrated into the daily activities at the center. Julie is at the center on a daily basis and she oversees the implementation of those programs. She works with the center staff to explain the communication goals and provides them with materials for training the targeted communication behaviors during the day. She also collects and compiles data on the frequency with which goals were addressed by the staff and the effectiveness of the program for a resident.

Julie's duties are fairly typical of support personnel. They include clerical work, making materials for intervention programs, and implementing the programs planned by the certified clinician. Julie's contribution on a daily basis increases frequency of services to the residents beyond what Kendall could provide on her own. Effective use of support personnel may mean that the certified clinician has to rethink the components of his or her job and how to best carry them out.

> "One of the things that has been very important for me in working with my aide was learning to prioritize," said Kendall. "I had to decide which tasks were critical for me to complete and let Julie do the rest."

As Kendall's experience shows, support personnel can make a positive contribution to the professions. However, the use of support personnel in clinical settings is not without controversy. Some clinicians are concerned that bureaucratic decisions will be made that increase the duties of support personnel beyond their training and abilities, eroding the quality of services. Professionals who have had experience working with support personnel have offered guidance for others who might also have the opportunity (Kimbarow, 1997). Their advice includes the following:

- Establish clear guidelines for use of support personnel.
- Establish minimum competencies for the work setting.
- Learn how to supervise and train support personnel.
- Allow for a training period for developing competencies before working with patients.
- Explain the rationale behind therapy procedures so that they are implemented correctly.
- Do not assign support personnel to work with new clients or with certain types of complex disorders.
- Establish a plan of supervision and feedback.

Employment Outlook

Speech-language pathology and audiology are relatively young professions that continue to grow. The U.S. Bureau of Labor Statistics (2010) estimates that employment of speech-language pathologists will increase by about 19 percent from 2008 to 2018. Job prospects are also favorable for individuals who obtain the AuD degree (U.S. Bureau of Labor Statistics, 2010). Among the job settings that will see the biggest demand are colleges and universities seeking teaching and research-oriented faculty in communication sciences and disorders. Data from the Council on Graduate Programs (2002) suggest that job openings for those with research doctorates will exceed the number of doctoral graduates for much of this decade.

The outlook is good for the professions, given factors such as increased awareness of communication disorders; early detection of hearing, speech, and language disorders in children; the aging of the population and associated increased prevalence of age-related communication impairments; and increased concern over occupation-related hearing disorders (ASHA, 1998). These trends suggest continued growth of the professions well into the future. Although work settings and models of service delivery are likely to change over time, the professions will remain devoted to increased understanding of the nature and treatment of communication disorders.

REFERENCES

American Academy of Audiology (2011). Academy information. Retrieved on 10/1/11 from www.audiology.org/Pages/default.aspx.

American Speech-Language-Hearing Association (ASHA). (2004). *Guidelines for the training, use, and supervision of speech-language pathology assistants.* Available at www.asha.org/members/deskref-journals/deskref/default

American Speech-Language-Hearing Association (ASHA). (1998, Spring). Position statement and guidelines for support personnel in audiology. *Asha, 40* (Suppl. 18), 19–21.

American Speech-Language-Hearing Association (ASHA). (2005). *Membership and certification handbook of the American-Speech-Language-Hearing Association.* Rockville, MD: Author.

American Speech-Language-Hearing Association. (2008). *Bylaws of the American Speech-Language-Hearing Association* [Bylaws]. Available from www.asha.org/policy.

American Speech-Language-Hearing Association. (2010a). *Code of Ethics* [Ethics]. Available from www.asha.org/policy

American Speech-Language-Hearing Association (ASHA). (2010b). *Highlights and trends: ASHA counts for Year End 2010.* Retrieved October 1, 2011, from www.asha.org/uploadedFiles/2010-Member-Counts.pdf#search=%222011%22

American Speech-Language-Hearing Association. (2009). *2009 Membership Survey summary report: Number and type of responses.* Rockville, MD: Author.

Cherry, R., & Giolas, T. G. (1997). Preface to aural rehabilitation with adults. *Seminars in hearing, 18,* 75.

Council on Graduate Programs in Communication Sciences and Disorders. (2002). *Demographic survey of undergraduate and graduate programs in communication sciences and disorders.* Minneapolis, MN: Author.

Johnson, A. F., & Jacobson, B. H. (2007). *Medical speech-language pathology: A practitioner's guide* (2nd ed.). New York: Thieme.

Kimbarow, M. L. (1997). Ahead of the curve: Improving services with speech-language pathology assistants. *Asha, 39,* 41–44.

Paden, E. (1970). *A history of the American Speech and Hearing Association, 1925–1958.* Bethesda, MD: American Speech and Hearing Association.

U.S. Bureau of Labor Statistics, United States. Department of Labor. (2010). *Occupational outlook handbook 2010–11.* Retrieved October 1, 2011, from www.bls.gov/oco/pdf/ocos099.pdf and www.bls.gov/oco/pdf/ocos085.pdf

acoustic neuroma A nonmalignant tumor that involves the myelin sheath of the VIIIth nerve.

acquired Describes conditions in which the onset occurs after a period of normal function.

addition error A type of speech articulation error characterized by adding a sound to the target phoneme or word; for example, for the word *blue*, a child pronounces it *bolu*.

affricate A consonant that begins with a plosive phoneme and ends with a fricative, such as *ch*, written phonetically as /T/.

agraphia An acquired impairment of writing caused by brain damage.

air conduction audiometry Testing hearing by introducing the tone into the ear canal, with the sound waves then traveling to the ear drum at the end of the canal (as opposed to bone conduction).

alerting devices Devices to warn a hearing-impaired person to sounds in the environment (e.g., a telephone ringing, a doorbell, a baby's cry, or an emergency alarm) through vibration, a light signal, or a combination of these.

alexia An acquired impairment of reading caused by brain damage.

alexia with agraphia An acquired impairment of reading and writing due to brain damage.

alexia without agraphia An acquired impairment of reading that is not accompanied by a writing impairment; also called pure alexia.

allophone One of the variant forms of a phoneme that is recognized by the listener as the target phoneme.

alveolar ridge The ridge of bone just behind the upper front teeth.

Alzheimer's disease The most common form of dementing illness; a chronic, progressive disease that results in intellectual decline affecting language, memory, and cognition.

anarthria A severe impairment of motor control for speech resulting in complete lack of articulate speech.

anomia A reduced ability to name objects or retrieve desired words.

anomic aphasia A fluent aphasia that is characterized by relatively good verbal expression and auditory comprehension but notable difficulty coming up with the names of things.

APGAR A five-point evaluation system for identifying the status of newborns.

aphasia An acquired impairment of language due to damage to the language-dominant hemisphere, typically the left.

aphonia Attempts to produce a voice that results in a whisperlike sound. This usually occurs with voice disorders that prevent the vocal folds from vibrating to produce sound.

apraxia of speech An impairment of motor planning for the movements for speech so that voluntary control for speech is disrupted.

arcuate fasciculus A bundle of nerve fibers (white matter) that originate in cell bodies in the superior temporal gyrus and project anteriorly to the frontal lobe.

articulation Production of speech sounds.

arytenoid cartilage The paired, pyramid-shaped cartilages that sit on the posterior portion of the cricoid cartilage and aid in abduction and adduction of vocal folds.

aspiration Inhalation of fluids or other matter into the airway.

assimilation The influence of one sound on a neighboring sound, so that the sounds become more similar, or the same.

assistive listening device (ALD) Any device designed to reduce the effects of distance, background noise, and reverberation on the perception of speech.

ataxia A motor disorder characterized by marked loss of coordination, often associated with cerebellar disease.

athetosis A form of cerebral palsy characterized by twisting and flailing of the extremities, neck, and trunk.

audibility index   An estimation of what percent of acoustic energy from speech will be audible to a particular person.

audiogram   A graphic representation of the results of a hearing test with axes for hearing level and frequency.

audiologist   A professional who is concerned with the prevention, evaluation, and rehabilitation of auditory, balance, and related disorders.

audiology   The study of normal and disordered hearing.

audiometer   An electronic instrument used to evaluate the auditory system.

auditory brainstem response   An electrophysiological response to sounds that results in five to seven peaks that appear within 10 ms after the presentation of a signal (usually a click).

auditory training   The training of a hearing-impaired individual to make use of residual hearing abilities.

auricle   The external ear, also known as pinna.

autosomal   Describes chromosomes other than the X and Y sex chromosomes.

autosomal dominant   A genetic condition in which one copy of a chromosome other than the X or Y sex chromosome is sufficient to cause a condition (e.g., hearing loss, mental retardation) to manifest.

autosomal recessive   A genetic condition in which two copies of a chromosome other than the X or Y sex chromosome is sufficient to cause a condition (e.g., hearing loss, mental retardation) to manifest.

basal ganglia   A collection of subcortical gray matter structures, including the putamen, globus pallidus, and caudate, that contribute to control of motor behavior.

basilar membrane   A thin tissue layer found within the cochlea on which the organ of Corti rests.

bolus   A cohesive mass of some substance, such as food.

bone conduction audiometry   In hearing testing, introducing the sound waves directly into the cochlea via the bones of the skull.

brainstem   The brain structures at the base of the brain excluding the hemispheres above, the cerebellum, and the spinal cord below.

Broca's aphasia   A nonfluent aphasia with relatively preserved auditory comprehension, associated with damage to the inferior portions of the left frontal lobe.

canonical babbling   Consonant-vowel or consonant-vowel-consonant-vowel combinations produced by babies.

carcinoma   A cancer or malignancy.

carrier   An individual whose genetic makeup includes one of two copies of a gene that causes a genetic condition (e.g., hearing loss) in cases where one copy of the gene is insufficient for the condition to manifest.

central auditory processing disorder   Difficulties understanding speech as a result of structural changes in the central auditory nervous system. The difficulties are most pronounced in background noise and other difficult listening situations (e.g., reverberation).

central nervous system   The brain and spinal cord, exclusive of the cranial and peripheral nerves.

cerebellum   A brain structure that sits below the cerebral hemispheres and above the pons, playing an important role in muscular coordination.

cerebral localization   A theory of brain function that associates particular functions and behaviors to particular sites of the brain.

cerebral palsy   A developmental motor disorder related to brain injury; the most common forms are spasticity, athetosis, and ataxia.

cerebrovascular accident   *See* stroke.

cerebrum   The largest division of the brain, containing the cerebral hemispheres and corpus callosum.

cerumen   A waxy substance produced by glands that lie within the skin of the ear canal.

childhood apraxia of speech   A development disorder of speech whereby the motor programming for speech is disturbed, but there is not muscle weakness.

chromosome   A structure containing genes that transmit genetic information.

cilia   Hairlike structures that extend from the surface of a cell.

circumlocution   Talking with an excess number of words; or talking around the topic rather than being direct because of a failure to retrieve desired words, as in anomia.

closed caption decoder   An electronic device that decodes the captioned signals that are often broadcast with television programs. It enables captions to appear on the television screen and helps hearing-impaired individuals to understand the dialogue of television programs and movies.

cluttering A disorder of fluency characterized by rapid speech, breaks in fluency, and faulty articulation.

coarticulation The simultaneous production of two or more consonants or vowels in normal speech production of a word, such as the word *tram*—the first three phones (/t/ /r/ /æ/) might overlap in production.

cochlea The snail-shaped part of the inner ear containing the sensory organs of hearing.

cochlear implant A coil and electrodes surgically placed in the inner ear and connected to an external transmitter/signal processor. It is intended to produce sensations of sound for those with profound hearing impairments.

code switching Shifting by speakers among one or more dialects or languages to accommodate social rules or situational demands.

cognate A pair of sounds, such as /p/ and /b/, produced similarly except that one (/p/) is unvoiced and one (/b/) voiced.

communication An interaction or exchange of one's feelings, ideas, thoughts, and wants among two or more people by such modes as speech, writing, facial expression, gesture, or touch.

co-morbid Co-existing but independent. Used to refer to when two disorders or conditions co-exist in the same individual, but one condition does not cause the other.

conduction aphasia A fluent aphasia characterized by relatively good auditory comprehension and poor verbal repetition.

conductive hearing loss A loss of hearing related to obstruction or disease in the outer or middle ear in which sound transmission fails to reach the cochlea in the inner ear.

congenital Present at birth.

content The elements of language that carry meaning; also called semantics.

continuant A speech sound that can be continued or prolonged, such as /m/ or /s/.

corpus callosum A large band of fibers that joins the two hemispheres of the brain.

cortex The surface layer of the brain that contains the bodies of neurons.

cranial nerves Twelve paired peripheral nerves that derive from or come into the cranial cavity, such as cranial nerve I, olfactory, or II, optic.

cricoid cartilage The ring of cartilage that forms the base of the larynx.

criterion-referenced test A type of measure that is used to compare a child's performance against a standard, or criterion, for behavior.

decibel (dB) A logarithmic unit of measurement of sound intensity.

delayed auditory feedback An event produced when a device presents the listener's own speech or voice after a time delay. One effect of delayed auditory feedback is fluency enhancement in individuals who stutter.

dementia A behavioral syndrome of generalized intellectual deficit that results from a number of diseases.

denasality Insufficient nasal resonance; hyponasality.

developmental language disorder A condition involving poor language skills that appears during childhood.

diadochokinesis The rapid, alternating movements of a body part, such as in the lips and tongue rapidly saying puh-tuh-kuh repeatedly.

diagnosogenic theory of stuttering Theory that posits stuttering begins when normal disfluencies are labeled as stuttering.

diaphragm The muscular-tendonous partition that separates the thorax from the abdomen, serving as the primary muscle of respiration.

diphthong A blending together of two vowels in the same syllable, such as heard as /aI/ in the word *right*.

diplophonia A voice that has two pitches occurring at the same time.

distortion error The production of a target phoneme utilizing a sound that is not in the language, such as in a lateral lisp.

dyslexia An impairment of reading due to developmental or acquired brain damage.

dysphagia An impairment of the ability to swallow.

dysphasia An acquired impairment of language (more commonly referred to as *aphasia*).

dysphonia A disorder of voice, such as hoarseness, breathiness, or harshness.

effusion Fluid that has exuded into the middle ear space.

electrolarynx An electronic device that creates sound that can be used as a substitute for the voice (usually because the larynx has been surgically removed).

endogenous Caused by genetic factors.

epiglottis An oblong cartilage that sits at the top of the larynx and covers its opening during swallowing.

Eustachian tube The air tube that connects the middle ear with the nasopharynx.

evidence-based practice Clinical procedures and methods that are based on scientific study of their effectiveness.

exogenous Acquired or caused by factors outside the genes.

external ear canal The external opening into the ear.

false negative An incorrect conclusion that a condition is not present when it is.

false positive An incorrect conclusion that a condition is present when it is not.

fluent aphasia An aphasia profile that is characterized by spoken output of relatively normal utterance length, ease of production, and prosodic variation.

FM system A device that uses a transmitter to send the desired signal to a receiver using a radio wave. The receiver is coupled to the listener via earphones or a hearing aid.

form The phonological, syntactic, and morphological elements of language.

four kilohertz (4 kHz) notch An increase in hearing impairment in the 3000 to 6000 Hz region with recovery of hearing at 8000 Hz. This pattern is associated with noise-induced hearing impairment.

frequency The number of cycles per second of a sound wave; perceived as pitch.

fricative A sound produced by forcing air through a narrow opening of the articulators so as to produce a sibilant sound quality. Examples include /s/ and /z/.

frontal lobe The anterior part of each cerebral hemisphere, from the Rolandic fissure forward.

global aphasia A nonfluent aphasia characterized by marked impairment of verbal expression and auditory comprehension, typically caused by large lesions to the perisylvian region of the left hemisphere.

glossectomy The surgical removal of the tongue.

glottis The opening between the vocal folds.

habilitation Services designed to assist a child in maximizing their capabilities as they develop. See also rehabilitation.

habituate Exhibit gradual decrease in responsiveness following repeated exposure to a stimulus.

handicap A disadvantage resulting from an impairment or disability that limits the fulfillment of a role that is normal for an individual.

hearing The perception of sound.

hearing assistance technology A range of devices that enhance communication or media access for deaf and hard of hearing persons.

hearing disability The restrictions in daily activities that result from a hearing impairment.

hearing impairment Any loss or abnormality of structure or function of the auditory system.

hearing loss The degree of hearing impairment.

hemiparesis Weakness of one side of the body.

hemisphere Literally, half circle. In reference to brain anatomy, hemisphere indicates the half of the cerebrum or cerebellum to each side of midline.

Hertz (Hz) Unit of measure that reflects cycles per second.

hyperlexia A reading disorder characterized by strong phonological decoding despite poor or very poor reading comprehension.

hypernasality Excessive nasal resonance.

hypertension A medical condition in which blood pressure is abnormally high

iatrogenic Describes a condition that is inadvertently caused by the medical treatment of another condition.

immittance audiometry Air-pressure and air-volume differences measured in the external and middle ear as a method of detecting conductive hearing loss.

incidence The number of new cases that appear in a population over a set period of time.

incus An anvil-shaped bone found in the middle ear.

IDEA Individuals with Disabilities Education Improvement Act. This law mandates a free and appropriate education for all handicapped children. It covers children from birth to 21 years of age.

idiopathic Without known cause.

intensity A measure of the magnitude or pressure of a sound wave; perceived as loudness.

involuntary repetitions A form of stuttering characterized by unexpected syllable or word repetitions.

jargon aphasia An acquired impairment of language characterized by meaningless utterances.

language The coding of meaning into a system of arbitrary symbols that are recognized by members of the community. Language may be spoken, written, or manual (signed).

learning disability Educational difficulties in reading, writing, listening, speaking, or arithmetic, believed to be related to some kind of central brain dysfunction.

left neglect Reduced awareness or responsiveness to sensory input from the left side of the body (intrapersonal space) or left half of the environment (extrapersonal space) that cannot be attributed to sensory or motor defects.

lesion Damage to the nervous system.

lexicon The words that make up one's vocabulary.

malleus A hammer-shaped bone attached to the tympanic membrane within the middle ear.

mandible The lower jaw.

Ménière's disease A disease of the inner ear thought to be associated with an overproduction of endolymph. Symptoms include tinnitus, vertigo, and hearing loss.

mental retardation Reduced cognitive abilities, confirmed by measured intelligence quotients of 70 or below and poor adaptive abilities.

metalinguistics The ability to reflect on components of language form, content, or use. Subcomponents of metalinguistics include *metaphonology* (to think about speech sounds), *metasemantics* (to think about word meanings), *metasyntax* (to think about sentence structure), and *metapragmatics* (to think about the social rules and functions of communication).

middle ear The air-filled space located in the temporal bone containing the three small middle-ear bones, incus, malleus, and stapes.

misarticulations Speech articulation errors of omission, addition, substitution, or distortion.

mitochondrial (genetic) Genetic effects linked to genes contained in the mitochondria of cell bodies.

mixed hearing loss A hearing loss caused by both conductive and sensorineural problems.

morpheme Words or the smallest unit of a word that has meaning. For example, the word *cat* is one morpheme; in the plural form *cats*, the *s* is an added morpheme.

morphology The study of words and word forms; the study of morphemes.

multi-infarct dementia A form of dementia related to many small strokes (or infarcts).

myofunctional therapy Muscle training of the tongue to reduce tongue pressures on dentition, that is, therapy for reverse swallow and tongue thrust.

nasals Sounds that are produced with an open airway between the throat and nose, so that sound resonates through the nasal passages.

nasoendoscope A scope used during a videoendoscopy examination of the larynx. This scope is a long, thin flexible tube. It is placed through the nose to view the soft palate and can also be positioned in the pharynx to view the larynx.

neologism A nonword, or literally "new word," produced by an individual with aphasia.

neuron Cell within the brain that supports activity through the conduction of chemical-electrical signals.

nonfluent aphasia An aphasia profile that is characterized by effortful speech production, reduced grammatical complexity, and short utterance length.

nonsyndromic Describes a condition (e.g., hearing loss, cleft palate) that occurs in the absence of other abnormalities.

normative sample A representative sample of individuals whose performance on a test or measure serves as a reference against which a single individual's performance can be compared.

norm-referenced test Test designed to allow comparisons between an individual's performance and a group of individuals of similar age.

occipital lobe The posterior part of each cerebral hemisphere.

omission error One of the four types of articulatory errors, in which the sound is totally omitted.

oral mechanism examination An examination of the structure and function of the face, mouth, and oral cavity, intended to assess the integrity of the articulatory mechanisms of speech.

organ of Corti Area within the cochlea containing the tectorial membrane and hair cells.

ossicles The three small bones (incus, malleus, stapes) that form the ossicular chain in the middle ear.

otitis media Inflammation of the middle ear.

otoacoustic emissions Sounds produced by the inner ear.

otosclerosis A disorder of the ear that is characterized by increased vascularity and bone resorption of the stapes. It results in a progressive, conductive hearing loss when it interferes with the movement of the stapes.

otoscope A lighted device with a speculum on the end used to visualize the tympanic membrane and ear canals.

ototoxicity Sensory damage to the cochlear or vestibular systems from exposure to a chemical.

oval window A membrane-covered opening of the vestibule of the cochlea that is attached to the footplate of the stapes. Vibration of the stapes footplate sets the oval window in vibration.

palate The roof of the mouth. Anteriorly, the hard palate is bone, covered with a membrane; posteriorly, the soft palate (velum) is muscle covered with a membrane. The palate separates the oral and nasal cavities.

paraphasia An erroneous word or a nonword that reflects disorders of word choice (e.g., *man* for *woman*) or sound substitution errors (e.g., *tike* for *bike*).

parietal lobe One of the four lobes of the cerebral hemisphere, extending posteriorly from the Rolandic fissure to the occipital lobe.

perinatal The period surrounding birth; between the twenty-ninth week of gestation to one to four weeks after birth.

peripheral nervous system The nervous system that extends beyond the brain and the spinal cord, including peripheral sensory nerves that send impulses to the central nervous system and motor nerves that carry effector impulses to peripheral structures.

peristaltic contractions In the esophagus, the sequential action of muscles as they squeeze together starting at the top and moving downward. Each neighboring segment squeezes together to push food toward the stomach.

perisylvian region The region of the brain that surrounds the sylvian fissure, which is the primary horizontal fissure for each cerebral hemisphere.

perseveration Involuntary repetition of a word, phrase, sentence, or idea.

pharynx The tube-shaped cavity at the back of the mouth that extends from the posterior nasal cavity to just above the larynx and trachea.

phone A speech sound.

phoneme The smallest sound unit of speech represented by a symbol of the International Phonetic Alphabet.

phonemic regression Poor auditory comprehension often associated with advanced age.

phonological process The systematic simplification by children of the production of adult-modeled articulation, such as deleting the final consonant of words or deleting a syllable within a word.

phonology The study of the sounds of spoken language, including the rules of phoneme use, phonemes, phonetic production, and voicing characteristics.

Pick's disease A dementing disease that is associated with atrophy of the frontal and temporal lobes.

pinna The visible outer ear, also known as the auricle.

pitch The perceptual correlate of the frequency of a sound as heard by the ear.

plosives A speech sound produced by impounding air behind an articulator and suddenly releasing it, as in /p/ or /b/.

postnatal Occurring after birth.

prelingual Before the development of speech.

prenatal Preceding birth.

presbycusis Hearing impairment associated with the aging process.

prevalence The total number of cases present in a population in a given period of time.

primary progressive aphasia An acquired impairment of language that follows a slowly progressive, rather than abrupt, onset and is not associated with dementia.

prosody The melody, flow, and rhythm of a spoken language; melodic changes in syllable stress, pitch, loudness, and duration.

protoword Early form of an actual word that usually contains some of the sounds of the target word.

pure alexia An acquired brain disorder in which the patient is unable to read, but is still able to write.

pure tone A periodic sound wave of a particular frequency that is generated in the audiometric testing of hearing.

recessive Describes genetic conditions that are only expressed when two copies of the gene causing the condition are present.

reflux Backward movement of food during swallowing. Often, reflux refers to acid from the stomach spilling upward into the throat, causing irritation to the tissues.

rehabilitation Services designed to restore capabilities lost after illness or injury.

reliability Quality of providing consistent information.

retrocochlear Anatomical location that is behind the cochlea.

rolandic fissure The central fissue that divides the posterior frontal lobe from the anterior parietal lobe.

rollover A phenomenon in which word recognition scores decrease as the presentation level of the stimuli increases.

round window An opening in the vestibule of the cochlea beneath the oval window on the cochlea, permitting the displacement or movement of fluid within the cochlea.

seizures The convulsions of an epileptic attack; epilepsy.

semantics The study of the history and meaning of words.

sensorineural hearing loss A hearing loss caused by disease of the inner ear or eighth cranial nerve.

sex-linked (genetic) Genetic effects linked to genes on the X or Y chromosomes.

signal-to-noise ratio (SNR) For our purposes SNR in a classroom is the relative difference between spoken instruction and unwanted competing noise. An SNR of 0 dB means that speech and noise are equal in intensity (strength). A SNR of 10 dB means that the speech signal is 10 dB more intense (stronger) than the competing noise. A SNR of –10 means that speech is 10 dB weaker than the competing noise.

site of lesion the location of an abnormality or damage that causes a condition (e.g, hearing loss, aphasia).

sound–symbol correspondence The ability to associate individual sounds with printed letters.

spasticity A paralysis characterized by extreme tension and hypercontraction of muscles with hyperactive tendon reflexes.

specific language impairment A diagnosis of a child who demonstrates impairment in understanding spoken language, speaking, reading, and writing with no other demonstrable impairment.

spectrogram A visual display of the sound frequencies of a spoken utterance.

speech Sound production via changes in the vocal mechanism and oral structures to form words and sentences in auditory-oral communication.

speech-language pathologist A professional who specializes in the diagnosis and treatment of communication and swallowing disorders.

speech-language pathology A profession that specializes in the diagnosis and treatment of communication disorders related to problems of hearing, articulation, language, voice, fluency, and swallowing.

speechreading The use of visual cues from a talker's face to identify his or her speech.

spinal cord The lower portion of the central nervous system, originating at the medulla and extending down within the spinal vertebra.

spinal nerves Thirty-one pairs of nerves that enter or exit the spinal cord.

spondaic words Two-syllable words pronounced with equal stress on each syllable.

stapedectomy An operation in which the stapes is removed and replaced with a prosthesis in an attempt to improve a hearing impairment that was caused by otosclerosis.

stapes A stirrup-shaped bone within the middle ear that attaches to the round window of the inner ear.

stimulability testing In testing articulation, a determination of how well the client can produce the target sound when the sound has been repeatedly presented (visually and auditorially).

stroke Sudden onset of disturbed neurological functioning caused by disruption of blood flow. Also called a cerebrovascular accident (CVA), usually one of three types: thrombosis, embolus, or hemorrhage.

stuttering The involuntary repetition, interruption, and prolongation of speech sounds and syllables, which the individual struggles to end.

subglottal air pressure The air pressure within the airway below the vocal folds; outgoing air moves between the vocal folds when pressure below the folds is greater than air pressure above them.

substitution error A type of articulation error characterized by an incorrect phoneme used in place of a target phoneme, such as /w/ said for /r/.

sylvian fissure The horizontal fissure that divides the inferior border of the frontal and parietal lobes from the superior temporal lobe.

syndrome A collection of physical features that co-occur and characterize a disorder or condition.

syndromic Describes a condition (e.g., hearing loss) that occurs in the context of other abnormalities.

syntax The grammatical structure and word order of a language.

telecommunication device for the deaf (TDD) A keyboard that attaches to a telephone to allow typewritten communication with other TDDs. It enables individuals with hearing difficulties to communicate using the telephone.

telegraphic speech Spoken communication that consists primarily of content words and is lacking functor words, such as pronouns, auxilary verbs, and articles.

temporal lobe One of the four lobes of a cerebral hemisphere, lying below the sylvian fissure.

teratrogen An agent that causes a developmental disorder or malformation.

thalamus A large gray mass of sensory nuclei deep within the hemisphere, bordering the third ventricle.

thyroid cartilage The shield-shaped outer cartilage protecting the larynx; popularly called the Adam's apple.

tinnitus Noises in the ear(s) usually described as ringing, hissing, or roaring.

tongue thrust Abnormal tongue positioning, particularly during swallowing, that may have an adverse effect on the anterior dental bite.

tracheostoma A permanent opening in the neck that is surgically created. This is usually done because the larynx has been surgically removed or is not able to open enough to allow breathing, such as with bilateral vocal fold paralysis or injury to the larynx.

transformer A device or mechanism that changes the nature or properties of a signal or substance.

traumatic laryngitis A dysphonia related to excessive use of harmful voicing behaviors such as yelling and screaming.

tympanic membrane The round membrane between the ear canal and middle ear, also known as the eardrum.

tympanometry An audiological test that evaluates the compliance of the tympanic membrane of the ear.

use The rules for communicative interactions, including the social-interactive aspects of language, sometimes called pragmatics.

validity The quality of providing accurate or true information.

velum The soft palate.

vestibular schwannoma A benign tumor of the cells of the VIIIth cranial nerve that can result in hearing loss.

vestibulotoxic Describes substances (e.g., medications, teratogens) that cause damage to the vestibular system.

videoendoscopy A procedure using special fiber-optic equipment to obtain views of the internal structure of the larynx.

videofluoroscopy The process whereby X-ray images of motion are recorded on videotape for the purpose of examination of function, such as in the study of swallowing.

video otoscopy A system that provides enlarged images that can be viewed on a monitor, stored on disk, or printed. Applications include visualization of the outer ear, tympanic membrane, and middle ear and counseling regarding hearing instrument insertion, operation, and hygiene.

vocal nodules   Benign growths on the vocal folds, usually bilateral, which are typically the result of laryngeal abuse and voice misuse.

vocal polyps   Benign growths on the vocal folds that usually occur unilaterally and are soft and compliant fluid-filled bags. These occur as a result of excessive use of harmful vocal habits such as yelling and screaming.

vocalization   Voicing or phonation.

voice   The production of sound by vibration of the vocal folds.

waveform   A graph of the oscillations corresponding to the frequency of a sound.

Wernicke's aphasia   A fluent aphasia characterized by poor auditory comprehension and errors in the selection of words or sounds that make up words, so that spoken utterances may not make sense.

Photo credits: pp. 1, 3, 13, 17, 18, 24, 30, 46, 59, 62, 66, 70, 92, 98, 99, 105, 134, 137, 138, 141, 142, 148, 158, 165, 174, 178, 185, 197, 217, 227, 243, 244, 256, 259, 263, 273, 275, 278, 281, 296, 301, 304, 309, 312, 313, 320, 336, 337, 339, 349, Courtesy of the Department of Speech, Language, and Hearing Sciences, The University of Arizona; p. 33, B. Story, The University of Arizona.